THE **CARE** AND **FEEDING** OF AN **IACUC**

The Organization and Management
of an Institutional Animal Care
and Use Committee

SECOND EDITION

THE **CARE** AND **FEEDING** OF AN **IACUC**

The Organization and Management of an Institutional Animal Care and Use Committee

SECOND EDITION

EDITED BY

Whitney Kayla Petrie
Ph.D., R.L.A.T.G., C.P.I.A.
UNIVERSITY OF CALIFORNIA, DAVIS, CA

Sonja Lea Wallace
B.A., R.V.T., R.L.A.T.G., C.P.I.A.
STANFORD UNIVERSITY, PALO ALTO
CALIFORNIA, USA

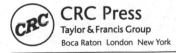

CRC Press
Taylor & Francis Group
Boca Raton London New York

CRC Press is an imprint of the
Taylor & Francis Group, an **informa** business

CRC Press
Taylor & Francis Group
6000 Broken Sound Parkway NW, Suite 300
Boca Raton, FL 33487-2742

First issued in paperback 2020

ISBN 13: 978-0-367-57584-7 (pbk)
ISBN 13: 978-1-4822-0110-9 (hbk)

Library of Congress Cataloging-in-Publication Data

The care and feeding of an IACUC : the organization and management of an institutional animal care and use committee / editors, Whitney Petrie and Sonja L. Wallace. -- Second edition.
    p. ; cm.
Includes bibliographical references and index.
ISBN 978-1-4822-0110-9 (hardcover : alk. paper)
    I. Petrie, Whitney, editor. II. Wallace, Sonja L., editor.
    [DNLM: 1. Animal Care Committees--organization & administration--United States. 2. Animals, Laboratory--United States. 3. Ethics Committees--organization & administration--United States. 4. Laboratory Animal Science--standards--United States. QY 54]

HV4708
179'.4--dc23

2014040865

Visit the Taylor & Francis Web site at
http://www.taylorandfrancis.com

and the CRC Press Web site at
http://www.crcpress.com

Contents

Chapter 1
Introduction to the IACUC: Its Purpose and Function 1

Cyndi Rosenblatt and Patrick Sharp

Chapter 2
Role of the IACUC, Bioethics and Scientific Review, Essential Environment
for IACUC Success 21

Jerry Collins

Chapter 3
Institutional Policies, Guidelines, and Procedures 37

Mary Jo Shepherd

Chapter 4
Protocol Processing: From Submission to Approval 43

Melinda S. Hollander

Chapter 5
Elements of the Protocol Form: How to Complete and Review 63

Monte Matthews

Chapter 6
Semiannual Program Evaluation, Facility Inspections, and Postapproval
Monitoring: All Part of the Same Thing 83

Deborah A. Frolicher

Chapter 7
IACUC Oversight of Training and Qualification in Animal Care and Use 101

Nicole Duffee

Chapter 17
Taylor Bennett and Andrew D. Cardon

Chapter 18

CONTENTS

Foreword

The excitement, as well as the challenges, of working in biomedical research is that it never stands still; it is a field of constant change and progress. What was the standard a few years ago may be past history, and it is imperative for those who perform and support research to stay abreast of new developments and seek opportunities to implement quality improvements whenever possible. This is certainly true for those performing research and equally true for those who work with and serve on an Institutional Animal Care and Use Committee (IACUC).

The IACUC plays a pivotal role at every institution where animals are used in teaching and research. The committee's first and foremost responsibility is to oversee and ensure the welfare of all animals under its authority. To fulfill this critical responsibility, compliance with the federal Animal Welfare Act, the Public Health Service Policy on Humane Care and Use of Laboratory Animals, and the Institute for Laboratory Animal Research *Guide for the Care and Use of Laboratory Animals* is a must. While the essence of these regulations and guidelines has not changed substantially since my coeditor Lawrence Podolsky and I produced the first edition of *The Care and Feeding of an IACUC* in 1999, reinterpretation and refinement of these documents has resulted in many changes. Principal investigators and IACUC members and staff continually need to adapt to these changes and improve on their processes. This second edition addresses how to meet ever-evolving expectations in an easy to understand format that is practical and extremely thorough.

I personally know and have worked with the editors of this edition and I am extremely impressed with the distinguished chapter authors that they have assembled to write the book. The editors and authors have worked in the IACUC trenches and thus know exactly what is important for readers to understand, without burdening them with excessive information. It will definitely help principal investigators improve the quality of their protocols and, in the end, expedite the review process. For IACUC committee members and staff, it will clarify their responsibilities and help them focus on the important issues.

I had the honor and pleasure of serving with Dr. Podolsky on an IACUC for several years. I was the attending veterinarian and he was our public member. He had a remarkable and distinguished career as a pediatrician and the first edition of *The Care and Feeding of an IACUC* was his brainchild. If he was still with us, I am sure he would be extremely proud that this second edition has been published, and that it will continue to advance the importance of animal welfare in research and teaching.

Victor S. Lukas
University of California, Davis

Acknowledgments

This edition has benefited greatly from several experts who conducted an outside review of the chapters and appendices for compliance with federal guidelines and regulations, as well as voluntary accreditation and assessment requirements. We would like to thank Carol Clarke and Robert Gibbens from the U.S. Department of Agriculture Animal and Plant Health Inspection Service Animal Care, and the staff of the Animal Welfare Information Center for reviewing the book for concordance with the federal Animal Welfare Act Regulations, the U.S. Department of Agriculture Animal and Plant Health Inspection Service Animal Care policies, and the interpretive rules that help regulated entities comply with existing Animal Welfare Act regulations and standards (http://www.aphis.usda.gov/animal_welfare/policy.php). The Animal Welfare Information Center is mandated by the Animal Welfare Act to provide information for improved animal care and use in research, testing, and teaching (http://awic.nal.usda.gov/).

We also thank Patricia Brown, Susan Brust Silk, and Lori Hampton from the National Institutes of Health Office of Laboratory Animal Welfare for reviewing the book for concordance with the Public Health Service Policy on Humane Care and Use of Laboratory Animals (http://grants.nih.gov/grants/olaw/references/phspol.htm), as well as John Bradfield from the Association for Assessment and Accreditation of Laboratory Animal Care (AAALC) International for reviewing the information regarding AAALAC accreditation that is included in Chapter 1. AAALAC International is a private, nonprofit organization that promotes the humane treatment of animals in science through voluntary accreditation and assessment programs (http://www.aaalac.org/).

We would also like to extend a special thanks to Laurie Brignolo of the University of California, Davis, for contributing to tables of blood withdrawal guidelines, including estimated total blood volume, recommended sampling sites, and recovery periods for single/multiple sampling (see Appendix E) and of recommended good practice compound administration volumes (see Appendix F) for common laboratory species.

Editors

Whitney Petrie is an Institutional Animal Care and Use Committee (IACUC) specialist at the University of California, Davis, where she is responsible for protocol and amendment review and facility and laboratory inspections. Dr. Petrie also sits on various subcommittees within the IACUC. She received a bachelor's degree in biochemistry, summa cum laude, from the University of New Mexico in 1994. As an undergraduate, she worked in a laboratory within the Toxicology and Pharmacology Department where she researched skin cancer. She remained at the University of New Mexico until 2008, at which time she completed her PhD in biomedical sciences concentrating on cell biology within the Department of Molecular and Cellular Biology. Again, her interests remained in the cancer research field but shifted toward cancer of the endometrium. From 2008 to 2013, she worked as a postdoctoral fellow in the Animal Science Department at the University of California, Davis, where she investigated both normal breast development and the transition from normal breast development to cancer. Dr. Petrie is currently one of the many staff members within the IACUC office at the University of California, Davis. She is a member of the Sacramento Valley American Association for Laboratory Animal Science and Public Responsibility in Medicine and Research. She is certified as an American Association for Laboratory Animal Science (AALAS)-registered laboratory animal technologist and a certified professional IACUC administrator.

Sonja L. Wallace is the training specialist in the Veterinary Service Center in the Department of Comparative Medicine at Stanford University, responsible for the development and implementation of animal care and use training programs for faculty and staff. Ms. Wallace received an AAS in animal health technology from Colorado Mountain College in 1981 and a BA in biological science from California State University East Bay in 2000. After completing an externship in Yale University's Section of Comparative Medicine, she began her research career as a veterinary technician in 1987, providing surgical support for cardiovascular studies at Syntex Research in Palo Alto, California. She started working as a biologist in cardiovascular pharmacology at Syntex in 1989 and helped the company to establish a good laboratory practice safety pharmacology laboratory in 1993. After working briefly as a toxicology biologist testing drug delivery systems at ALZA in Mountain View, California, she moved to Roche Bioscience, Palo Alto, CA, to supervise the company's veterinary technician staff and set up an IACUC training program in 1997. She transitioned into being a senior compliance analyst with Roche's IACUC and later the IACUC manager and training coordinator, chairing both the IACUC training and enrichment subcommittees. In 2009, she became the associate director of Stanford's Institutional Animal Care and Use Program, serving as an *ex officio* member of the university's IACUC and managing the IACUC staff in the Research Compliance Office under the vice provost and dean of research. She is currently in charge of training programs in Stanford School of Medicine's Department of Comparative Medicine. Ms. Wallace's certifications include registered veterinary technician in the state of California, AALAS-registered laboratory animal technologist, and certified professional IACUC administrator. She served as president of the Northern California Branch of the AALAS board of directors in 2007 and 2013 and has served on the California Society for Biomedical Research board of directors since 2007.

Contributors

Taylor Bennett
National Association for Biomedical
 Research
Washington, DC

Linda N. Brovarney
Institutional Animal Care and Use
 Program
University of California
San Francisco, California

Marcy Brown
Comparative Medicine
Worldwide Research and Development
Pfizer, Inc.
La Jolla, California

Andrew D. Cardon
National Association for Biomedical
 Research
Washington, DC

Jane Chambers
Drug Safety Research and Development
Worldwide Research and Development
Pfizer, Inc.
La Jolla, California

Mark S. Christensen
Department of Philosophy
Lourdes University
Sylvania, Ohio

Jerry Collins
Department of Anesthesiology
Yale University
New Haven, Connecticut

Nicole Duffee
Education and Scientific Affairs
American Association for Laboratory
 Animal Science
Memphis, Tennessee

Stephen A. Felt
Department of Comparative Medicine
Stanford University School of Medicine
Stanford, California

Deborah A. Frolicher
IACUC Office
The Scripps Research Institute
La Jolla, California

Sherril L. Green
Department of Comparative Medicine
Stanford University School of
 Medicine
Stanford, California

William G. Greer
Office for Research Protections
Pennsylvania State University
University Park, Pennsylvania

Melinda S. Hollander
Office of Research Integrity and
 Compliance
West Virginia University
Morgantown, West Virginia

Michael Kreger
Division of Bird Habitat Conservation
U.S. Fish and Wildlife Service
Falls Church, Virginia

Monte Matthews
Animal Care Services
University of Oregon
Eugene, Oregon

Kathleen A. Murray
Preclinical Laboratory Animal
 Medicine
Charles River Laboratories
Wilmington, Massachusetts

Cyndi Rosenblatt
Office of Research Integrity
Medical University of South Carolina
Charleston, South Carolina

Patrick Sharp
Animal Resources Authority
Murdoch, Australia

Mary Jo Shepherd
IACUC Office
Columbia University
New York, New York

Mary W. Wood
Center for Animal Alternatives
  Information
Carlson Health Sciences Library
University of California
Davis, California

Bill Yates
Departments of Otolaryngology and
  Neuroscience
University of Pittsburgh School of
  Medicine
Pittsburgh, Pennsylvania

CHAPTER 1

Introduction to the IACUC
Its Purpose and Function

Cyndi Rosenblatt and Patrick Sharp

CONTENTS

1.1 INTRODUCTION

It can be reasonably intuited that most of you did not randomly choose this book as a possible bit of bedtime reading just because the title was so catchy. That leaves the likely conclusion that you are reading this book because you already have some sort of interest in or involvement with an Institutional Animal Care and Use Committee, commonly referred to as an IACUC (pronounced 'ī-ə-ku'k). There are many types of individuals who may play a role in the Animal Care and Use Program (ACUP), and myriad routes by which they came to that role, so the purpose and function of the IACUC will be addressed first. Later chapters will discuss specific IACUC responsibilities in more detail, and by the end of the book you will know everything you need to know about the care and feeding of an IACUC.

Like the types of research and work that we do, and the species and models we utilize in that work, IACUCs come in all shapes and sizes. Although not all IACUCs are operating under the same set of expectations and regulations, they all share the same aim—to ensure that the highest ethical and humane standards are applied to the care and use of the animals that we are privileged to utilize in our various undertakings.

To understand the current role of the IACUC, it is helpful to know some of the history that eventually led to the creation of, and often mandates for, local regulatory committees in the form of the IACUC. It is a fascinating history, notable for the great minds that developed new ways to think about and attempt to alleviate human suffering, as much as for the great souls who sought to ensure that the welfare of the animals was not overlooked in the process.

1.2 HISTORY OF ANIMAL SUBJECTS RESEARCH

The concept that animal models can provide insight into the human condition appeared in the ancient Greek writings of Aristotle, but it was not until the mid-1800s that the systematic use of animals in biomedical research took root (Lennox 2011, Horner and Minifie 2011). With the increasing use of animals came a collective concern for how such use was being conducted, though this concern was rather sharply divided between two distinct ideological lines. Those approaching the issue of animal protection from the side of animal welfare were supportive of animal use in research, as long as it was carried out in the most ethical and humane ways possible. On the other side of the animal protection push were animal rights advocates who asserted that animals were never acceptable as research subjects, regardless of the potential benefit to human or animal health. Some of the oldest animal welfare and animal rights groups are still active today, and their histories can be traced to the same time frame (Horner and Minifie 2011). While there is a fundamental difference between animal welfare and animal rights, the activity of both of these groups led to significant changes over time in how animals were utilized (Horner and Minifie 2011).

Animal laboratory medicine as a specialized field was initiated in 1915 and started to gain general acceptance in the late 1940s, as laboratory research was coming under pressure from animal rights groups (Steneck 1997). Beginning in the early 1950s, a more formal approach to the care of laboratory animals was developed, with laboratory animal care programs proliferating and working to improve the conditions under which research animals were housed and used (Steneck 1997). By 1985, additional public pressure ushered in what Steneck describes as the "era of IACUCs," when "officials at the local, state, and especially federal levels revised once more the rules and regulations for the care and use of research animals." Since that time, aided by a growing cadre of dedicated IACUC and animal care personnel, the field of animal research has continued to evolve, complying with increasingly stringent regulations and detailed standards (Table 1.1).

Table 1.1   Selected Events and Publications in the Field of Animal Research

Year	Event or Publication	Additional Data
1950	Animal Care Panel organized	Veterinarian initiated
1950	National Society for Medical Research	American Association of Medical Colleges advocacy organization
1952	Institute for Laboratory Animal Research	National Academy of Sciences
1963	First Report of the AVMA Panel on Euthanasia	American Veterinary Medical Association
1963	*Guide for the Care and Use of Laboratory Animals* (1st edn)	Animal Care Panel
1966	Animal Welfare Act, as amended	Pub. L. No. 89-544
1967	American Association for Laboratory Animal Science	New iteration of Animal Care Panel
1973	Grants Administration Manual required adherence to the *Guide for the Care and Use of Laboratory Animals*	Public Health Service
1979	Research Animal Alliance	Animal research advocacy group
1985	Health Research Extension Act of 1985	Pub. L. No. 99-158
1985	U.S. Government Principles for the Utilization and Care of Vertebrate Animals Used in Testing, Research, and Training	Interagency Research Animal Committee
1986	Public Health Service (PHS) Policy on Humane Care and Use of Laboratory Animals (revision of the 1979 Policy)	Public Health Service under Health Research Extension Act Authority
1996	Association for Assessment and Accreditation of Laboratory Animal Care International	Name change reflected growing global presence
2002	*Institutional Animal Care and Use Committee Guidebook* (2nd edn)	Applied Research Ethics National Association and Office of Laboratory Animal Welfare
2006	Animal Enterprise Terrorism Act	Pub. L. No. 109-374
2007	Animal Care Policy Manual	Animal and Plant Health Inspection Service
2011	*Guide for the Care and Use of Laboratory Animals* (8th edn)	National Research Council
2013	AVMA Guidelines for the Euthanasia of Animals (8th rev)	American Veterinary Medical Association

1.3 FRAMEWORK FOR ANIMAL WELFARE OVERSIGHT

With privilege comes responsibility. The privilege of working with animals comes with the responsibility of adhering to applicable regulations and standards. That sounds like a straightforward task, but in the United States, our work might be covered under regulatory requirements at the federal, state, and local levels. In addition to the regulations, an individual program may receive funds from a funding source with its own set of standards, or it may choose to seek voluntary accreditation, further defining what must be done and how. The three-person program at a small biotech firm may be subject to the same standards and requirements as the hundreds-strong program at a major research university—or it may not. It depends on a number of factors, including the type of work, species, animal source, funding source, and accreditation status.

How did our system become so complicated? Contemporary animal care and use standards and requirements have developed over time, with laws and amendments passed in response to both chronic and acute concerns (Steneck 1997). Certainly, animal use is regulated in many other countries, and some of those regulations are substantially more stringent than the requirements in the United States. The primary complication with the U.S. system is that it is far more diverse, involving multiple agencies, overlapping authorities, and separate reporting mechanisms (Wynes et al. 2002). This stands in contrast to the more centralized oversight mechanisms in place in other Western countries (Paul 2002).

There are two primary federal laws covering the use of animals for research purposes. Exposés on the use of pet dogs in biomedical research were published by *Sports Illustrated* in late 1965 and *Life Magazine* in early 1966 (Adams and Larson 2007). The public rallied in response to the articles and heavily lobbied Congress, which passed the Animal Welfare Act (AWA) in August 1966. The Health Research Extension Act (1985) and subsequent amendments to the AWA were also brought about due to public pressure (Steneck 1997). Those two pieces of legislation cover a majority of the animal research that is conducted using vertebrate animals in the United States (Sandgren 2005). IACUCs hold a central role in the current iterations of both laws (Sandgren 2005).

1.3.1 U.S. Department of Agriculture: Animal Welfare Act

The AWA, as currently amended from the original 1966 law, specifies the standards of care and use for most species of warm-blooded vertebrate animals that are used in research, as well as many of those that are used in exhibits or are handled commercially in any way. As part of a 2004 amendment, the perennial mainstays of modern scientific research, mice (of the genus *Mus*) and rats (of the genus *Rattus*), are explicitly exempted from the provisions of the AWA (USDA 2004, 2013b) if they are bred for research. Birds also fall into this category and are only exempt if, like mice and rats, they are bred for use in research. In 2004, the U.S. Department of Agriculture (USDA) notified the public of the department's interpretation of the revised definition of *animal* and published an Advanced Notice of Proposed Rulemaking soliciting input for the development of regulations to cover birds (USDA 2004).

The interpretation and enforcement of the AWA were assigned to the USDA, which placed the oversight duties under its Animal and Plant Health Inspection Service (APHIS) (USDA 2013b). The standards established in the AWA are the basis for additional regulations developed by the USDA, known as the Animal Welfare Regulations (AWRs). The USDA is charged with performing annual unannounced inspections of research facilities, and inspectors (veterinary medical officers [VMOs]) utilize the standards as laid out in the AWRs to evaluate all registered research programs (USDA 2013a).

1.3.2 NIH: Public Health Service Policy

Prior to the Health Research Extension Act of 1985, research laboratories using animals not already covered by the AWA were largely unregulated. The Health Research Extension Act was an attempt to ensure that, regardless of the species, vertebrate animals that were used in research funded by the U.S. Public Health Service (PHS) agencies received similar standards of care to those already covered under the AWA (Wynes et al. 2002). There were several important distinctions in the new legislation. Among other things, the 1985 regulations covered purpose-bred rodents and birds, as well as cold-blooded vertebrates (Steneck 1997). A limitation in the new law was that, while the AWA was applicable based on species, the Health Research Extension Act only applied based on the funding source (Sandgren 2005). Any public or private institution that receives PHS funding must have a PHS Assurance (Wynes et al. 2002). An exception is the Department of Veterans Affairs (VA), which, under a memorandum of understanding, agrees to oversight by the Office of Laboratory Animal Welfare (OLAW) of all of its research activities with animals.

Oversight for the 1985 Health Research Extension Act was placed with the National Institutes of Health (NIH) (Wynes et al. 2002). The NIH placed enforcement responsibility on OLAW, formerly called the Division of Animal Welfare, Office for Protection from Research Risks (Horner and Minifie 2011). Part of this responsibility was to create and promulgate detailed guidance covering the care and use of vertebrate animals in research. In response, the NIH developed the PHS Policy for the Care and Use of Laboratory Animals (the PHS Policy) in 1986, and that policy is the basis for OLAW oversight under the 1985 Health Research Extension Act (Wynes et al. 2002).

To minimize the need for a complicated and evolving set of standards, the decision was made to defer detailed definitions of what constituted humane care and use to a nongovernmental body, the Institute for Laboratory Animal Research (ILAR). The *Guide for the Care and Use of Laboratory Animals* (the Guide) was originally published in 1963 by the independent Animal Care Panel, with subsequent editions published as a project of the ILAR under the National Academy of Sciences. The Guide thus forms the basis for expected laboratory practices in projects that are subject to the PHS Policy (NRC 2011, NIH 2002).

1.3.3 AAALAC International

Perceived as the "gold standard" of laboratory animal care, the Association for Assessment and Accreditation of Laboratory Animal Care International (AAALAC International) provides voluntary, peer review–based accreditation to institutions using animals in research, teaching, and testing. Established in 1965, AAALAC International is a private, nonprofit, and nongovernmental organization.

AAALAC International uses three primary regulatory standards: the Guide, the Guide for the Care and Use of Agricultural Animals in Research and Teaching, and the European Convention for the Protection of Vertebrate Animals Used for Experimental and Other Scientific Purposes, Council of Europe (ETS 123) (Appendices A and B). For U.S. institutions, the current version of the Guide along with other pertinent regulations apply. A given nation's rules and regulations apply to foreign institutions seeking AAALAC International accreditation; should there be a foreign regulatory "void" (e.g., occupational health and safety), the Guide or the associated regulation applies, and in the case of a regulatory conflict, the stricter regulation applies.

AAALAC International's functional components currently consist of a board of trustees, a council on accreditation, and *ad hoc* specialists/consultants. The board includes members of various eminent professional, scientific, and educational organizations that govern AAALAC International. Council members are animal care/use and research professionals selected worldwide who conduct program reviews; the subsequent council deliberations determine if an institution has achieved AAALAC International accreditation. The *ad hoc* specialists/consultants bring their unique expertise to each site-visit team.

AAALAC International's accreditation process requires an institution to submit a written (in English) program description (PD) highlighting institutional compliance with the pertinent regulatory standards. The PD format follows the Guide's subject headings and may be downloaded from AAALAC International's website. The AAALAC International site visitors review the PD before the site visit. Additional PD site-visit information may be found in Table 1.2. Institutions that are attempting accreditation include a nonrefundable fee with the application materials. The institution provides a new, updated PD before each triennial site revisit. Institutions that are seeking accreditation may choose to undergo a program status evaluation, which serves as a "pre-AAALAC site visit," (Sharp and Villano 2012) providing programmatic feedback to those institutions that may be unfamiliar with the AAALAC International accreditation process.

A minimum of two site visitors conduct the visit, with one being an AAALAC International council member and the other(s) being the AAALAC International *ad hoc* specialist(s)/consultant(s). The council member coordinates pre-site-visit communications with a designated institutional representative. The site-visit length and the number of site visitors vary with the size and complexity of the institution. The

Table 1.2   Program Description and Site-Visit Information

Program Description Due Date	Site Visit Occurs	AAALAC International Council Meeting Review[a]
December 1	January–March	May
April 1	May–July	September
August 1	September–November	January

[a] AAALAC International Council currently meets three times per year.

site visit involves an entrance briefing, a program review (including a PD review and clarification session), meetings with various institutional representatives (e.g., institutional official [IO], IACUC members/chair, attending veterinarian [AV]), document review (e.g., research protocols, compliance records), and facility review (e.g., animal housing, animal research areas).

At the end of the site visit, the site visitors will enter into an executive session to discuss, among themselves, their site-visit findings. After the executive session, the site visitors, led by the council member, conduct an exit briefing outlining their findings with institutional representatives. Their findings consist of *mandatory items* or *suggestions for improvement*. At the exit briefing, the site visitors can convey to the institutional representatives their intended AAALAC International accreditation category recommendation to the AAALAC International council. Institutions have the opportunity to respond to the site visitors' findings in a post-site-visit communication (PSVC) (Sharp and Villano 2012). The site visitors' findings, with the PSVC, will be presented at the next AAALAC International council meeting for deliberation and decision (Table 1.2). Council meeting results (Tables 1.3 and 1.4) are conveyed in writing.

Table 1.3   Possible AAALAC International Accreditation Categories for New Application Institutions

Accreditation Category	Considered Accredited?	Mandatory Item Correction Time
Full	Yes	N/A
Conditional	Yes	Correct mandatory item(s) by the AAALAC International annual report or as determined by AAALAC International Council
Provisional	No	Up to 24 months
Withhold	No	N/A

Table 1.4   Possible AAALAC International Accreditation Categories for Existing Accredited Institutions

Accreditation Category	Considered Accredited?	Mandatory Item Correction Time
Full	Yes	N/A
Conditional	Yes	Correct mandatory item(s) by the next AAALAC International annual report or as determined by AAALAC International Council
Deferred	Yes	Up to two months; uncorrected mandatory item(s) will result in Probation
Probation	Yes	Up to 12 months; uncorrected mandatory item(s) will result in Revoke
Revoke	No	N/A

AAALAC International–accredited institutions must complete an annual report. In mid-December, the accredited institution will be provided with an annual report form. It is currently up to the institution to decide its reporting period (e.g., fiscal year, calendar year, governmental regulatory report year). The annual report requests notification of research noncompliance and changes to animal facilities, the IACUC, and the ACUP. AAALAC International stipulates, "the accredited unit shall promptly notify AAALAC International (e.g., through copies of correspondence) of adverse events relating to the animal care and use program." *Adverse events* may include natural disasters, animal rights activities, and/or investigations by regulatory agencies.

1.3.4 Other Oversight by Agencies and Jurisdictions

Federal agencies are subject to the AWA but have the option of developing their own standards with the AWA as the baseline. As federal research programs, the VA and the Department of Defense (DOD) must follow the AWA and the PHS Policy but do not operate under the direct oversight of the USDA (USDA 2013b). Instead, they have developed their own strict sets of rules and policies governing the use of vertebrate animals in research: DOD Directive 3216.1, Use of Animals in DOD Programs (DOD 2010); the 1995 Army Regulation 40-33/ SECNAVINST 3900.38C/AFMAN 40-401(I)/DARPAINST 18/USUHSINST 3203, The Care and Use of Laboratory Animals in DOD Programs (DOD 2005); and the VA Handbook 1200.07 Use of Animals in Research (VA 2011). Research conducted with VA funds must be approved through a VA IACUC, while extramural research conducted with DOD funds must still adhere to most provisions of the DOD research regulations, regardless of what other regulatory requirements may be applicable to a given research project (DOD 2005, VA 2011). Table 1.5 summarizes the various institutional and IACUC requirements that are stipulated by the PHS Policy, the AWA, the DOD Directive and Army Regulations, and the VA Handbook.

Other federal agencies have also developed their own regulations or policies for the conduct of vertebrate animal research. In addition, many local and state entities have passed laws related to the use of animals in research (NABR 2014). These regulations vary widely between localities, but may include additional reporting and inspection requirements or specific restrictions on use (NABR 2014).

Table 1.5 is a comparison of the differences and similarities between the PHS Policy, AWA, DOD, and Veterans Health Administration (VHA) regulations with regard to the use of laboratory animals in research, testing, and teaching.

1.3.5 Institutional Animal Care and Use Committees

The one overriding commonality among all of the different sets of rules and regulations governing animal research is the central role of the IACUC. Conceptually, the IACUC is intended to ensure high ethical standards, humane treatment, and accountability in all use of research animals. The details of an IACUC composition differ, but the scope of its authority and responsibility is consistent.

Table 1.5 Regulatory Agencies

Regulatory Agency	PHS Policy	AWA	DOD[b]	VA
Species covered	III A. Any live, vertebrate animal used or intended for use in research, research training, experimentation, or biological testing or for related purposes.	§ 2132. (g) any live or dead warm-blooded animal, as the Secretary may determine is being used, or is intended for use, for research, testing, experimentation, or exhibition purposes, or as a pet; but such term excludes (1) birds, rats of the genus *Rattus*, and mice of the genus *Mus*, bred for use in research purposes, and (3) other farm animals, such as, but not limited to livestock or poultry, used or intended for use as food or fiber, or livestock or poultry used or intended for use for improving animal nutrition, breeding, management, or production efficiency, or for improving the quality of food or fiber.	Glossary. Part II.[b] 1.*b*.[c] Any living or dead vertebrate animal including birds, cold-blooded animals, rats of the genus *Rattus* and mice of the genus *Mus*. With respect to avian and other egg-laying vertebrate species, their offspring are considered animals only after hatching. With respect to fish and amphibians, their larval offspring are considered animals. For the purpose of the definition "dead" is defined as animals killed for the direct purpose of conducting RDT&E or training. However it does not include dead animals or parts of dead animals purchased at grocery stores or slaughterhouses.	3.c. Any live vertebrate animal used or intended for use in research, research training, experimentation, or biological testing, or for a related purpose. An animal for purposes of compliance with the AWAR means any live or dead dog, cat, non-human primate, guinea pig, hamster, rabbit or any other warm-blooded animal which is being used or is intended for use in research, teaching, testing, experimentation, exhibition purposes, or as a pet. The term excludes birds, rats of the genus *Rattus* and mice of the genus *Mus* bred for research, horses not used for research and other farm animals used or intended for use as food or fiber, or livestock or poultry used or intended for use in improving animal nutrition, breeding, management, or production efficiency, or for improving the quality of food or fiber.

(continued)

Table 1.5 (Continued)   Regulatory Agencies

Regulatory Agency	PHS Policy	AWA	DOD	VA
IACUC membership composition	IV. A. 3. b. The IACUC committee must contain no less than 5 members (one DVM, one practicing scientist, one non-scientist, and one non-affiliated member). An individual who meets the requirements of more than one of these categories may fulfill more than one requirement. However, the committee must be composed of at least 5 members.	§ 2.31. b. The Committee shall be composed of a Chairman and at least 2 other members, one a doctor of Veterinary Medicine and one a nonaffiliated member. If the Committee is composed of more than three members, not more than three members shall be from the same administrative unit of the facility. § 2.33 a. 3. The AV shall be a voting member of the IACUC *provided however* that a research facility with more than one DVM may appoint to the IACUC another DVM with delegated program responsibility for activities involving animals at the research facility.	Enclosure 3. (3) c. 1-2.[b] 5. *f.f.*[c] The IACUCs of DOD institutions shall consist of at least 5 members with various backgrounds to promote complete and accurate review of RDT&E and training activities including one DVM, one non-affiliated member and one non-scientist. The IACUC must delegate an alternate member(s) for the non-affiliated member. To have a quorum at least one veterinarian and one non-affiliated member (or his or her alternate) must be present. When a compelling reason exists, the IACUC may request approval from the Head of the OSD or DOD Component to waive this requirement in order to meet without the non-affiliated member.	8. a. The medical facility Director who must serve as the IO must officially appoint members in writing to the IACUC. A minimum of 5 members are required to serve as voting members of the IACUC including a Chairperson, the AV, one scientist with animal research experience, a non-affiliated member, and a lay member.
Internal accreditation, registration, and assurance requirements	IV. A. Animal Welfare Assurances shall be signed by the IO and submitted to OLAW. Assurances are approved for a specified period of time (Domestic Assurances are approved for up to 4 years, Interinstitutional and Foreign Assurances are approved for up to 5 years) at which time a new Assurance must be submitted to OLAW.[a]	§ 2.30. Each research facility other than Federal research facilities shall register with the Secretary the proper form which will be furnished by request, by the AC Regional Director and filled with the AC Regional Director of the State. Registrations must be updated every three years. (For a full description of registration requirements, see §2.30a 1-3.)		

| Outside agency accreditation, registration, and assurance requirements | IV.A.2. Each institution must assure that its program and facilities are in one of the following categories: Category 1, Accredited by the AAALAC. All of the institution's programs and facilities (including satellite facilities) for activities involving animals have been evaluated and accredited by AAALAC, or another accrediting body recognized by PHS. All of the institution's programs and facilities (including satellite facilities) for activities involving animals have also been evaluated by the IACUC and will be reevaluated by the IACUC at least once every six months. Category 2: Evaluated by the Institution. All of the institution's programs and facilities (including satellite facilities) for activities involving animals have been evaluated by the IACUC and will be reevaluated by the IACUC at least once every six months. The most recent semiannual report of the IACUC evaluation shall be submitted to OLAW with the Assurance.[a] | Enclosure 3. (3) b.[b] 4. e.[c] All DOD institutions housing animals for RDT&E or training shall attain and maintain AAALAC accreditation with these exceptions: (1) DOD institutions housing animals for RDT&E or training for less than 8 continuous calendar days, however they shall have animal facilities inspected and approved by a DOD veterinarian. (2) Additional exemptions as the DDR&E determines appropriate. Enclosure 3. 2. b. Non-Federal institutions conducting DOD-supported RDT&E or training in the United States must be registered with the USDA, unless otherwise exempt. | 4. b. All VA animal research must be covered by a PHS Assurance. Local VA medical facilities may be covered by their affiliate's PHS Assurance in lieu of having their own PHS Assurance. The text in the affiliate's Assurance document must make it clear that the VA medical facility animal research program is covered as part of the affiliate's Assurance. 7. e. All VA animal facilities and affiliates, or other animal facilities that house animals purchased with VA funds, or used for VA or VA research and education corporation projects must be accredited by AAALAC. |

(continued)

Table 1.5 (Continued) Regulatory Agencies

Regulatory Agency	PHS Policy	AWA	DOD	VA
Semiannual program review requirements	IV. B. 1-3. The IACUC must review at least once every six months the institution's program and inspect all of the institution's animal facilities using the Guide as the basis for evaluation. The IACUC must prepare semiannual program review and facility inspection reports that are submitted to the IO.	§ 2.31 c. The IACUC shall review at least every six months the research facility's program and inspect all of the animal facilities including animal study areas (any building room, area, enclosure, or other containment outside of a core facility or centrally designed or managed area in which animals are housed for more than 12 hours). The IACUC may use subcommittees composed of at least two members in conducting animal facility and study area evaluations. Reports of the semiannual evaluations shall be signed by a majority of the IACUC, and be submitted to the IO.	Enclosure 3. (3) e.[b] 4. f., 8. a.[c] All DOD institutions using or housing animals for RDT&E or training for more than 12 hours shall conduct a program review, including facility inspections, at least annually using DOD Form 2856 which must be signed by a majority of the IACUC's members and submitted to the IO. This review shall also be submitted to the DOD Component headquarters oversight office.	8.f.1.The designated VA IACUC must perform a self-assessment review of the program of animal care and research use, and an inspection of the animal facilities and husbandry practices at least every 6 months. The review team, consisting of at least 2 voting members of the IACUC, must include all facilities and investigator areas where laboratory animals purchased with local VA funds are used in procedures, or housed for longer than 12 hours. As part of the Program review, the IACUC must randomly review IACUC records representing at least 5% of the total active projects (a minimum of 5). The compliance items found in the VA IACUC Program and Facility Self-Assessment Checklist must be covered by the IACUC. The OLAW Semiannual Program and Facility Review checklist, or a similar checklist incorporating all the elements found in the VA checklist need to be completed within 1 month of the self-review. The report must be approved by a majority vote of the IACUC, discussed with the medical facility Director by the

IACUC Chairperson, veterinarian and one or more other research administrators. The medical facility Director must sign the report which must be sent to the CVMO through the medical facility Director within 60 days of the self-review date.

8.f.2. The IACUC must review proposed research at convened meetings at which a quorum is present. The use of designated review systems may be used where each new protocol must be assigned to at least 2 voting members. VA policy stipulates that all IACUC members receive complete copies of all protocol forms to aid them in deciding whether or not to request full committee review. The research office must provide packets to the IACUC members no later than 3 business days before the IACUC meeting.

Enclosure 3. 2. a-d.^{b} 4. f.^{c} At a minimum, the DOD Component headquarters oversight office must conduct an administrative review and approve of all DOD-supported RDT&E and training, which shall be submitted to the IACUC using the DOD Standard Animal Use Protocol Format. A DOD veterinarian shall conduct the review. When an IACUC approves significant changes to an approved protocol the Component must review and approve the changes before they are implemented. For DOD- supported but not conducted RDE&T or training, RDE&T and training must be approved by the performing institution's IACUC, a veterinarian working under the

§ 2.31. d. 2. Prior to IACUC review each member of the Committee shall be provided with a list of proposed activities to be reviewed. Any member of the IACUC may request full Committee review. If full Committee review is not requested, at least one member of the IACUC, designated by the Chairman shall review those activities.

Initial protocol review

IV. C. 2. Prior to review each IACUC member shall be provided with a list of proposed research projects to be reviewed with the option of requesting full committee review of a research project. If full committee review is not requested, at least one member of the IACUC, designated by the chairperson, shall review the research project.

(continued)

Table 1.5 (Continued)   Regulatory Agencies

Regulatory Agency	PHS Policy	AWA	DOD	VA
			authority of the IACUC must oversee the animals approved in a protocol or under an IACUC policy referenced in the protocol, significant changes must be approved by an IACUC before they are implemented and all RDE&T and training must be reviewed by the IACUC annually. Non-DOD institutions are not required to use the DOD standard Animal Care and Use Protocol Format.	
Continuing protocol review	IV. C. 5. The IACUC shall conduct continuing review of each previously approved, ongoing activity at appropriate intervals as determined by the IACUC, including a complete review at least once every three years.	§ 2.31. d.5. The IACUC shall conduct continuing review of activities involving animals at appropriate intervals as determined by the IACUC, but not less than annually.	Enclosure 3. 2.c.[b] All RDT&E and training approved by an IACUC must be reviewed by the IACUC at least annually.	8. g. The IACUC must review the conduct of all animal protocols annually. Prior to the third anniversary, the IACUC must conduct a complete re-review of the protocol.
Suspension of animal activities	IV. C. 7. If the IACUC suspends an activity involving animals, the IO in consultation with the IACUC shall review the reasons for suspension, take appropriate corrective action, and report that action with a full explanation to OLAW.	§ 2.31. d.7. If the IACUC suspends previously approved activities involving animals, after review of the matter at a convened meeting with a quorum present and a majority vote of the IACUC, then through the IO, the reason for suspension, corrective actions taken and a full explanation must be submitted to APHIS and any Federal agency funding that activity.	Enclosure 3. 6. C.[b] 8. a.[c] Records that document extramural compliance or noncompliance shall be made accessible for inspection and copying by authorized representatives of the DOD at reasonable times in a reasonable manner as determined by the supporting DOD Component.	8.i. The VA Central Office expects that the IACUC and institutional administrators will avoid any appearance of hiding or suppressing deficiencies. Any serious or continuing non-compliance with PHS Policy (including any serious deviation or continuing non-compliance with the provisions of The Guide, as required by the PHS Policy) or USDA AWA or suspensions of

| Internal reporting requirements | IV. F. 1-2. At least every 12 months, the IACUC, through the IO, shall report to OLAW: any change in the institution's program or facilities that would place it in a different category than specified in the Assurance, any change in the description of the institution's program, changes to IACUC membership, and notice of the dates that the IACUC conducted its semiannual evaluations. If no changes have been made then this should be reported to OLAW including the dates of the required IACUC evaluations. | § 2.36 Each reporting facility shall submit an annual report to the AC Regional Director for the State where the facility is located on or before December 1 of each calendar year. The report should be signed and certified by the CEO or IO and shall cover the previous Federal fiscal year. | protocols previously approved or suspensions of procedures or studies never given approval must be reported.

8.l. The following reports and correspondence must be forwarded to the CVMO's office or ORD as indicated: USDA annual report, AAALAC annual reports (the triennial program description should not be submitted to ORDs or the CVMO, unless a copy is requested), IACUC semiannual self-assessment reviews (no later than 60 days after the self-assessment review date), annual VA VMU report for the previous fiscal year must be completed using the Web site designed for that purpose by January 15, new PHS Assurances (within 30 days of submission to PHS) and a copy of all correspondence between OLAW, USDA, AAALAC, and VA facilities must be forwarded to the CVMO and ORO within 15 business days of receipt or mailing. |

(continued)

Table 1.5 (Continued) Regulatory Agencies

Regulatory Agency	PHS Policy	AWA	DOD	VA
Other reporting requirements	IV. F. 3. The IACUC, through the IO, shall promptly report to OLAW with a full explanation of the circumstances and actions taken: any serious or continuing noncompliance with the PHS Policy, any serious deviation from the Guide, and any suspension of an activity by the IACUC.	§ 2.31. c. 3. If a program or facility notes a significant deficiency during the semiannual program review that remains uncorrected, it shall be reported in writing within 15 business days by the IACUC through the IO, to APHIS and any Federal agency funding the activity.	Enclosure 3. (3) g.[b] 5. c.[c] Institutions must notify the DOD Component when the institution is notified by the USDA that it is under investigation, notified by AAALAC that it has lost its accreditation status or when an institution has experienced any adverse events regarding the RDT&E or training. The institution shall notify their Component headquarters oversight office within 5 business days. Upon notification by the USDA or AAALAC when the issue is relevant to a DOD-supported activity, a DOD veterinarian shall perform a site inspection within 30 days of the notification.	8.i. Deficiencies meeting the criteria of any serious or continuing non-compliance with PHS Policy or USDA AWA, suspensions of protocols previously approved or suspensions of procedures or studies never given approval, and failure to correct a significant deficiency (identified during a semiannual IACUC program or facility self-assessment review) must be reported in writing within 15 business days of the self-imposed deadline by the IACUC through the IO, to USDA and any Federal agency funding that activity. This required 15 business day reporting period is extended to cover all categories of reportable deficiencies and must be reported to ORD, OLAW, USDA, AAALAC, the affiliate's IACUC, the VA ORO or any other Federal agency funding the activity that has been suspended.

Records retention requirements	IV. E. The awardee institution must maintain for at least 3 years: a copy of the Assurance; IACUC meeting minutes; records of applications, proposals, and proposed significant changes in the care and use of animals and whether IACUC approval was given or withheld; records of semiannual reports; and records of accrediting body determinations. Records related directly to applications, proposals, and proposed significant changes should be kept for an additional 3 years after completion of the activity.	§ 2.35 The research facility shall maintain for the duration of the activity and for an additional 3 years after completion of the activity the following records: IACUC meeting minutes, records of proposed activities and proposed significant changes in activities involving animals and whether IACUC approval was given or withheld, and records and forms required for cats and dogs.	Enclosure 3. 6.ᵇ 8. a.ᶜ DOD Components are to retain records for at least 3 years beyond the end of the RDT&E and training activity or the effective date of the record including; records from DOD-conducted or --supported RDT&E and training that are created by either the Government or the institution conducting the work, records regarding waivers, exemptions, and extensions and records that document extramural compliance or noncompliance.	8. f. The IACUC semiannual program review report must be retained on file for at least 3 years by the research office or as required by the VHA Record Control Schedule. Appendix E. c. Minutes of IACUC meetings and semiannual reports are kept for 3 years. IACUC documents are kept for 3 years after end of study. All PHS, USDA, ORO, AAALAC, and other reports and correspondence related to the animal care and research use program are maintained for at least 3 years.

(continued)

Table 1.5 (Continued)   Regulatory Agencies

Regulatory Agency	PHS Policy	AWA	DOD	VA
Institution inspections by regulatory agency	V. C. Institutions are subject to review at any time by PHS staff and advisors, which may include a site visit.	§ 2.38 a.-b. Each research facility shall during business hours allow APHIS officials to: enter its place of business, examine records required to be kept by the Act, make copies of records, and inspect the facilities, property, and animals. § 2.35 f. APHIS inspectors will maintain confidentiality and will not remove materials from the premises unless there has been an alleged violation, they are needed to investigate an alleged violation, or for enforcement purposes. Release of any such materials, including reports, summaries, and photographs that contain trade secrets or commercial of financial information that is privileged or confidential will be governed by the Freedom Of Information Act.	Enclosure 3. d. 5. [b] 5. c. [c] For all RDT&E using dogs, cats, nonhuman primates, or marine mammals and for all medical training using live animals the contractor must pass an on-site evaluation conducted by a DOD veterinarian within 30 days of the signed agreement with the DOD if the animals are already present at the institution or within 30 days of delivery of the animals if they are not. The onsite evaluation shall be repeated annually for the duration of the training agreement, as longs as animals are being used. If the institution is accredited by AAALAC or meets equivalent standards the DOD Component may waive the requirement for on-site inspection.	

Source: Data from NIH (National Institutes of Health). 2002. Public Health Service policy on humane care and use of laboratory animals. Bethesda, MD: Office of Laboratory Animal Welfare, NIH; USDA (U.S. Department of Agriculture). 2013a. Animal Welfare Act and Animal Welfare Regulations: Animal Care Blue Book. Code of Federal Regulations (CFR), Title 9, Chapter 1, Subchapter A, Parts 1–3.; VA, VHA (Department of Veterans Affairs, Veterans Health Administration). 2011. VHA Handbook 1200.07, Use of animals in research. VA, VHA, Washington, DC.

[a] OLAW. 2012. Obtaining an Assurance. Bethesda, MD: NIH. http://grants.nih.gov/grants/olaw/obtain_assurance.htm.
[b] DOD. 2010. Department of Defense Instruction 3216.01 Use of Animals in DOD Programs.
[c] DOD. 2005. Army Regulation 40-33/SECNAVINST/3900.38C/AFMAN 40-40(1)/DARPAINST 18/USUHSINST 3203 The Care and Use of Laboratory Animals in DOD Programs.

1.4 CONCLUSION

Navigating the myriad of external regulations, voluntary accreditation, and internal institutional policies can be a daunting task. Regulations, standards, and policies do change and evolve over time; hence, it is important to keep abreast of current developments. USDA Animal Care maintains a stakeholder registry, which is a venue to receive information on current events and to comment on proposed regulatory and policy changes (https://public.govdelivery.com/accounts/USDAAPHIS/subscriber/new). In addition, Regulations.gov (http://www.regulations.gov/#!home) is the general federal website where one can learn about pending legislation and proposals, as well as provide public comment.

This book will attempt to provide institutions with the necessary information and resources to organize and manage an effective IACUC, whether the institution is a large complex academic program or a small device company attempting to establish a program for safety testing of its product. Regardless of its size or complexity, a well-run animal care and use program is essential to ensure that animals used in research, teaching, and testing are afforded humane and appropriate treatment. When done correctly, the public's confidence is earned through a system of self-regulation, and keeping regulatory burden to a minimum. If done incorrectly, further regulation and regulatory oversight are certain to follow.

REFERENCES

Adams, B. and J. Larson. 2007 (updated 2014). *Legislative History of the Animal Welfare Act.* U.S. Department of Agriculture, Animal Welfare Information Center. Washington, DC: USDA. http://awic.nal.usda.gov/legislative-history-animal-welfare-act-table-contents.

DOD (Department of Defense). 2005. The care and use of laboratory animals in DOD programs. DOD, Washington, DC.

DOD (Department of Defense). 2010. DOD Instruction 3216.01. Use of animals in DOD programs. DOD, Washington, DC.

Horner, J. and F. D. Minifie. 2011. Research ethics I: Responsible conduct of research (RCR): Historical and contemporary issues pertaining to human and animal experimentation. *Journal of Speech, Language, and Hearing Research* 54 (1):S303–S329.

Lennox, J. 2011. Aristotle's biology. *Stanford Encyclopedia of Philosophy.* Stanford, CA: The Metaphysics Research Lab.

NABR (National Association for Biomedical Research). 2014. Animal Law Section. Washington, DC: NABR. http://www.nabranimallaw.org/

NIH (National Institutes of Health). 2002. Public Health Service policy on humane care and use of laboratory animals. Bethesda, MD: Office of Laboratory Animal Welfare, NIH.

NRC (National Research Council). 2011. *Guide for the Care and Use of Laboratory Animals,* 8th edn. Washington, DC: National Academies Press.

Paul, E. F. 2002. Why animal experimentation matters. *Society* 39 (6):7–15.

Sandgren, E. P. 2005. Defining the animal care and use program. *Lab Animal (NY)* 34:41–44.

Sharp, P. and J. Villano. 2012. *The Laboratory Rat,* 2nd edn. Boca Raton, FL: CRC Press.

Steneck, N. H. 1997. Role of the institutional animal care and use committee in monitoring research. *Ethics & Behavior* 7 (2):173–184.

USDA (U.S. Department of Agriculture). 2004. Rules and regulations, animal welfare: Definition of an animal. *Federal Register* 69 (108):31537.

USDA (U.S. Department of Agriculture). 2013a. *Animal Welfare Act and Animal Welfare Regulations* (Animal Care Blue Book). Code of Federal Regulations (CFR), Title 9, Chapter 1, Subchapter A, Parts 1–4.

USDA (U.S. Department of Agriculture). 2013b. Animal Welfare Act of 1966 intended to regulate the transport, sale and handling of dogs, cats, guinea pigs, nonhuman primates, hamsters and rabbits intended to use for research or other purposes. *Public Law* 89 (544):2131–2156.

VA, VHA (Department of Veterans Affairs, Veterans Health Administration). 2011. Use of animals in research, *VHA Handbook 1200.07*. VA, VHA, Washington, DC.

Wynes, D. L., G. Martin, and D. J. Skorton. 2002. Regulatory challenges in university research. *Issues in Science and Technology* 18:37–42.

CHAPTER 2

Role of the IACUC, Bioethics and Scientific Review, Essential Environment for IACUC Success

Jerry Collins

CONTENTS

2.1 THE IACUC PROCESS: WHY BOTHER?

Service as a member of an Institutional Animal Care and Use Committee (IACUC) is frequently viewed by the uninitiated as something to be avoided at any price. The workload is viewed as excessive, the responsibilities are judged to be onerous, and the IACUC process is thought to be another administrative burden. In spite of that "outsider's" view, it has been the experience of this author that once an individual with that view begins to serve on a well-functioning IACUC, they are very likely to change their opinion; they recognize that the IACUC process is essential to our ongoing use of nonhuman animal models (hereafter referred to as *animal models*) in research, teaching, and testing.

2.1.1 Living Beings Deserve Compassion and Benevolence

The Nuremberg Code (U.S. GPO, 1949) is a set of ethical principles promulgated after the Second World War in order to establish basic requirements for acceptable medical experiments on humans. One of those requirements, Point 3 of the Nuremberg Code, states in part, "The experiment should be so designed and based on the results of animal experimentation ... that the anticipated results will justify the performance of the experiment." In essence, humans should not be the subject of medical experimentation without first using animal models to establish the value of the proposed experiment. Basing human experimentation on the results of animal experimentation means that animal models not only provide us with knowledge of living systems but also act as surrogates for each of us and for all our friends and family. Nonhuman animals act as our surrogates for developmental studies of new drugs, new devices, and new procedures. The following quote from the National Aeronautics and Space Administration (NASA) Principles for the Ethical Care and Use of Animals is a wonderfully succinct statement about the responsibilities associated with the use of animal models:

> The use of animals in research involves responsibility—not only for the stewardship of the animals but to the scientific community and society as well. Stewardship is a universal responsibility that goes beyond the immediate research needs to include acquisition, care, and disposition of the animals, while responsibility to the scientific community and society requires an appropriate understanding of and sensitivity to scientific needs and community attitudes toward the use of animals. (NASA 1996)

Members of an IACUC are charged with giving final approval for our surrogates to be used in ways that almost always result in death and may involve distress or pain. As an IACUC member, each of us must ensure that compassion and benevolence underlie all decisions that relate to the use of animal models, and that those decisions are supportive of the scientific process and are informed by the attitudes of the community in which the research, teaching, and testing occur. Although IACUC service is challenging, the opportunity to serve community, science, and the living beings used as animal models is judged by many to be an honorable and important undertaking.

2.1.2 Society Expects Experiments to Be Regulated

Unfortunately, scientists are frequently portrayed as "mad scientists"—people who do horrible things behind closed doors. As with most professions, the vocabulary and complexity of procedures associated with the use of animal models in biomedical research, teaching, and testing make it difficult for the general public to understand the undertaking and add to the suspicion about what really happens in labs. A well-functioning IACUC process enables investigators and institutions to assure the public that there are rules and regulations in place.

In the United States, we are fortunate to be able to apply the Animal Welfare Regulations (USDA 2013a) and Public Health Service (PHS) Policy on Humane Care and Use of Laboratory Animals (NIH 2002) at the local level where the unique circumstances of each institution can be best understood. The Congressional Committee report accompanying the 1985 Health Research Extension Act included the following statement: "It is far preferable to place primary responsibility for assuring compliance with NIH guidelines on committees within institutions rather than relying on intrusive Federal inspections" (Wigglesworth 2006). Recognition of the value of local oversight led to the creation of the IACUC process. However, the opportunity to participate in local oversight carries with it a heavy responsibility to our own institution and also to the larger research enterprise. Each IACUC member must understand and willingly accept both the authority and responsibility vested in the IACUC. We are the ones who are charged with ensuring that rules and regulations pertaining to the use of animal models are understood and followed. If we fail to meet those obligations, then we can blame no one but ourselves for society's increasing unease with the use of animal models in research, teaching, and testing.

2.1.3 Efficient IACUC Processes Can Facilitate Science

Although investigators rarely view the IACUC process as facilitating science, Congress recognized that the undertaking that was to be overseen is essential to human and animal health. The Congressional Statement of Policy associated with the 1985 amendments to the Animal Welfare Act (AWA) (USDA 2013b) contains the following statement: "The use of animals is instrumental in certain research and education for advancing knowledge of cures and treatment for diseases and injuries which afflict both humans and animals." Federally mandated oversight created a means by which the public's representatives in Congress could be assured that legitimate concerns about inappropriate animal use would be addressed, while at the same time ensuring that essential animal-based research, teaching, and testing would proceed.

The IACUC process is complex and can unfortunately lend itself to bureaucratic growth without a concomitant overall improvement in animal welfare. Each of us must participate in meaningful program review that includes careful consideration of what we ask of our colleagues as they seek permission to use an animal model. We are in a position to facilitate science by reducing to an absolute minimum, in keeping with regulatory and policy requirements and humane animal care, the amount of work required of an investigator participating in the federally mandated IACUC process. In law, neither research utilizing United States Department of Agriculture (USDA)-covered species nor PHS-funded research with animals could proceed without IACUC approval. An IACUC facilitates science by doing its job well and efficiently.

2.2 INSTITUTIONAL CULTURE

Each institution, whether it is public or private, academic or industrial, has its own way of doing things and of viewing the world in which it operates. Those methods of operation and worldviews will, to a large extent, underlie the success or failure of an IACUC. In most institutions, the IACUC is only one of many regulatory processes that impact research, teaching, or testing. Chemical safety, biological safety, radiation safety, and the safety of human subjects are some of the additional issues to which investigators must attend before engaging in their work. The way that an institution enforces compliance, provides support to facilitate interactions with regulatory bodies, and encourages collegial interactions will greatly influence the IACUC's success.

2.2.1 Culture of Compliance

A fair and impartial IACUC that strives to make well-informed decisions is the ideal. If an institution's culture relies on a hierarchal process of leniency for the "big hitters," it is unlikely that that institution has a robust IACUC. At best, that IACUC will be fighting a constant battle with those with special interests who view their undertakings as too important to be bogged down by rules and regulations. In contrast, a "culture of compliance" will enable all involved to understand that compliance with the rules is expected of all concerned. We will consider below how individuals may contribute to an equitable process in which all are expected to meet the same standards.

2.2.2 Service Oriented

Anyone who has sought permission from an IACUC knows that the process is not instantaneous; it can't be! We all recognize that we may not come to work on

Monday with a new idea and immediately test it on an animal model. Having used animal models prior to the requirement for IACUC review, I am convinced that animal welfare has improved with the introduction of that review. By that same token, I have also experienced the frustration of having to wait for IACUC approval.

Institutions are required to provide resources necessary to enable an IACUC to function. But resources are not enough! We must recognize that IACUC review imposes delay and, perhaps more importantly, that IACUC review is seldom the only permission that an investigator must obtain before beginning a project. As an example, consider a pediatrician who is treating patients, conducting human studies of an investigational drug, and conducting animal studies in genetically modified animals that include radioactive markers, nanoparticles, magnetic resonance imaging, and newly developed monoclonal antibodies. That individual is faced with obtaining clearance from, at a minimum, a human subject institutional review board (IRB), an IACUC, a biosafety committee, and a radiation safety committee. That is not including agencies that oversee medical and drug licenses or protect the privacy of clinical data (HIPPA). We will consider below how individuals, by focusing on providing a service, may contribute to a reduction in that workload, at least from the IACUC perspective.

2.2.3 Collegial Decisions Made by a Majority

In my experience, efforts to reach a consensus on all items being discussed can be a source of great inefficiency for an IACUC. Each committee member brings a unique perspective to the table, and each opinion must be allowed full voice. That does not mean that each opinion should be repeated *ad nauseum*! Nor does it mean that discussions must continue until all parties are in agreement. An IACUC is frequently asked to make very difficult decisions that involve balancing the impact on individual animals with a greater anticipated good. It is reasonable to expect that an IACUC will not reach consensus on challenging issues. We will consider below how individuals may maintain collegial relationships in a setting where they are, at times, in the minority on issues of great importance to them.

2.3 SCIENTIFIC AND ETHICAL REVIEW BY AN IACUC

A well-functioning IACUC recognizes that scientific and ethical issues embedded within a research proposal deserve consideration and must be addressed as part of protocol review. The Animal Welfare Regulations (AWRs) and the PHS Policy each identify areas of inquiry that an IACUC should consider as it reviews a request to use an animal model for research, teaching, or testing (USDA 2013a, NIH 2002). The 8th edition of the Guide for the Care and Use of Laboratory Animals (the Guide) (NRC 2011) contains a slightly expanded version of topics that should be considered by an IACUC. Those lists should be the basis for questions contained in the forms that are used by an institution to provide an IACUC with information upon which to base a decision about requested animal usage, hereafter referred to as the "protocol" form.

Embedded within those topics are two areas, ethical review and scientific review, that are frequently claimed to be outside of the purview of an IACUC. A closer consideration of the degree of ethical and scientific review may help to clarify this issue.

2.3.1 Harm–Benefit Analysis

The term *ethical review* raises obvious questions about the meaning of ethics. A better term is *harm–benefit analysis*. The following is a quote from the U.S. Government Principles for the Utilization and Care of Vertebrate Animals Used in Testing, Research, and Training (NIH 1985) on the issue of harm versus benefit: "Procedures involving animals should be designed and performed with due consideration of their relevance to human or animal health, the advancement of knowledge, or the good of society." It is not enough for an IACUC to determine that adequate anesthesia and analgesia will be present when a group of animals undergoes a survival surgical procedure. A harm–benefit analysis must enter into the picture; is the likely benefit to other nonhuman or human animals or the advancement of knowledge important enough that animals be exposed to the planned procedures?

As society's gatekeeper, the IACUC is faced with deciding if an animal should be used in the proposed project. Animals may experience pain, distress, or both, and each member of an IACUC should continually ask if the benefit of the animal use is balanced by the harm that may impact the animal. We must always remember that although the IACUC process can quickly devolve into crossing *t*'s and dotting *i*'s, our focus *must* remain on the animals; and that at times, difficult decisions about harm versus benefit must be made. In a situation where animal testing of a drug that is likely to reverse rheumatoid arthritis is being proposed, the potential benefit to both nonhuman and human animals is obvious, and an aggressive model of rheumatoid arthritis might be approved. In contrast, if the proposal is to conduct an initial study of an as-yet untested drug that it is hoped will reduce symptoms of rheumatoid arthritis, it may be more appropriate to use a less aggressive arthritis model that has less harm associated with it than a more aggressive one.

2.3.2 Scientific Merit

Scientific review by an IACUC is not and never was intended to be equivalent to a peer-review process like that conducted for NIH grant applications. However, there are many aspects of the scientific process to which an IACUC should attend. Although the PHS Policy and the AWRs do not directly address this issue, they make statements including "Procedures with animals will avoid or minimize discomfort, distress, and pain to the animals, consistent with sound research design" (NIH 2002) and "No animal will be used in more than one major operative procedure from which it is allowed to recover unless justified for scientific reasons" (USDA 2013a). These two examples imply that part of the consideration of the humane nature of animal use must include attention to scientific principles. The Guide is more specific: "The IACUC should evaluate scientific elements of the protocol … e.g. hypothesis testing, sample size, group numbers, and adequacy of controls" (NRC 2011).

2.4 WHO DOES WHAT?

Before discussing some of the roles of members and how each may contribute to an advantageous institutional culture, there is value in considering the limits to the expectations placed on an IACUC. An IACUC is charged with responsibilities much greater than those assigned to other committees at most institutions. Fortunately, those responsibilities are delineated in the AWRs, the PHS Policy, and the Guide and should be referred to when administrators decide to add "just a few more tasks" to the IACUC. The following are two examples of concerns that may be identified by an IACUC, but should not be placed in an IACUC's portfolio.

2.4.1 Conflict of Interest

Each IACUC should have a means by which reviewers may recuse themselves from actions that may impact research in which they may have an interest, including both the success of the research and financial conflicts of interest; for example, a committee member should not review a spouse's protocol, nor should that member review any protocol associated with an entity in which the member has a significant financial interest. Beyond those actions, the IACUC should not become involved in determining or managing conflict-of-interest issues. If an IACUC encounters evidence of a possible conflict, that information should be passed on to the relevant entity within the institution for follow-up.

2.4.2 Scientific Misconduct

Given the broad charge imposed on an IACUC, it is possible that it may encounter evidence of scientific misconduct. While that information should be shared with the relevant entity within the institution, the IACUC should not be expected to investigate and recommend actions. An institutional culture of compliance should include individuals with adequate expertise in the various regulatory areas who are charged with focusing on those specific areas, rather than attempting to place additional burdens on an IACUC.

2.4.3 IACUC Roles and Responsibilities

If an IACUC functions best in a culture of compliance where there is a focus on service and collegial interactions, how may each member of an IACUC contribute to that environment in a meaningful way?

2.4.3.1 Institutional Official (IO)

Although not a member of the IACUC, the institutional official (IO) is a key figure in ensuring that an institution's culture is supportive of the IACUC process. Typically, an IO is well positioned within an institution's administration to provide input into how regulatory issues are addressed. In addition, an IO frequently has responsibility for other regulatory concerns (e.g., human investigations, conflicts of interest). In that leadership role, an IO has an opportunity to reinforce the need for the creation of a level playing field for all, a playing field that emphasizes the importance of maintaining compliance by everyone, irrespective of rank or seniority. The IO also is in a position to encourage ongoing training for all relevant members of the animal program to ensure that they understand both the regulatory requirements and the institution's expectations concerning compliance with those requirements.

The focus on the IACUC providing service is also within the purview of the IO, not only through leadership, but also through resource allocation. Typically, the IACUC staff is the "face" of the IACUC, and staff must be adequately trained and provided with the resources necessary to guarantee a smooth interaction among the various parties that rely on the IACUC. The IO can clarify an expectation that service is the goal and back that up with resources necessary for staff to participate in ongoing training in both regulations and office efficiency.

Given the far-reaching responsibilities of a CEO or IO they rely heavily on information from other sources to identify potential new members. That selection should take into account the need for fair and impartial oversight of the animal program by individuals who are concerned about animal welfare and recognize the importance of minimizing burdens on already overburdened investigators. A detailed description of the roles and responsibilities of the CEO or IO can be found in both the AWA (d)(8) and the Animal Welfare Regulations (9 CFR Subchapter A, Parts 1–4, Section 2.31 (c)(3), (d)(7), and (d)(8)) for USDA-regulated activities as well as the PHS Policy IV. B.3 and IV.C.7. for federally funded activities.

2.4.3.2 Attending Veterinarian (AV)

The PHS Policy states that one member of the IACUC shall be a "Doctor of Veterinary Medicine, with training or experience in laboratory animal science and medicine, who has direct or delegated program authority and responsibility for activities involving animals at the institution." The Guide says the following: "The attending veterinarian is responsible for the health and well-being of all laboratory animals used at the institution" (NRC 2011). The IACUC is charged with oversight of the entire animal program, and within that program the AV is in charge of the health and well-being of the animals. The need for collegial interactions is quite evident in the interface that exists between the AV and IACUC. That collegiality requires that the IACUC understand and respect the authority and professional judgment of the AV. It also requires that the AV recognizes and respects the authority vested in the IACUC to monitor the animal program. Those interactions can be strengthened by the IACUC's provision of a buffer between the AV and investigators, a buffer that functions to allow the AV to be seen as an essential resource rather than a regulator.

As with the IO, the AV frequently has access to higher levels of administration and therefore is in a position to encourage an institutional culture of compliance. The AV is the epitome of service that is at the heart of humane animal care. In addition to providing for animal health and well-being, the AV is also ideally placed to facilitate service to investigators. An efficiently run animal program provides healthy subjects that maximize the ability to obtain useful information.

AVs may face the challenging and potentially conflicting job of being responsible for the budget that provides for animal care and well-being while at the same time being responsible for the health and well-being of all laboratory animals used at the institution. The potential conflict arises when an institution pressures the AV to reduce expenses. The efficient, cost-effective management of a division is to be expected, but excessive demands for cost cutting can place animals at risk. The institution is responsible for providing the AV with resources to manage the program of veterinary care, and the IACUC is responsible for oversight of that care and of institutional support essential to that care. An IACUC must recognize that it has the authority, as part of program review, to partner with the AV in efforts to obtain resources needed for adequate humane animal care. The AV should never be placed in a position of being the only voice seeking those essential resources.

2.4.3.3 IACUC Chair

The IACUC chair has a unique role to play in ensuring a culture of compliance and delivery of service in a collegial atmosphere. Perhaps the most important thing that a chair can do to enhance a culture of compliance is to ensure that all committee opinions are openly expressed, and that all issues receive fair and impartial review. The chair is also positioned to work with the IACUC staff to maximize the efficiency of interactions with investigators. The chair should always challenge both the committee members and staff to minimize regulatory burden, while meeting the goal of humane animal care.

The chair has an opportunity to ensure collegial interactions in many ways. Among the most important are ensuring ongoing committee education and avoiding having one individual become the *de facto* IACUC. Collegial interactions can be challenging when some members of the committee lack a basic understanding of the issues under consideration. It is unlikely that any committee member is well versed in all topics of discussion. The chair should ensure that opportunities are provided for questions to be asked by all committee members in a supportive environment; at times, that will mean reminding talkative souls that their point has already been well expressed.

It is likely that the AV, chair, and director of the IACUC office have the best understanding of issues likely to be discussed by the committee. It is not uncommon for some committee members to withdraw from real interactions and simply assume that one of those individuals will solve the problem. The chair must constantly be attentive to the committee's inappropriate reliance on the opinion of any one individual and, if necessary, work with that individual to more fully engage the reticent members.

2.4.3.4 Scientist

Opportunities abound for the scientist members of an IACUC to contribute to a culture of compliance and delivery of service in a collegial atmosphere. It is likely

that the scientists will have close working relationships and friendships with individuals whose protocols are under review. That knowledge is a double-edged sword.
On the one hand, it provides expertise essential to the decision-making process, but
on the other hand it can lead to "reading between the lines" when all necessary information has not been provided in a protocol. Each reviewer must remember that an
approved protocol defines the limits of the project. If important details are missing
from an approved protocol because the reviewer "knew" what a colleague meant,
the stage has been set for noncompliance! If it is not described in the protocol, it has
not been approved!

It is this author's opinion that the best thing a scientific member of an IACUC
can do to provide service, beyond ensuring humane animal care, is to constantly
ask why a particular question is being asked of an investigator. An IACUC can be
the worst source of "regulatory creep." Every committee member should review
both the questions being asked and the process by which they are asked, and in
addition ask themselves what will be done with the information when an answer is
provided. Avoid doing something just because that is how it has always been done.
Investigators deserve to receive clear, precise, relevant questions, just as they are
expected to provide clear, concise, relevant answers.

As stated above, ongoing committee education is very important, and scientific
members of a committee are well placed to contribute. Each committee member
has recognized expertise, and when those areas are under discussion, the relevant
member should endeavor to provide all members of the committee with at least a
summary of the technical points. In today's rapidly changing research environment,
it is not just the nonscientists who may be challenged to understand what has been
proposed. Each of us should consider it an obligation to ensure that all colleagues
serving on the committee are making informed decisions, recognizing that the depth
of understanding will vary from individual to individual.

2.4.3.5 Nonscientist, Unaffiliated Member

These two positions are perhaps the most challenging for the individuals who are
willing to take on the responsibility, and at times are filled by the same individual.
Meaningful on-the-job training is especially important for them if they are to be
fully engaged committee members. In an earlier part of this chapter, we raised the
issue of the public view of a scientist. The nonscientist and unaffiliated member,
because of their separation from the language and process of the science under discussion, provide an important reality check. Their contribution to a culture of compliance is best evidenced when they ask why; they will not read between the lines.
Their insistence on being provided with an explanation of issues under discussion
forces all of us to set aside assumptions and base decisions on the information with
which we are presented.

Their very presence on the committee provides an opportunity for the encouragement of a collegial environment. We need to take time to enhance their understanding of the challenging issues we all face. After all, they can serve as a conduit
for dissemination of the fact that humane care is important to our institutions.

2.5 SOME THOUGHTS ON THE EIGHT IACUC FUNCTIONS

Although an IACUC is frequently thought of as a group of people who only review protocols and inspect facilities, in reality the heavy responsibilities placed on this group of volunteers extend far beyond those two activities. Other authors will provide in-depth considerations of IACUC functions, but the following are some issues that deserve repetition.

2.5.1 Inspect Facilities, Review Program, Report Findings to the IO

The first responsibility—to inspect facilities—is fairly straightforward; enter an animal room or laboratory and use your senses (sight, hearing, smell) to determine if there is a problem. If a problem is identified during an inspection, it is the responsibility of the IACUC to determine the seriousness of the issue. A significant deficiency is one judged as such by the IACUC and the IO and defined by both the PHS Policy and the AWRs as a deficiency that is or may be a threat to the health or safety of the animals (USDA 2013a, NIH 2002). Note that the IO must be involved in this decision. The IACUC is also responsible for determining appropriate corrective action and an associated schedule for correction. Obviously, corrections will frequently involve collegial interactions with other members of the institution; however, the IACUC, not other entities, should define both the schedule for correction and the limits of the correction. Keep in mind that a mechanism should be in place to confirm that the correction occurred and that it was adequate. Trust but verify!

Reporting results to the IO is also fairly straightforward, keeping in mind that departures from the Guide must be included in the report, and that a majority of the committee must review and sign the report. It should be noted that minority reports are not simple votes against the approval of a protocol; rather, they represent the times when a committee member disagrees on the findings of a facility inspection or program review or has expressed a recommendation to the IO. Additional Semi-annual Program Review reporting requirements can be found in Chapter 6.

I am of the opinion that program review is the greatest challenge faced by an IACUC; I believe that the IACUC is responsible for the oversight of everything that may influence the health and well-being of live vertebrate animals and for many issues that may influence the health and well-being of humans working with those animals. This means that we are charged with overseeing the work of others. For example, if fire suppression systems exist in animal facilities, the IACUC should know that they are tested as required. An IACUC needs to know that emergency power that is required for animal survival is tested at appropriate intervals. It does not, however, mean that members of the IACUC should be responsible for the testing of emergency power or fire suppression systems! Unfortunately, some IACUCs or institutions confuse oversight with actually doing the work. Program review requires close working relationships between the IACUC and all offices that may have an impact on the animal program. As uncomfortable as it may sometimes be, we must ensure that others meet their responsibilities to the animal program.

2.5.2 Review and, If Warranted, Investigate Concerns

As described in 9 CFR §2.31 (c)(4) of the AWRs section IV.B.4. of the PHS Policy, the IACUC must "review, and if warranted investigate concerns involving the care and use of animals at the research facility resulting from public complaints received and from reports of noncompliance received from laboratory or research facility personnel or employees" (USDA 2013a). This is an IACUC responsibility that is likely to require close cooperation with other entities within the institution. It is also one for which plans should be in place. An important partner in this endeavor is likely to be a member of the institution's legal group. If an investigation reveals a problem, it is likely that institutional actions beyond those vested in the IACUC may be required. It is essential that all involved recognize that the IACUC has responsibility for ensuring the welfare of the animals, and that IACUC actions may trigger necessary actions by other groups. As an example, if the IACUC determines that an individual has failed to demonstrate an ability to work with animals, what happens to that person's employment status? Although each event will be unique, an agreed-upon approach that identifies roles and responsibilities will facilitate what can be a very difficult IACUC function.

2.5.3 Make Recommendations to the IO

Another function of the IACUC as described in the AWRs (Section 2.31(c)(5)) and the PHS Policy (Section IV.B.5) is to make recommendations to the IO regarding any aspect of the animal program, animal facilities, or training of the personnel (USDA 2013a). This function is at the heart of a well-functioning program. It is not the act of making a recommendation that is of the greatest importance, but rather the collegial environment in which positive, productive interactions between the IO and the IACUC are taken for granted. Too frequently we hear of IOs who have no interest in, or understanding of, animal research and of the animal program at their institution. Much less frequently we hear of the IO who "runs" the IACUC. Both extremes are problematic. The expectation that an IO is appropriately placed in an organization to find solutions for problems identified by the IACUC means that that person is likely to be engaged in many important and demanding activities within the institution's administration. The IACUC must work to provide the IO with a reasonable understanding of the nature of the animal work being conducted and of the likely challenges that the institution may face. The IO and IACUC chair should know each other on a first-name basis and each should feel comfortable in knowing that their time will be used wisely by the other. Make sure that the IO is aware of the species and relative numbers of animals housed in each facility. Provide the IO with opportunities to make efficient inspections of key facilities. Encourage senior scientists, especially those serving on the IACUC, to avail themselves of opportunities to discuss the animal program with the IO.

2.5.4 Review of Proposed Research

Protocol review is the activity that most often comes to mind when one thinks of what an IACUC does. Protocol review is at the heart of the IACUC process since it is through that review and, if warranted, the approval of described procedures that the IACUC indicates that the proposed procedures are of great enough value scientifically and ethically to be performed at the IACUC's institution. The AWRs (Section 2.31(c)(7)) and PHS Policy (Section IV.B.6) indicate that one of the many responsibilities of the IACUC is to review and approve, require modifications in (to secure approval), or withhold approval of those components of proposed activities related to the care and use of animals (protocol review) as well as proposed significant changes regarding the care and use of animals in ongoing activities (amendment review) (USDA 2013a). As described elsewhere in this book, the protocol review process is complex and demanding. My comments are limited to two aspects of that process.

The first issue relates to the use of designated member review (DMR). DMR is an efficient process that makes it possible for institutions to provide timely review, but one that can devolve into a process that weakens committee function if all reviews are conducted by DMR. An animal program is best served by the participation of well-educated, involved members. In the absence of participation by all members in open, detailed discussion of protocols and the local issues of importance to the research portfolio, it is difficult to understand how new members of an IACUC receive on-the-job training; it is also difficult to understand how all members continue to develop a better understanding of the ongoing institutional view that is essential to consistent review across protocols. Any institution that relies heavily on DMR must ensure that both of those needs—on-the-job training and consistency—are met. They also need to make sure that the members of the committee consider themselves as part of the whole, rather than individual reviewers acting on their own behalf without an understanding of how other committee members would address similar proposals.

The second issue is how a committee reaches a decision. While consensus is a desirable end point, the challenges of protocol review will at times make reaching consensus difficult if not impossible. Majority rule facilitates the process, but only if the committee insists that all viewpoints are given fair hearing.

2.5.5 Suspend an Activity

Suspension of an activity is an important tool in the IACUC's toolkit but one that must be wielded in a fair and reasonable way. According to the AWRs,

> The IACUC may suspend an activity that it previously approved if it determines that the activity is not being conducted in accordance with the description of that activity provided by the principal investigator and approved by the Committee. The IACUC may suspend an activity only after review of the matter at a convened meeting of a quorum of the IACUC and with the suspension vote of a majority of the quorum present.

The PHS Policy has almost identical wording, contained in Section IV.C.6, Review of PHS-Conducted or Supported Research Projects, and would apply to those facilities receiving PHS funds. Section IV.C.7 discusses the IO's role and reporting requirements whenever the IACUC votes to suspend a PHS-supported activity involving animals.

In the event of a suspension, the IACUC in conjunction with the IO must review the reason for the suspension, take corrective action, and report the corrective action along with a full explanation to APHIS. If federally funded, the agency funding the project must also be notified (USDA 2013a, NIH 2010).

It is the responsibility of the IACUC to ensure the humane treatment of animals under their purview and to also protect humans working with those animals. It is *not* the responsibility of an IACUC to punish an individual who fails to meet humane expectations. There will be times when reeducation and increased oversight do not address significant problems, and suspension is required. Each committee member must be willing and able to vote in favor of suspension, even of a friend's protocol, if the situation warrants. Any committee member who is reluctant to do so would do the IACUC process a favor by asking to be removed from the committee.

2.6 SUMMARY

As stated above, I believe that the IACUC is responsible for oversight of everything that may influence the health and well-being of live vertebrate animals and for many issues that may influence the health and well-being of humans working with those animals. In order to do the job well, each of us must understand the authority vested in an IACUC and accept responsibility for an IACUC process that provides humane care for our surrogates, while supporting efforts to improve the health and well-being of future generations of both human and nonhuman animals. Service on an IACUC is a challenging but noble endeavor.

REFERENCES

NASA (National Aeronautics and Space Administration). 1996. NASA principles for the ethical care and use of animals. NASA. http://quest.nasa.gov/neuron/events/habitat/NASAprin.html.

NIH (National Institutes of Health). 1985. US government principles for the utilization and care of vertebrate animals used in testing, research and training. Office of Laboratory Animal Welfare, NIH, Bethesda, MD. http://www.grants.nih.gov/grants/olaw/references/phspol.htm#USGovPrinciples.

NIH (National Institutes of Health). 2002. Public Health Service policy on humane care and use of laboratory animals. Office for Protection from Research Risks, NIH, Bethesda, MD.

NIH (National Institutes of Health). 2010. NOT-OD-07-044: NIH policy on allowable costs for grant activities involving animals when terms and conditions are not upheld. NIH, Bethesda, MD. http://grants.nih.gov/grants/guide/notice-files/NOT-OD-07-044.html.

NRC (National Research Council). 2011. *Guide for the Care and Use of Laboratory Animals.* 8th edn. National Academies Press, Washington, DC.

USDA (U.S. Department of Agriculture). 2013a. *Animal Welfare Act and Animal Welfare Regulations* (Animal Care Blue Book). Code of Federal Regulations (CFR), Title 9, Chapter 1, Subchapter A, Parts 1–4. USDA.

USDA (U.S. Department of Agriculture). 2013b. Animal Welfare Act of 1966 intended to regulate the transport, sale and handling of dogs, cats, guinea pigs, nonhuman primates, hamsters and rabbits intended to use for research or other purposes. Public Law 89-544, pp. 2131–2156. Washington, DC: U.S. GPO.

U.S. GPO (U.S. Government Printing Office). 1949. *Trials of War Criminals before the Nuremberg Military Tribunals under Control Council Law No. 10*, Vol. 2, pp. 181–182. Washington, DC: U.S. GPO.

Wigglesworth, C. 2006. Development of public health service animal welfare policy. *ALN Magazine*, 30 September. http://www.alnmag.com/articles/2006/09/development-public-health-service-animal-welfare-policy.

CHAPTER 3

Institutional Policies, Guidelines, and Procedures

Mary Jo Shepherd

CONTENTS

3.1 INTRODUCTION

Institutional policies, guidelines, and procedures are essential to the health of an organization. They provide a framework for daily operations and help foster compliant and consistent behavior. Institutional Animal Care and Use Programs (ACUPs) and Institutional Animal Care and Use Committees (IACUCs) benefit greatly from the creation and use of policies, guidelines, and procedures, since such institutional guidance documents assist with maintenance of compliance and assurance of animal welfare. Although the development and maintenance of the guidance documents discussed in this chapter are not a record-keeping requirement of the Animal Welfare Act (AWA), the Animal Welfare Act Regulations (AWRs), or the Public Health Service Policy on Humane Care and Use of Laboratory Animals (PHS Policy) (USDA 2013a and USDA 2013b, NIH 2002), they can be an integral part of a successful program that provides individuals with the information they need to perform tasks properly and can facilitate consistency in the program. According to the Guide for the Care and Use of Laboratory Animals (the Guide), "Establishing standard operating procedures can assist an institution in complying with regulations, policies, and principles as well as with day-to-day operations and management" (NRC 2011). This chapter will explore the purposes and use of such documents and will suggest mechanisms for their organization and maintenance.

3.2 DEFINITIONS

The following definitions have been established for this entire volume and will be utilized in this chapter:

*   Policies: Practical statements of collective wisdom, convention, or management direction that may be internal to the institution. They are often the means by which an implementing agency (e.g., Office of Laboratory Animal Welfare [OLAW] or USDA) interprets existing statutes (e.g., the PHS Policy or USDA animal care policies).
*   Guidelines: A recommended practice that allows some discretion or leeway in its interpretation, implementation, or use; for example, the American Veterinary Medical Association Guidelines for the Euthanasia of Animals: 2013 Edition.
*   Procedures: A detailed, step-by-step process meant to ensure the consistent application of institutional practices. Often called *operating procedures* or *standard operating procedures* (SOPs), they are intended to assist an institution in complying with regulations, policies, and principles as well as day-to-day operations and management.

Policies, guidelines, and procedures facilitate the conduct of animal research. Research staff that are well educated as to what is expected of them by the veterinarians, the IACUC, and the regulatory agencies are empowered with the knowledge to conduct research with animals humanely, consistently, and compliantly. For example, a policy or guideline on rodent survival surgery along with a strong training program ensure that good surgical technique is practiced at all times. Good surgical technique equates with good animal welfare.

3.3 STANDARD PROCEDURES FOR IACUC PROTOCOLS

Animal welfare can also be enhanced with standard procedure descriptions created by the veterinary staff. Written templates for standard methods used in animals (e.g., blood draws, genotyping, and perfusion) may be made available to the research community for insertion into IACUC protocols. According to OLAW FAQ D.14, "IACUCs may approve SOPs that can be cited by investigators in their protocols in order to avoid needless repetition. SOPs should be reviewed by the IACUC at appropriate intervals (at least once every three years) to ensure they are up-to-date and accurate" (NIH 2014a). Although there is no record-keeping requirement to maintain SOPs, the USDA's perspective is that if an institution uses SOPs to document procedures (i.e., animal manipulations, routine animal care, or administrative processes), it needs to have a defined process in place for developing and reviewing those SOPs, including a schedule for frequency of review. The IACUC should verify the institution's adherence to this schedule as part of the program review. This provides a customer service to the research community and facilitates protocol review, potentially reducing protocol review turnaround time. It is important that institutions and IACUCs assure that personnel are trained and experienced in any SOP/template procedures such as these in order to ensure compliance. It may be tempting for investigators to put the prepared procedure descriptions in their protocols to facilitate protocol approval, when they and their staff may not be properly trained or experienced in the techniques described.

3.4 IACUC ADMINISTRATION SOPs

Other types of guidance documents also allow committees to be transparent in their operations, which can improve the research community–IACUC relationship. Committees may wish to post SOPs for their routine operations, such as protocol review and facility inspections, on a website available to the research community. Having those procedures freely available to animal users helps to educate those individuals on institutional and regulatory requirements and helps them to understand the ins and outs of IACUC processes, such as protocol review. Committees should assure that any posted SOPs or guidance are entirely aligned with the institution's NIH-OLAW Animal Welfare Assurance and its Association for Assessment and Accreditation of Laboratory Animal Care (AAALAC) program description (if applicable), to assure compliance and consistency in IACUC operations. Posting links to the AWA, the AWRs, the PHS Policy, the Guide, and so on assures the research community that the standards they are held to and the procedures that they must adhere to are required by federal law and regulation and are not just promulgated at the whim of the institution or the IACUC. A solid training component at the institution that covers regulatory requirements also backs this up.

Transparency of IACUC operations and expectations is essential for creating and maintaining a collegial and healthy relationship between the IACUC and the research community. Regulatory requirements regarding protocol review and facility and laboratory inspections may sometimes serve as a source of contention between the two groups. The IACUC may be perceived as an obstruction to necessary and beneficial biomedical research. IACUC staff members can particularly benefit from transparency in operations given that they are generally on the front lines of interaction with members of the research community. The IACUC staff serves as a liaison between the committee and the investigative community. Investigators sometimes become unhappy with protocol turnaround time and questions raised during protocol review, and that frustration is often taken out on the IACUC staff. Institutions may enhance the perception of their IACUC by ensuring the committee conducts business with consistency during operations such as protocol review and investigation of animal welfare/compliance concerns if guidance documents exist. Likewise, the IACUC staff can then provide more consistent customer service to the research community.

An IACUC may wish to create guidance and training on protocol preparation, as this will assist in reducing protocol review turnaround time. Since inconsistency during protocol review is a frequent criticism of IACUCs, the IACUC can improve on the consistency of review by utilizing guidelines and policies as appropriate, and by ensuring IACUC members adequately understand those guidelines and policies. If reviewers are familiar with institutional veterinary standards for the conduct of common procedures (e.g., tumor monitoring, regulation of food/fluid administration), their personal biases and previous laboratory practices should not come into play when they review protocols. When an IACUC stays compliant with its own procedures, such as those for investigating animal welfare and compliance concerns, it is more apt to treat each case uniformly and fairly among members of the research community, and investigators know more fully what to expect. Examples of subjects that IACUCs could cover to enhance IACUC operational transparency and customer service are details of who may serve as a principal investigator, the procedure for comparing grants to protocols, collaborations, significant protocol modifications, and field studies.

3.5 IACUC POLICIES

According to the OLAW Semiannual Program Review Checklist (Institutional Policies and Responsibilities, Item 5, IACUC Membership and Functions) (NIH 2014b), the committee may assess whether policies are in place for special procedures listed in the Guide (N RC 2011, 27–32). The OLAW program review checklist is provided to assist IACUCs in conducting semiannual program assessments as required by the PHS Policy, Section IV.B.1.-2 (NIH 2002). OLAW does not require IACUCs to use the checklist, but the Guide lists the following procedures or approaches that may require special consideration during protocol review: experimental and humane end points, unexpected outcomes, physical restraint, multiple survival surgical procedures, food and fluid regulation, use of non-pharmaceutical-grade chemicals and other substances, field investigations, and agricultural animals. IACUCs may wish to assure that policies and guidelines exist for these special procedures to assist committee members during protocol review and to assist the research community in preparing protocols and conducting procedures.

3.6 ANIMAL FACILITY SOPs

The details in the SOPs standardize the processes that personnel conduct and provide step-by-step, how-to instructions that enable them to perform tasks in a consistent manner. An animal care staff will perform tasks correctly, consistently, humanely, and safely if it is provided with clear and easily understood written SOPs and trained to perform tasks according to those SOPs. Very simply, SOPs are written instructions that define the who, what, where, why, and exactly how of every task in a facility. The SOPs serve as an instructional resource that allows employees to act without having to ask for directions, reassurance, or guidance after they have received the initial training. Since expectations are documented and employees' actions can be measured against the SOPs, the step-by-step written procedures can also help hold employees accountable. Communicating procedures that anyone in the operation can follow with consistent results will ensure that operations continually provide high-quality service and animal care.

3.7 WRITING POLICIES, GUIDELINES, AND PROCEDURES

These documents can be developed by individuals or groups of individuals. An individual with specific expertise in a certain area may wish to draft guidance in that area, but groups of people generally generate more variety in thought. Pairing an expert with an IACUC member and a veterinarian could improve the process over that achieved when one person works alone. A process to maintain these guidance documents should be created and could be described in SOP style such that all of the documents are handled, formatted, and reviewed consistently. The SOPs could include steps for formatting the documents for example, font, header/footer, and numbering. Numbering of documents should be sequential. The header/footer may include the institution/IACUC logo or brand, approval date, version number (updated for each revision), and page number. Past versions of each document could be archived for future reference. Each document should include consistent sections (as applicable), such as title, purpose, definitions, applicability, and references. An example of an IACUC guideline is included in Appendix F of this book.

The documents should be kept up to date with current best practices and published information, and they should be reviewed and revised by the appropriate group, IACUC, or veterinary staff on a regular basis, with the frequency of review spelled out in the procedure on SOPs, but no less than once every three years. Document developers should not "reinvent the wheel," so to speak, as many examples of guidelines and policies are already available online. Involving members of the investigative community during the development and revision of guidance documents could help foster a collegial relationship among all the individuals in the ACUP. Investigators with expertise and experience in certain areas, such as antibody production, may be more than willing to participate in the development and maintenance of guidance in that area.

3.8 DOCUMENT ROLLOUT

New guidance documents or updates and changes to existing documents should be promptly communicated to the research community via e-mail, newsletters, websites, training sessions, and so on. The guidance should be readily available at all times for reference. Links to guidelines and policies may be placed in electronic protocol forms to assist investigators with protocol creation and compliance.

The research community should be educated as to the difference between policies, guidelines, and procedures (see Section 3.2), as there are generally different expectations associated with each. For instance, policies generally must be complied with, whereas deviations from guidelines may be permitted by the IACUC when adequate justification is provided.

3.9 CONCLUSION

Instructional documents ensure that the ACUP is run efficiently, consistently, and appropriately. They remove any ambiguity and set the bar for what is expected to be the standard of care in an institution. Policies, guidelines, and procedures provide a framework for the research staff when drafting proposals and a checklist of sorts for the IACUC reviewer who is trying to determine if the proposal can be approved. Guidance documents take the guesswork out of performing day-to-day tasks in a humane and responsible manner, ensuring animal welfare compliance is preserved.

REFERENCES

NIH (National Institutes of Health). 2002. Public Health Service policy on humane care and use of laboratory animals. Office of Laboratory Animal Welfare, NIH, Bethesda, MD.

NIH (National Institutes of Health). 2014a. Frequently asked questions: PHS policy on humane care and use of laboratory animals: May standard operating procedures (SOPs) or blanket protocols that cover a number of procedures be utilized in lieu of repeating descriptions of identical procedures in multiple protocols? Office of Laboratory Animal Welfare, NIH, Bethesda, MD. http://grants.nih.gov/grants/olaw/faqs.htm#proto_14.

NIH (National Institutes of Health). 2014b. Semiannual program review and facility inspection checklist. Office of Laboratory Animal Welfare, NIH, Bethesda, MD. http://grants.nih.gov/grants/olaw/sampledoc/cheklist.htm.

NRC (National Research Council). 2011. *Guide for the Care and Use of Laboratory Animals*, 8th edn. Washington, DC: National Academies Press.

USDA (U.S. Department of Agriculture). 2013a. *Animal Welfare Act and Animal Welfare Regulations* (Animal Care Blue Book). Code of Federal Regulations (CFR), Title 9, Chapter 1, Subchapter A, Parts 1–4. USDA.

USDA (U.S. Department of Agriculture). 2013b. Animal Welfare Act of 1966 intended to regulate the transport, sale and handling of dogs, cats, guinea pigs, nonhuman primates, hamsters and rabbits intended to use for research or other purposes. *Public Law* 89 (544):2131–2156.

CHAPTER **4**

Protocol Processing
From Submission to Approval

Melinda S. Hollander

CONTENTS

4.1 INTRODUCTION

One of the first things that comes to mind for most people involved in animal research or teaching at institutions is writing or reviewing animal use protocols. While writing a protocol is not specifically required by any federal or regulating agency, this is the method that most institutions use to comply with the required documentation for the descriptions of all proposed uses of animals to (1) ensure that all required information is provided and (2) maintain consistency in all documentation, which helps with the review process.

A review of activities using animals in research, testing, or teaching is the responsibility of the Institutional Animal Care and Use Committee (IACUC). The requirement that all proposed activities involving animals in research, testing, and teaching be reviewed and approved by the IACUC before those activities can begin is found in some form in external guidelines and regulations: the Public Health Service (PHS) Policy on Humane Care and Use of Laboratory Animals (NIH 2002b), U.S. Government Principles for the Utilization and Care of Vertebrate Animals Used in Testing, Research, and Training (NIH 1985), the U.S. Department of Agriculture (USDA) Animal Welfare Act (AWA) (USDA 2013b), the USDA Animal Welfare Act Regulations (AWRs) (USDA 2013a), *Veterans Health Administration Handbook 1200.07, Use of Animals in Research* (VHA 2011), *Guide for the Care and Use of Laboratory Animals* (8th edn.; the Guide) (NRC 2011), *Guide for the Care and Use of Agricultural Animals in Agricultural Research and Teaching* (FASS 2010), and the *IACUC Guidebook* (NIH 2002a).

This chapter describes the submission, review, and approval of protocols and modifications to approved protocols. It should be noted that institutions each have their own way of accomplishing these activities, thus this chapter focuses on what is required and provides an insight regarding the different methods of fulfilling these requirements.

4.2 PRESUBMISSION CONSULTATIONS

To begin writing a protocol, it is often helpful for principal investigators (PIs) to initiate various consultations, depending on the content of the protocol. Consulting specialists and/or applicable institutional entities can ensure that the appropriate information is documented in the protocol, which can expedite the review and approval process.

A consultation with a veterinarian is not necessarily required, but can be invaluable to PIs during the preparation of protocols. According to the AWRs (USDA 2013a), consultation with the attending veterinarian (AV) or his or her designee is required when procedures are proposed that may involve more than momentary pain or distress (i.e., USDA pain categories D and E; see Appendix G). The AWRs (USDA 2013a) state that this consultation should include guidance regarding anesthesia, analgesia, handling, immobilization techniques, euthanasia, and pre- and postprocedural care. A veterinary consultation can be performed by the AV; however, other veterinarians or experts can be designated by the AV to avoid delays in the event that the AV is unavailable, or where other veterinary expertise is more appropriate.

An additional consultation that can be beneficial is with a librarian, or information scientist, who is experienced with database searches and can assist with searches for alternative approaches to potentially painful or distressful procedures carried out on animals. This is important because PIs must document the methods and sources that were used to identify potential alternatives, and this is often done using a database search. In fact, the USDA requires database searches (USDA 2013a, Ch. 1; USDA 2013b, 7 U.S.C. Ch. 54). This can be a very difficult requirement for a PI to fulfill, and a consultation with a librarian experienced with web or database searches can often be helpful. Personnel in these positions are often well versed in various databases and how to conduct useful searches using appropriate keywords and Boolean operators.

Another important part of a protocol is defining and justifying the number of animals to be used for a study. Advice from a biostatistician is useful when it comes to deciding on the number of animals needed to obtain statistically relevant data. A consultation with a biostatistician is particularly useful for basic science research, as biostatisticians specialize in analyses involving several conditions, treatments, and/or groups and have a strong understanding of how to estimate the size of an effect based on several independent variables. Biostatisticians will also be able to help animal researchers provide sufficient detail so that the IACUC can easily understand how the numbers of animals were calculated.

Finally, consulting other institutional committees or offices (the Institutional Biosafety Committee [IBC], the Radiation Safety Committee [RSC], the Environmental Health and Safety [EHS] Committee, etc.) for animal studies requiring the use of hazardous agents is necessary. To begin with, institutions should have specific policies and standard operating procedures (SOPs) for using hazardous agents in or with animals. These written policies and procedures help PIs to determine what agents are defined as hazardous. When a PI plans on using hazardous agents in animal research, meeting with appropriate committees or officers before submitting the IACUC protocol can ensure that the proper information is included and that other special approvals (e.g., biosafety and radiation) are received or are in the process of being reviewed.

4.3 PROTOCOL SUBMISSION

Once a PI has consulted with the appropriate experts to ensure that they have provided all of the necessary information, they must submit their protocol for review by the IACUC. Before a protocol is sent to the IACUC, a preview by an IACUC administrator and a veterinarian is often done and can result in a faster approval time.

An administrative preview of a protocol is not required in the submission and review process. It can, however, prove to be invaluable to the reviewers and the PIs. Typically, IACUC administrators are well versed in what information is required in a protocol and can conduct a quick preview to ensure that essential information has been included in the protocol. An administrative prereview often consists of the following (PRIM&R 2013):

1. Check for completeness.
2. Check that any attachments (copies of grants, approval letters from collaborating sites, etc.) have been included.
3. Ensure that the three Rs (replacement, refinement, and reduction) have been addressed.
4. Verify that training requirements have been completed by study personnel.
5. Check for additional required approvals (e.g., biosafety and radiation).
6. Verify that the pain category is appropriate.
7. Check for and note potential exceptions to the Guide.
8. Ensure that the number of animals adds up and the justification seems appropriate.
9. Decide the appropriateness for a review determination query to the IACUC members (see Section 4.5).

It is important for the person who is performing the administrative prereview work with the PI to address substantial changes required before the final review can be conducted by the IACUC members. IACUC members can conduct a much more thorough and efficient review of the protocol when basic problems or issues have already been addressed and corrected.

All protocols will undergo a thorough review by members of the IACUC who may not have the expertise to comprehensively evaluate veterinary issues. Therefore, it is imperative that the veterinary review is focused and thorough. In fact, the AV or his or her designee plays a key role in reviewing activities involving animals. There is no explicit requirement as to when a veterinary review is conducted, but many institutions require a veterinary evaluation of a protocol before the protocol reaches the IACUC to avoid unnecessary delays in approval (Silverman et al., 2006). Having the veterinary review done before a committee review of a protocol also ensures that the general review and discussion are focused on important issues, such as the harm–benefit analysis, the three Rs, exceptions to the Guide, or the appropriateness of the species to be used. The position of the American College of Laboratory Animal Medicine (ACLAM) is that the AV or his or her designee be involved in the review of all protocols to ensure that procedures meet veterinary standards, that adequate measures for the alleviation of pain/distress are in place, and that the drugs to be administered are appropriate (Silverman et al., 2006).

If a consultation has occurred between a veterinarian and the PI prior to submission, the veterinary review should be relatively straightforward. Nonetheless, a formal veterinary review should still be performed to ensure that the issues discussed during the consultation were correctly understood by the PI and incorporated into the protocol appropriately. The specific points to be considered during a veterinary review are

- A description of any procedures, especially surgical procedures, to ensure that they meet veterinary standards
- An adequate plan to monitor and intervene in the alleviation of potential pain or distress, including an evaluation of experimental and humane end points

- The method of euthanasia and the secondary method to ensure death
- The drugs to be used (anesthetics, analgesics, sedatives, experimental drugs, etc.)
- The appropriateness of the drug
- The dosage of the drug
- The frequency of use

The veterinary review should focus on protocol issues with the potential to impact the health, well-being, and care of animals, rather than the scientific or teaching parts of the protocol, such as the number of animals, the rationale for the use of animals, and the experimental design; these matters can be evaluated by other IACUC members.

To ensure a complete and focused veterinary review, many institutions use a checklist. This also helps veterinarians save time by listing the specific topics that should be reviewed, pointing the veterinarian to the appropriate location in the protocol where that information will be located, and ensuring that sections that should contain relevant information for the veterinary review are not overlooked.

4.4 TYPES OF SUBMISSIONS

Protocol submissions can be either new protocols or renewal protocols, and they should describe the animal activities that a researcher or instructor is requesting for a research project or for an academic course, respectively. Protocol submissions should address all essential information that the IACUC is required to gather and review for all animal care and use activities. The difference between a new protocol and a protocol renewal is that a new protocol is describing a new study or course using animals, and a protocol renewal involves a three-year *de novo* review of a currently or previously approved project. A *de novo* review of protocols is required every three years per the PHS Policy for federally funded proposals (NIH 2002b), but institutions deal with this process differently. For example, whereas some institutions require that PIs completely rewrite the protocol, including a progress report summarizing their findings, publications, and so forth resulting from the use of animals in the previous three-year protocol, other institutions require that PIs amend their current protocol to include changes that will occur in the next three years. The critical requirements are that (1) every protocol is completely and thoroughly reviewed every three years, and (2) work is not unnecessarily duplicated.

Another type of submission that is made is to request changes in ongoing research. This type can be termed differently at different institutions (e.g., amendment, addendum, revision, or modification). For the purposes of this chapter, a request for changes to a protocol will be referred to as an *amendment*. The changes can be considered minor or significant, and each institution specifically defines minor changes versus significant changes. Minor changes are typically reviewed and approved by the IACUC administrator or chair without prior notification to the IACUC (e.g., non-PI personnel changes and funding changes). All significant changes (e.g., change in the species or the approximate number of animals used, surgical procedures, and new treatment groups), however, must be reviewed and approved by the IACUC before the changes can be implemented by a PI or a course instructor (NIH 2002b). Some institutions' IACUCs have agreed to allow a total increase in animal numbers for animals not regulated by the USDA that does not exceed 10% of the number reviewed and approved by the IACUC. In regard to USDA requirements, any increase in the number of regulated species would require an amendment in accordance with the AWRs (USDA 2013a).

4.4.1 Continuing Review

The AWRs state that "The IACUC shall conduct continuing reviews of activities covered by this subchapter at appropriate intervals as determined by the IACUC, but not less than annually" (USDA 2013a, 9 CFR §2.31 d5). The PHS Policy states "The IACUC shall conduct continuing review of each previously approved, ongoing activity covered by this Policy at appropriate intervals as determined by the IACUC, including a complete review in accordance with IV.C.1.- 4. at least once every three years."

While the AWRs and the PHS Policy differ in terms of review intervals, the Office of Laboratory Animal Welfare (OLAW) has indicated that a continuing review, subject to the AWRs, may be performed annually as a best practice and monitoring function by the IACUC. The intent of a continuing review is to monitor animal activity to ensure compliance with the protocol and with regulations and guidelines. It is important for individual IACUCs to establish a system for continuing review of all animal activity that fits into the requirements of the AWRs and the PHS Policy. Typical time frames are every six months to coincide with the semiannual inspections, or annually as required by the AWRs.

The method for a continuing review varies among institutions, but many initiate the review with a form that is to be completed by the PI, which provides such information as

- PI name
- Protocol title and number
- Personnel
- Species
- Number of animals approved
- Approval and expiration dates

This form would also request information from the PI, such as

- Personnel to be added or removed
- Unexpected outcomes
- Surgical updates
- Handling of drugs and chemicals
- Changes that have occurred
- Changes that are needed

Any changes noted by the PI, however, must receive IACUC review and approval, as described in Section 4.5, before they can be implemented. If the PI has already instigated significant changes to an animal activity, the IACUC must investigate the matter and determine if noncompliance occurred. If it is a PHS-funded activity, the IACUC must report the noncompliance to OLAW.

4.5 METHOD DETERMINATION FOR IACUC REVIEW

"Prior to IACUC review, each member of the Committee shall be provided with a list of proposed activities to be reviewed" (USDA 2013a). There are only two recognized methods for reviewing a protocol or amending a protocol: a full committee review (FCR) or a designated member review (DMR). An FCR involves a review of a protocol (or an amendment to a protocol) during a convened meeting of a quorum (greater than 50% of voting members in attendance) of the IACUC. A DMR involves a review of a protocol (or an amendment to a protocol) by one or more members of the IACUC after every member has had the opportunity to call for an FCR. The specifics of each method are described in this chapter, but it is important to mention that any other review or a hybrid of either an FCR or a DMR is not an acceptable method of review, and for USDA-regulated species, the method must be in accordance with 9 CFR §2.31 (d)(2) (USDA 2013a). It is also important to note that the methods should be agreed on in advance by the IACUC and must be detailed in the institution's PHS Assurance and/or Association for Assessment and Accreditation of Laboratory Animal Care (AAALAC) Program Description. A guidance document or SOP is also helpful in this regard.

An FCR of protocols must be conducted at a convened meeting of a quorum of the IACUC. Typically, a primary and a secondary reviewer are assigned to review each protocol that is to be discussed at the meeting. The assignment of specific reviewers for an FCR is not required because, technically, the full committee is conducting the review. Many institutions, however, assign IACUC members as primary or secondary reviewers to protocols to ensure that someone can lead an effective discussion of the protocol at the meeting.

If the IACUC follows the rules of order or parliamentary procedure in its deliberations, once a protocol is reviewed and discussed at a meeting (see Section 4.4 for review topics), one member will make an initial motion to approve, and another member will second that motion. The chair will then call for a vote, and those members present at the meeting may vote. The actions that may be taken by an IACUC after a review of a protocol are to approve, require modifications to secure approval, withhold approval, or disapprove. It is not appropriate to poll members who are not in attendance individually via e-mail or telephone for a vote when conducting the FCR method. However, members who attend via video- or teleconference may vote as long as they have access to the documents that are necessary to fully participate and have the opportunity for real-time verbal interaction (NIH 2006).

The approval of a protocol being reviewed via an FCR can only be granted with an approval vote of a majority of the quorum present at that meeting (USDA 2013a, NIH 2002b). If a protocol requires modifications to secure approval, the IACUC can do one of two things. The committee can vote to have the protocol returned to an FCR after modifications have been completed, or it can vote to have the modified protocol reviewed via the DMR method (this is referred to by OLAW as a DMR subsequent to an FCR). This method is allowed if all IACUC members have agreed in advance in writing that a quorum of voting members present at a convened meeting may unanimously vote to have a modified protocol reviewed via a DMR. If a single voting member objects, the modified protocol must come back for review at the next convened committee meeting. This withholding of approval is referred to as *tabling* a protocol by some IACUCs. If all members are not present, and the IACUC lacks a written standard procedure as described, the committee has the option to vote to return the protocol for an FCR at a convened meeting, or to employ a DMR, but only after the revised protocol has been made available to all the members, including the members not present at the meeting, and all have had the opportunity to call for an FCR. Only after all the members of the committee have had an opportunity to request an FCR, and none has done so, may the protocol be reviewed and approved by a DMR. It is important to note that, regardless of the method of review, any member of the IACUC may, at any time, request to see the revised protocol and/or request an FCR of the protocol.

The second process of review is a DMR, which is probably more commonly used at many institutions, especially larger ones, due to the sheer number of protocols being reviewed in a given period. The first requirement for the DMR process is a review determination. A review determination is the process of notifying all voting IACUC members of the submission, be it a full protocol or an amendment to an already approved protocol, allowing them access to the submission and providing them with the opportunity to call for an FCR (NIH 2002b, USDA 2013a). The members are typically given a deadline to submit their response; if an IACUC determines that a nonresponse from a member is a vote for a DMR, this must be explicitly stated in writing. Typically, the IACUC administrator follows guidelines determined by each institution stating what type(s) of submissions are eligible for a DMR. For example, because of the potential severity of the procedures that are carried out on an animal, an institution may decide that all pain category E protocols (see Appendix G for an explanation of USDA pain categories) must be reviewed via a full committee. In other words, each institution has guidelines to determine what type of review a particular protocol submission must undergo.

The golden rule with the DMR process is that any voting member, for any reason, may request that a particular protocol or protocol amendment be reviewed via an FCR. Once it has been determined that a protocol will be reviewed via a DMR, the chair must assign at least one qualified committee member to conduct the review (USDA 2013a, NIH 2002b). Many institutions assign more than one reviewer as a best practice. The AWRs and the PHS Policy require that the chair is the person who assigns designated member reviewers (NIH 2002b).

Some institutions might describe the DMR process as an "expedited review," but this is not necessarily accurate. The process may take less time than if the protocol were reviewed via an FCR, especially if the protocol had been submitted several weeks before the regularly scheduled IACUC meeting; however, reviews by the designated member(s) must be as thorough and rigorous as an FCR of a protocol or a protocol amendment.

The actions that can be taken by designated member reviewers regarding a protocol or an amendment to a protocol are approval, require modifications to secure approval, or referral to full committee. Designated member reviewers cannot disapprove a protocol. Disapproval or withholding approval of a protocol or an amendment can only be done by a majority vote by a quorum of members at a convened meeting.

4.6 PROTOCOL REVIEW TOPICS

The following topics must be described in detail in a protocol for review via one of the two review methods covered in Section 4.5. A discussion of these topics here is limited to a brief introduction, because Chapter 5 provides an in-depth look into each of these as well as additional topics.

4.6.1 Justifications

A number of justifications are required when writing an animal care and use protocol, such as species, number of animals to be used, and exceptions to the Guide.

A vast number of different species across the phylogenetic scale may be used for research, testing, and teaching. Depending on the nature of the activities proposed, it is important that an appropriate species be used, even if that species happens to be higher on the phylogenetic scale. The IACUC reviewers must scrutinize the scientific justification for the use of the particular species being requested and ensure that the species chosen is the most appropriate for the work being proposed.

The number of animals to be used for a particular study must also be justified to ensure that no animals are wasted. While most people agree that it is nearly impossible to predict the exact number of animals needed to obtain statistically significant results, the protocol must include the method used to predict the minimum number of animals that the PI expects will be needed. This is often done using statistical methods such as power analyses. Another common method is to refer to published peer-reviewed journal articles in which similar studies were undertaken and cite the number of animals necessary to gain statistically meaningful outcomes in those articles. For example, if a publication indicates that eight mice per group were needed to measure the effectiveness of a therapeutic drug in a procedure performed to measure cardiac function in mice, and a PI plans to look at another type of treatment while using an identical or similar procedure in mice, it would be reasonable for the PI to request the use of eight mice per group. Whatever method is used, it is imperative for the PI to give a succinct and understandable justification for the number of animals that he or she plans to use to answer the scientific question. This again is a way to ensure that no animals are being utilized unnecessarily.

In the Guide, there are a number of "must" and "should" statements, and these can only be deviated from if there is (1) a specifically described Guide exception,

(2) an IACUC-approved scientific justification or veterinary or animal welfare reason, or (3) a locally established performance standard. These include, but are not limited to

- Prolonged restraint
- Multiple survival surgical procedures
- Food or fluid restriction
- Use of non-pharmaceutical-grade compounds

A departure from the guidelines specified in the Guide for any of these areas requires close scrutiny by the IACUC (NIH 2012).

The use of prolonged restraint must be scientifically justified and should be avoided or minimized unless it is absolutely necessary for the objectives of the research. Common examples of prolonged restraint that have been used in research with proper justification and IACUC approval are chairing of nonhuman primates and tail suspension of rats. The term *prolonged restraint* is difficult to specifically define as it relates to the time of restraint. The critically important point is that the following considerations are applied when justifying prolonged restraint (Silverman et al., 2006):

- The method of restraint that is used
- The prior experience of the animal (e.g., acclimation to the restraint device)
- The lack of availability of less stressful methods

If alternative methods are available, the PI must give scientific justification as to why the alternative method cannot be used. The Guide (NRC 2011) has a number of points addressing the important guidelines for using restraint that the IACUC should reference when reviewing the use of prolonged restraint to ensure that scientific justification is adequate, that the use of prolonged restraint will meet the goals of the study, and that less painful or distressful alternative methods have been fully investigated.

Multiple survival surgeries are generally defined as any type of surgical procedure performed on a single animal under separate administrations of anesthesia. Such procedures require scientific justification and include those animals that have already been surgically manipulated before they are ordered from a vendor (e.g., ordering ovariectomized animals). Multiple survival surgical procedures in animals are generally discouraged and must be specifically justified and approved by the IACUC. If the species is a USDA-regulated species, the institutional official (IO) must first submit a request to the USDA's Animal and Plant Health Inspection Service for approval for the animal to undergo multiple major survival surgeries for different, unrelated projects or protocols (NRC 2011, USDA 2011). The AWRs define a major operative procedure as "any surgical intervention that penetrates and exposes a body cavity or any procedure which produces permanent impairment of physical or physiological functions" (USDA 2013a). Although there is no requirement to distinguish between minor or major surgical procedures in a protocol form, the PI is required to provide scientific justification regarding the need for multiple surgeries and to prove that this need is essential for the research project. It is important that the IACUC examines this justification carefully while keeping in mind the potential impact on the animal's well-being. The Guide states that "conservation of scarce animal resources" may be an appropriate justification, but cost considerations alone are not (NRC 2011). The Guide also encourages IACUCs to be diligent about following up with PIs who have been approved to conduct multiple survival surgical procedures to evaluate the outcomes. An effective way to accomplish this is through the postapproval monitoring process, which is discussed in more detail in Chapter 6.

The regulation or restriction of food or fluid intake can be used in many different research and teaching protocols and must also be scientifically justified. The regulation of food or fluid often refers to animals being fed on a fixed schedule, so that they eat/drink at regular intervals, typically as much food/fluid as they want to consume within a specified window of time. The restriction of food or fluid is defined as strictly monitoring and controlling the total volume of food or fluid consumed (NRC 2003, FASS 2010). When it is reviewing food or fluid regulation or restriction, the IACUC must consider the scientific justification for regulation or restriction, the potential impact on the animals' well-being, and potential adverse effects. The PI must provide specific information about how the health of the animals will be monitored to ensure adverse effects are avoided, and a log must be kept documenting the monitoring of these animals. Typically, daily to weekly recording of animal body weights is required, along with the amount of food/fluid consumed. The IACUC must be sure that the PI has a specific monitoring plan such that changes in the well-being of the animal can be promptly detected.

Scientific justification is also required for the use of non-pharmaceutical-grade drugs. Pharmaceutical-grade drugs or compounds should be used whenever possible to ensure that no unwanted or toxic side effects occur as a result of their use in animals. Often, however, experimental compounds/drugs are not available in a pharmaceutical preparation. In such instances, the PI must justify the use of non-pharmaceutical-grade drugs, even if only to document for the record that pharmaceutical-grade equivalents are not available. If a pharmaceutical-grade alternative is available, the PI must provide scientific justification for the use of non-pharmaceutical-grade drugs (i.e., use is necessary to meet the research goals of the project) satisfactory to the IACUC. The IACUC must take into consideration the potential problems that might arise from the use of non-pharmaceutical-grade compounds and requires that the PI provide a detailed plan to monitor the animals for unwanted side effects while using that compound. It is also best practice to require the PI to provide as much information as possible about the non-pharmaceutical-grade compound, such as purity, sterility, pH, osmolality, stability, site and route of administration, formulation, and pharmacokinetics (NRC 2011).

4.6.2 Harm–Benefit Analysis

The harm–benefit analysis is the consideration of the potential pain or distress that animals on a study may experience in light of the potential benefit that the study results may produce. This analysis is especially important if it is known that the study animals will endure pain or distress. The review of all animal activities should include discussion and/or documentation of the potential benefit of the work being proposed and the pain or distress that the animals may endure. The PI's rationale for the use of animals and relevance to human or animal health must justify any potential harm to the animal. The way in which IACUC reviewers conduct the harm–benefit analysis, however, differs from institution to institution. The critical issue is that the IACUC or designated member reviewer(s) critically evaluate the ratio of benefit to harm, especially if the project involves more than momentary pain or distress without relief.

4.6.3 Experimental Design

The experimental design of a project is likely the most important part of a protocol for understanding how a PI plans to answer the question(s) for which the research described is being undertaken. A clear statement to convey the purpose of the experimental design and how to write and evaluate it is found in the Guide: "a clear and concise sequential description of the procedures involving the use of animals that is easily understood by all members of the committee" (NRC 2011, 25). This statement eloquently sums up what is needed in an experimental design: the reviewer(s) must understand what procedures are being carried out on each animal and when (i.e., over the course of the study) those procedures are being done. It is also important for the PI to differentiate what procedures are being done to different groups of animals since there is typically more than one study group (e.g., experimental groups and control groups).

4.6.4 The Three Rs

Replacement, refinement, and reduction, better known as the three Rs, are principles espoused by the IACUC to ensure that animal use is performed ethically. W.M.S. Russell and R.L. Burch published strategies for researchers to use when designing studies using animals (Russell et al., 1959), and all three of these principles should be addressed by PIs.

The first principle, replacement, addresses methods that involve the use of nonanimal models or techniques, or a species which is phylogentically lower. Consideration of replacement methods refers to both absolute replacement (i.e., replacing animals with nonanimal alternatives, such as *in vitro* cell models or computer simulations) and relative replacement (i.e., replacing one species with another species lower on the phylogenetic scale) (Russell et al., 1959). Refinement is the second principle. This addresses modifications to ameliorate pain or distress or improve the animal's well-being. This can be accomplished using modifications of experimental procedures (e.g., using a bioluminescence imaging system to determine tumor growth rather than removing the tumor for measurement) or husbandry practices (e.g., changing dirty bedding more often in a cage containing diabetic mice) (Russell et al., 1959). While it is important that animals do not suffer unnecessary pain or distress, IACUCs must keep in mind that some studies will require that animals suffer some degree of pain or distress to successfully answer a scientific question. The committee's responsibility is to ensure that there is appropriate scientific justification for that pain or distress and that it is minimized as much as possible.

The third principle, reduction, addresses the maximization of data obtainable from the smallest number of animals. This principle was discussed in Section 4.6.1. The PI must be sure to design an experiment using the appropriate number of animals to provide statistically meaningful data. The Guide defines reduction as "strategies for obtaining comparable levels of information from the use of fewer animals or for maximizing the information obtained from a given number of animals (without increasing pain or distress) so that in the long run fewer animals are needed to acquire the same scientific information" (NRC 2011).

4.6.5 End Points

When reviewing protocols, especially those that propose procedures that may cause more than momentary pain, it is essential that the PI specifically describes humane end points that will be adhered to while conducting his or her study. The IACUC should ensure that criteria are provided to determine when an animal will be removed from the study. Removal may be in the form of simple removal from the study, clinical intervention, or humane euthanasia. Specifically stating when intervention will occur ensures that animals will not suffer unnecessarily. This information should be kept in the log or laboratory notebook by the PI and periodically reviewed to determine the effectiveness of the stated end point. The IACUC should review these logs and work with the PI to determine if end points need to be modified during the course of the study.

4.6.6 Unexpected Outcomes

In a typical protocol, expected outcomes are addressed by PIs. However, with the increased use of genetically modified animals, unexpected outcomes are an increasing concern. When creating genetically modified animals, a specific targeted change is made in the genome of an animal with the intention to change a specific phenotype in some way. However, the creation of these specific changes can and does sometimes change other phenotypes unexpectedly. Many times these unexpected changes are not significant or do not affect an animal's well-being. Nonetheless, these unexpected outcomes can cause problems in the animal. A PI creating a new genetically modified animal, or using a genetically modified animal that has not been fully characterized, should provide a specific plan for how he or she will monitor the animals for unanticipated problems that might affect their well-being. Examples include, but are not limited to, embryonic lethality, newborns that fail to thrive, or increased stress/anxiety. The IACUC must be comfortable that the PI understands that unanticipated problems can occur with genetically modified animals, or any species or strain, and that he or she needs to inform the IACUC when unexpected problems occur. In this way, immediate interventions may be provided to alleviate matters that negatively affect animal well-being.

Unexpected outcomes might also occur when new approaches are used with animals or if a PI is using a particular technique for the first time. It is also important for these to be justified and reviewed by the IACUC. It is appropriate for a committee to request that a PI conduct a pilot study to determine if there might be any unexpected outcomes.

4.6.7 Scientific Merit

A review of scientific merit is often challenged and vehemently contested by PIs. The IACUC, however, is required to ensure that animals are not being used unnecessarily. In order to do this, scientific merit should be considered by the IACUC (Prentice et al., 1992).

Neither the AWA nor the AWRs explicitly discuss scientific merit; however, regarding the review of scientific merit, the AWA states, "except as provided in paragraphs (7) of this subsection, shall be construed as authorizing the Secretary to promulgate rules, regulations, or orders with regard to the design, outlines, or guidelines of actual research or experimentation by a research facility as determined by such research facility" (USDA 2013b, §2143 (a)(6)(A)(i)). Furthermore, the AWRs state, "Except as specifically authorized by law or by these regulations, nothing in this part shall be deemed to permit the Committee or IACUC to prescribe methods or set standards for the design, performance, or conduct of actual research or experimentation by a research facility" (USDA 2013a). These statements suggest that the IACUC should not dictate how research is done. However, the PHS Policy, the Guide, and the USDA require that PIs conduct research in a way that is consistent with sound research design, that the animal species chosen are appropriate models, that the number of animals be appropriate and justified, that previous work not be duplicated, that procedures conducted produce scientifically valuable results, and that scientific elements of a protocol relating to the welfare of animals are evaluated. In addition, the Guide states that members may seek advice from outside experts when reviewing scientific merit.

Finally, although research projects described in a protocol that is extramurally funded on a competitive basis are considered to have passed scientific review, IACUCs may still want to evaluate the proposed science with specific attention paid to potential animal welfare concerns. If a formal scientific merit review of the proposal has not been performed, which is often the case with some nonfederally or internally funded projects, the IACUC may consider conducting or requesting such a review.

4.7 REVIEW OF PROTOCOLS AT CONVENED IACUC MEETINGS

At a convened meeting of the IACUC, a quorum must be present to conduct official business. A quorum is defined as greater than 50% of the total voting members, regardless of which voting members are present. A chair should be present to run the meeting unless a designee is formally appointed to conduct official IACUC business. A good way to avoid potential problems with this issue is to designate a vice-chair and state ahead of time that the vice-chair will perform the chair's duties in the absence of the chair.

One primary responsibility of an IACUC at a convened meeting is the review of animal care and use protocols. Discussion and review of protocols typically involve two parts: (1) a brief summary of the projects/studies proposed in the protocol, and (2) recommended modifications.

Even though all members should be provided with access to a copy of every protocol that is to be discussed at a convened meeting, all members may not review each protocol in depth. Therefore, the assignment of primary, and sometimes secondary, reviewers ensures that at least one or two members are prepared to lead a detailed discussion of each protocol. Reviewers typically provide the following information in their summary of a protocol:

- Species
- Number of animals
- Purpose of the studies
- Summary of experimental design
- Harm–benefit analysis

Once a summary has been presented, reviewers typically list any problems found in the protocol, along with recommended modifications that might be needed. It is always a good idea to have more than one person review each protocol, as this increases the likelihood that all potential problems are noted. For protocols discussed at a convened meeting, it is also a good idea to have the IACUC administrator or chair summarize what modifications are being requested before a vote is taken to ensure all issues that need to be resolved have been documented.

4.7.1 Meeting Minutes

Recording the minutes of convened meetings is essential, and the AWRs and PHS Policy require that the minutes of an IACUC-convened meeting include:

- Records of attendance
- Activities of the IACUC
- IACUC deliberations

The first things that should be recorded in the minutes are the presence of a quorum and a list of meeting attendees. It should be noted that listing member codes instead of names is appropriate for the documentation of attendance and is encouraged. Recording the presence of a quorum and the attendance is important since no official business—that is, voting—can be done without a quorum.

Once it has been determined that a quorum is present, committee discussions and deliberations should be noted. Deliberations can include, but are not limited to, discussion of inspection reports, investigations regarding adverse events or noncompliance, policies and procedures, protocol submissions, protocol amendment submissions, and postapproval monitoring reports.

Decisions regarding these deliberations should also be detailed in the minutes. Decisions might include whether items in an inspection report are minor or significant; whether an adverse event needs to be reported; whether a new policy or procedure should be accepted and implemented; whether a protocol or protocol amendment should be approved, require modifications to secure approval, withheld, disapproved, or suspended; and whether any actions need to follow a postapproval monitoring report.

Most of these decisions require a vote, and a passing vote is defined as an affirmative vote from greater than 50% of the quorum. Members can vote for or against an issue, or they can abstain from voting. All votes, including abstentions, must be recorded in the minutes to accurately document a majority vote. It should be noted that no entities can overturn a decision of the IACUC. For example, an IO cannot allow a PI to conduct research that has been disapproved by the IACUC. An IO may, however, decide that certain activities approved by an IACUC cannot be supported by the university or institution. Such decisions are typically financially motivated (i.e., because the resources needed to conduct the activity cannot be provided to the PI).

When preparing the minutes, it is important to determine what type of information should be omitted from the minutes. The question of what information should not be included in the minutes typically centers on issues regarding the Freedom of Information Act (FOIA) (The Freedom of Information Act 5 U.S.C. § 552 signed into law 1966, and amended by Public Law No. 104-231, 110 Stat. 3048 in 1996). It is important to be aware of the FOIA and any state open record or meeting laws (Silverman et al., 2006). The FOIA does not require the direct release of information to the public, but information submitted to federal agencies can be requested through the FOIA. For this reason, care should be taken to prevent the inclusion of information that is sensitive to public disclosure (Silverman et al., 2014). To protect personal safety, it is best practice to avoid the inclusion of specific names in the minutes. All federal, regulatory, and accrediting agencies understand this and accept coded references to specific individuals in the minutes. The exceptions, however, are the names of the chair and the AV, which should be made available in the public domain. Chapter 17 provides additional information regarding meeting minutes with respect to FOIA requests and regulatory inspections.

The key point is to make sure that the appropriate information is included in the minutes, namely, the discussions, deliberations, decisions, and votes of the committee, in a way that would maintain researcher anonymity and prevent the disclosure of personally identifiable and sensitive information.

4.8 ACTIONS TAKEN BY THE IACUC

There are a number of actions that can be taken by an IACUC with regard to protocols reviewed at a convened meeting according to the PHS Policy IV. B.6 and AWRs 9 CFR §2.31 (c)(7). They are

- Approval
- Require modifications (to secure approval)
- Withhold approval
- Disapprove
- Suspend

If no concerns are raised by members of the IACUC, a protocol can be approved at a meeting with a majority affirmative vote. At any time, any member of the IACUC has the right to file a minority report if he or she disagrees with the actions taken by the committee. Often, to secure approval the IACUC requires that the PI make modifications. In this case, the IACUC will send the PI a list of required modifications that need to be addressed before a protocol can be approved. A review of these changes and the subsequent approval of the protocol are often completed via a DMR after an FCR (see Section 4.5). A DMR after an FCR must be part of the vote on the protocol during the meeting, and an affirmative unanimous vote authorizes a single IACUC member or subset of members to review the changes and grant approval. If the designated member or members are not satisfied with the modifications made to the protocol, they must refer the protocol back to the IACUC, since withholding approval and disapproval are not allowed during a DMR.

A vote for withholding approval (or *disapproving a protocol*) can only be done at a convened full committee meeting. Typically, this action is taken if insufficient information has been provided for an appropriate review of a protocol, or if the described procedures will not be allowed by the IACUC, respectively. The PI should be provided with feedback as to the reason(s) for withholding approval or disapproving his or her protocol, as he or she may choose to make major changes and resubmit.

Alternately, the IACUC may request and approve a pilot study before a larger study is considered for approval. When requesting a pilot study, the IACUC should discuss its concerns with the PI and work with the PI on proposing a pilot study that will address those concerns. Oftentimes, the veterinary staff will work with the PI on these pilot studies. It is imperative that the IACUC receives a report following the pilot study to determine if its concerns have been alleviated. Once a pilot study has been successfully carried out, the PI may submit a new protocol, or an amendment to his or her pilot study protocol, so that the full study can be accomplished.

Another action that can be taken by the IACUC is to suspend a protocol. The suspension of a protocol usually occurs when the IACUC has serious concerns about the activities, usually noncompliant activities, occurring under that protocol. Once an IACUC votes for a suspension, only the IACUC may overturn the decision. It should be noted that the suspension of a protocol requires a report to OLAW, USDA, or both, if applicable.

Whatever the decision or action taken by the IACUC, it is important that the notification to the PI be in writing. Written approvals should include the initial approval date, species, number of animals, period of approval (i.e., expiration date), and conditions of approval, if any (2013).

4.9 PROTOCOL FORMAT

There is no required format for protocols, so long as the proposed activities to be conducted are documented (see Section 4.6) and reviewed by the IACUC. Ideally, the format should be relatively easy and straightforward for researchers to complete and for IACUC members to review.

The two most common formats are form-based systems and database systems (i.e., paper and electronic, respectively). The purpose of both formats is the same: to gather the information that is required for a thorough review of the activities carried out with animals and to gather the information required in reports to federal agencies and accrediting organizations.

Fillable form-based protocols with drop-down boxes and web links (PRIM&R 2013) are relatively easy to create, implement, and use. To assist with regulatory reporting, ideally the forms should be searchable so that relevant data can easily be extracted. Form-based protocols do not require a lot of user training on how to use the actual form (although training may be required to assist PIs with the content of the form), and they are easy to manipulate. It is important, however, that there is good communication with PIs to ensure that they are informed when the forms are altered and know where to get the most recent version.

Electronic-based protocols can be very useful for reporting purposes, as they are typically a relational database and have the capability to extract needed information, but it is imperative that the system is user-friendly to both PIs and reviewers. When choosing or developing a commercially available electronic protocol system, it is necessary to know what attributes are important to the IACUC and ensure that the system has those attributes. While commercially available systems are typically ready to use out of the box, they usually cannot be easily customized and require a service contract with the developing company for troubleshooting and maintenance. Developing an institution-specific electronic system will ensure that an IACUC/institution gets the type of system it wants, but it takes a long time for development and testing to be completed before implementation.

4.10 PROTOCOL RECORD KEEPING

The PHS Policy and the AWRs require that protocols describing the use of animals in research, teaching, or testing are kept for at least three years after the activity is completed. The record should include documented reviews, whether protocols were reviewed by an FCR or a DMR, decisions, and votes. In addition, significant and minor amendments should be documented and kept for the same period of time. If a protocol is renewed at the three-year mark via *de novo* review, the renewal is still considered to be part of the same animal activity and must be retained for an additional three years after completion.

It should be noted that even though a protocol/activity can be approved for three years, it may be closed at any time. Therefore, records can be destroyed three years from the inactivation date of a protocol. Since some federally funded grants can be approved for up to five years, the institution may consider keeping associated IACUC records for three years beyond the expiration of the grant.

4.11 CONCLUSION

Although the regulations are very specific regarding the requirements for the review and approval of animal care and use protocols, it is important to note that the methods for accomplishing these can vary from institution to institution based on each institution's unique situation and research mission. Methods should be clearly laid out in the institution's internal guidelines and its PHS Assurance and/or AAALAC Program Description, as applicable. Clear and transparent communication is essential to remove any ambiguity and will ensure that all research proposals are given fair and thoughtful consideration by the IACUC.

REFERENCES

FASS (Federation of Animal Science Societies). 2010. *Guide for the Care and Use of Agricultural Animals in Agricultural Research and Teaching*, 3rd edn. Consortium for Developing a Guide for the Care and Use of Agricultural Animals in Agricultural Research and Teaching. FASS, Champaign, IL.

The Freedom of Information Act 5 U.S.C. § 552 signed into law 1966, and amended by Public Law No. 104-231, 110 Stat. 3048 in 1996.

NIH (National Institutes of Health). 1985. U.S. government principles for the utilization and care of vertebrate animals used in testing, research and training. http://grants.nih.gov/grants/olaw/references/phspol.htm#USGovPrinciples.no.13. NIH, Bethesda, MD.

NIH (National Institutes of Health). 2002a. *Institutional Animal Care and Use Committee Guidebook*, 2nd edn. Office of Laboratory Animal Welfare, NIH, Bethesda, MD.

NIH (National Institutes of Health). 2002b. Public Health Service policy on humane care and use of laboratory animals. Office of Laboratory Animal Welfare, NIH, Bethesda, MD.

NIH (National Institutes of Health). 2006. NOT-OD-06-052: Guidance on use of telecommunications for IACUC meetings under the PHS Policy on Humane Care and Use of Laboratory Animals. NIH, Bethesda, MD.

NIH (National Institutes of Health). 2012. NOT-OD-12-148: Guidance on departures from the provisions of the guide for the care and use of laboratory animals. Office of Laboratory Animal Welfare, NIH, Bethesda, MD. http://grants.nih.gov/grants/guide/notice-files/NOT-OD-12-148.html.

NRC (National Research Council). 2003. *Guidelines for the Care and Use of Mammals in Neuroscience and Behavioral Research*. National Academies Press, Washington, DC.

NRC (National Research Council). 2011. *Guide for the Care and Use of Laboratory Animals*, 8th edn. National Academies Press, Washington, DC.

Prentice, E. D., D. A. Crouse, and M. D. Mann. 1992. Scientific merit review: The role of the IACUC. *ILAR Journal* 34 (1–2):15–19.

PRIM&R (Public Responsibility in Medicine and Research). 2013. Essentials of IACUC administration, at IACUC Conference, Baltimore, MD, March 18–19.

Russell, W. M. S., R. L. Burch, and C. W. Hume. 1959. *The Principles of Humane Experimental Technique*. London: Methuen.

Silverman, J., M. A. Suckow, and S. Murthy (eds). 2006. *The IACUC Handbook*, 2nd edn. Boca Raton, FL: CRC Press.

Silverman, J., M. A. Suckow, and S. Murthy. 2014. *The IACUC Handbook*. Boca Raton, FL: CRC Press.

USDA (U.S. Department of Agriculture). 2013a. *Animal Welfare Act and Animal Welfare Regulations* (Animal Care Blue Book). Code of Federal Regulations (CFR), Title 9, Chapter 1, Subchapter A, Parts 1–4.

USDA (U.S. Department of Agriculture). 2013b. Animal Welfare Act of 1966 intended to regulate the transport, sale and handling of dogs, cats, guinea pigs, nonhuman primates, hamsters and rabbits intended to use for research or other purposes. Pub. L. 89 (544):2131–2156.

USDA (U.S. Department of Agriculture). 2011. Animal Care Resource Guide Policies. 14: Major survival surgery dealers selling surgically-altered animals to research. Animal and Plant Health Inspection Service, USDA, Washington, DC.

VHA (Department of Veterans Affairs, Veterans Health Administration). 2011. Use of animals in research. *VHA Handbook 1200.07*. VA, Washington, DC.

CHAPTER 5

Elements of the Protocol Form
How to Complete and Review

Monte Matthews

CONTENTS

5.1 INTRODUCTION

All institutions, whether academic or private, develop animal use applications or protocols that request information based on the elements that are required by the Animal Welfare Act Regulations (AWRs), the Public Health Service Policy on Humane Care and Use of Laboratory Animals (PHS Policy), the Guide for the Care and Use of Laboratory Animals (Guide), and the U.S. Government

Principles for the Utilization and Care of Vertebrate Animals Used in Testing, Research, and Training (U.S. Govt. Principles) (NIH 2012b, 2014a, 2014h, 2014i, U.S. DHHS 2013). Although the National Institutes of Health (NIH) Office of Laboratory Animal Welfare (OLAW), the NIH office responsible for enforcing the PHS Policy for institutions that receive PHS funding, has provided a sample protocol form for use (NIH 2011), most institutions continue to create their own protocol form or tailor commercially available protocol forms to their own needs.

Additionally, all of the questions and the requested information contained in protocols are organized differently across institutions. Part of the reason for this is that there is no universally adopted or standardized protocol across all institutions in the United States. Although this allows for greater flexibility in designing a protocol form for one's own institution, it is challenging to be constantly changing and updating the form based on new rules, regulations, and policies that affect not only the elements required in a protocol, but also how they are to be integrated into the Animal Care and Use Program (ACUP). There is a segment of the research community that is neither PHS-funded nor uses species regulated by the United States Department of Agriculture (USDA) (i.e., privately funded institutions that only use mice of the genus *Mus* and rats of the genus *Rattus*, or institutions funded by government agencies other than the Department of Health and Human Services); hence many of the protocol sections and questions discussed in this chapter, as well as those included on the sample form provided in the appendices of this book, may not apply. Even though an institution may not be subject to these rules and regulations, it might be in their best interest to include many of these sections and questions on their institution's protocol form in the event their program undergoes an unexpected change (i.e., they recruit an investigator that has a PHS-supported grant from their former institution, or an investigator wants to start using USDA-regulated species).

This chapter will provide information on the basic elements required for protocol review and best practices. The following 11 sections, which are bolded, contain many of the protocol elements that the author has reviewed from several sample protocol forms across academia and industry. Some of these protocol elements are self-explanatory and require no further explanation. In many cases, references are made to AWRs, PHS Policy, the Guide, and the U.S. Govt. Principles.

How a protocol form is designed determines whether or not all of the protocol elements are addressed and the quality and detail of the answers. There is no single, correct way of organizing the elements of a protocol as long as the information that is requested is easily understood and organized in a way that makes it relatively easy and painless for the investigator to complete, and for the members of the Institutional Animal Care and Use Committee (IACUC) to review. Answers to many of the questions and requested information can be provided through drop-down tables, radio buttons, checkboxes, and so on. Often, this makes it easier for the investigator to fill out a standard set of answers. Detailed examples of these are not given here but can be seen in the sample protocol form found in Appendix 1.

5.2 GENERAL INFORMATION

Identification of Protocol: This section is typically filled out or assigned by the IACUC office. This information is important for keeping track of regulatory or policy requirements, such as the USDA's requirement for no less than annual review or the PHS Policy's requirement for *de novo* review every three years (NIH 2002). Additionally, an institution may choose to develop metrics for assessing the effectiveness of the protocol review process, such as how long it takes a protocol to be approved once it is submitted.

A. Name of institution, date submitted, protocol number, approval date, and expiration date.
B. Protocol title: Helpful to indicate the species to be used and be descriptive of the procedures/surgery involving animals.
C. Protocol type: Initial submission, three-year renewal, annual renewal, and amendment.
D. Protocol purpose checklist: It is helpful to give the IACUC and IACUC staff an idea of what the purpose of the protocol is in order to provide a general framework for the review. Some protocols may have more than one purpose and all of them should be identified. This can be accomplished by providing a simple checklist like the following:
   1. Research
   2. Teaching/training
   3. Pilot project
   4. Protocol specific breeding
   5. Antibody production
   6. Behavioral
   7. Colony health surveillance
   8. Use of animals for food
   9. Holding protocol
   10. Field study

5.3 PERSONNEL: QUALIFICATIONS AND TRAINING

The AWRs (9 CFR §2.31 [d][1]), PHS Policy, the Guide, and the U.S. Govt. Principles require all those who care for and use animals in research, testing, or teaching to be adequately trained and qualified to perform the duties described in the protocol. The Guide also requires that personnel training is documented (NRC 2011). Non–principal investigator (PI)/protocol director (PD) personnel can be added to protocols as a minor amendment as long as the institution has developed a mechanism to assure that all individuals associated with the project have been identified, are adequately trained and qualified, and have enrolled in the institution's occupational health and safety program (OHSP) (NIH 2014f).

A. **Principal Investigator**: Every protocol should have an individual who acts as the PI who is responsible for the project or activities associated with the protocol. The PI's responsibilities are described in 9 CFR §2.31 (d)(1) (ii-iii) of the AWRs.
   1. PI name
   2. Title/rank

3. Department/division/unit
4. Contact information, such as office phone, emergency phone, e-mail, office address, and fax

B. **Protocol Personnel**: Name, position, department, work location, work phone, emergency phone, and e-mail (multiple ways to reach in an emergency if possible).
   1. Identify which personnel are the co-PI, administrative contact, or other roles (i.e., research associates, data analysts, lab technicians, etc.).
   2. Qualifications/training.
      a. Credentials/background/experience: A detailed list of the individual's qualifications and training should be provided—especially that experience related to the species-specific procedures that the individual will be performing as part of the study.
      b. List of procedures they will be performing as part of the protocol: This description is important to assess the adequacy of training.
      c. List of procedures that will require additional training: All of the procedures that the individual will require additional training before performing should be listed so that the institution can fulfill its responsibility for providing training.
      d. List of individuals who will be performing the training: Trainers should also be identified so that the IACUC knows who is providing their training and whether or not they are qualified to do so.
   3. Occupational health considerations and clearances: Institutions can develop different mechanisms to assure that all of those who are working with or are exposed to animals are enrolled in the OHSP. The author's institution has chosen to document the individual's OHSP participation as part of the protocol's personnel qualifications and training section. Information in this section could include
      a. OHSP category: typically based on species the individual will be working with
      b. OHSP training date
      c. Medical evaluation clearance date

C. **Personnel Assurance**: Each individual associated with the protocol should sign off on their personnel page assuring that the information is correct and that they have read the protocol and understand their responsibilities.

D. **PI Assurance**: Given the broad authority and responsibility given to the PI to direct the project, the author believes it is a good idea to have the PI sign off on the personnel page for each individual working on the protocol.

5.4 FUNDING, COLLABORATIONS, CONFLICT OF INTEREST

A. **Funding Information**: How a project is funded is important for many reasons, such as assuring adequate funds for the project; determining scientific-merit review (NIH 2014d); identifying all grants, contracts, or subawards if there is more than one funding component associated with a single protocol; and cross-referencing with other departments, such as a grants or sponsored-projects office.
   1. Proposal type: New, continuation, renewal, or revision
   2. External funding agency, title, grant/contract number, dates of funding, and any internal funding or accounting number if applicable
   3. Other funding, such as departmental funds, gifts, or fellowships

B. **Protocol/Grant Congruency**: Although federal regulations do not require institutions to perform a side-by-side comparison of the protocol with the grant application or proposal, institutions are responsible for assuring that all animal care and use procedures that the IACUC reviews and approves are congruent with all of the animal care and use information contained in the grant application (NIH 2010, 2014c).

   1. List mechanism for establishing congruency: This is often a checkbox that is part of an IACUC standard operating procedure (SOP).
   2. Peer review of unsponsored research: Some IACUCs choose to develop mechanisms for scientific review for those protocols that do not undergo a rigorous peer review. Examples would include departmental review of research protocols and curriculum review for teaching protocols.
      a. Internal funds
      b. External funds with no scientific merit review
      c. Teaching protocols

C. **Collaborations**: Institutions that are involved in collaborations are expected to have a formal written understanding, such as a memorandum of understanding (MOU), that defines their respective responsibilities. NIH requires that both awardee and performance site institutions have a PHS Animal Welfare Assurance to conduct PHS-funded activities (NIH 2012a). Although there is no federal requirement that each institution review each protocol separately, it is recommended that the review should be maintained by both institutions (NIH 2014g).

   1. External collaborations
      a. Vendor
      b. Other institutions
   2. Internal collaborations

D. **Conflicts of Interest**: Although not a required protocol element, some institutions choose to have the PI disclose actual or potential conflicts of interest that are or may be associated with the protocol. A conflict of interest occurs when an individual's professional actions or decisions are influenced by personal financial gain. Examples of potential conflicts of interest for an individual in relation to a sponsoring company, vendor(s), provider(s) of goods, or subcontractor(s) can include, but are not limited to, consulting arrangements, responsibilities, serving as a member of an advisory board, or having equity holdings; having a financial relationship (including the receipt of honoraria, income, gift funds, or stock/stock options as payment); or having an ownership or royalty interest in any intellectual property utilized in the project. Conflicts of interest may not be limited to the PI; they can include anyone listed on the protocol, an immediate family member (spouse, dependent child as defined by the IRS, or domestic partner), or anyone in a supervisory role to personnel listed on a protocol.

5.5 RATIONALE AND PURPOSE OF STUDY

Sometimes referred to as the "lay summary," this section and its associated questions provide the ethical framework for the IACUC to formulate its harm–benefit analysis of the protocol. Although there are no specific requirements to list separately all of the benefits and harms of the proposal, there is an expectation that the IACUC "will weigh the objectives of the study against potential animal welfare concerns" (NRC 2011). The information provided below should be written in terms that a nonscientist would understand and should not be a copy and paste of the aims from the grant.

    A. What are the study objectives or aims of the study?
    B. How are the procedures and design of the study relevant and important for human or animal health, the advancement of knowledge, or the good of society? (NIH 1985)

5.6 ANIMAL USE JUSTIFICATION

This section also extends the ethical framework for the harm–benefit analysis by justifying the use of animals; choice of species; numbers of animals to be used; refinement techniques for minimizing pain, distress, and discomfort; and addressing the unavailability of alternatives.

A. Addressing the three Rs: Replacement, reduction, and refinement are commonly referred to as the three Rs. These principles were derived from William Russell and Rex Burch's 1959 publication *Principles of Humane Experimental Techniques.*
    1. Replacement: Justification for the use of animals and choice of species.
        a. Use of animals: This section should describe why it is necessary to use animals and what non–live animal models (such as isolated organ preps, cell or tissue culture, or computer simulation) were considered.
        b. Choice of species: This section should justify the particular species that was chosen, which also should be the lowest possible on the phylogenetic scale. What biological characteristics of this species make it the most appropriate for this project? This section could also include a justification for the particular developmental stage of animal.
    2. Reduction: Justification for the number of animals proposed. The number of animals proposed should be the minimum number required to obtain scientifically and statistically valid results (NIH 1985). Whenever possible, the number of animals and experimental group sizes should be statistically justified (NRC 2011). What statistical test was used to determine n and experimental group size? The number of animals required for breeding (both parents and projected offspring necessary to produce animals expressing the desired genotype) should also be included. In some cases, group size may depend on the amount of tissue required.
    3. Refinement: This section should describe how procedures are designed for minimization of pain, distress, and discomfort.
B. Alternatives: The AWRs (9 CFR §2.31 (d)(1) (ii)), PHS Policy, the Guide, and the U.S. Govt. Principles require the consideration of alternatives to animal use activities. By addressing the three Rs above, the PI has already discussed those aspects of:
    1. Assurance that all animal use activities do not unnecessarily duplicate previous experiments.
    2. Written narrative description of the methods and sources used to determine that alternatives are not available for the study in question. USDA Policy 12 (Consideration of Alternatives to Painful/Distressful Procedures) provides further guidance. (USDA 2014)

a. Was a database search used as a means for fulfilling this requirement? If so, please list:
   i. Name(s) of the databases searched
   ii. The date the search was performed
   iii. The time period covered by the search
   iv. The search strategy used (including keywords used in the search and scientifically relevant terminology)

5.7 ANIMAL SUBJECTS INFORMATION

A. Common name/scientific name/strain or substrain.
B. Age, sex, number, (weight, size, developmental stage): The number of animals has already been justified previously. A list here of the number of animals needed per year or per three years is helpful for vivarium planning purposes. Some institutions choose to have the number of animals listed here by USDA pain category. Pain categories are addressed in Section 5.12 and in Appendix G.
C. Source of animal: For example, name of vendor, transfer from another institution, transfer from another PI from same institution, bred in-house.
D. Health status: For example, specific pathogen free (SPF), germfree, and so on.
E. Acclimation period: Identify the minimum duration the animal will be allowed to acclimate once it arrives and before it is used in the study.
F. Animal identification: The method used to identify animals should be listed, such as ear notches/punches/tags, tattoos, collar, cage card, subcutaneous implants, fin clips, and so on. Toe clipping of small rodents, particularly neonatal mice, should be adequately justified here and used when no other individual identification method is feasible (NRC 2011).
G. Genetic information: For genetically modified animals, some of this information will be captured for Institutional Biosafety Committee (IBC) approval.
   1. Will genetically modified animals be used?
   2. For each strain, what is the inserted or knocked-out gene?
   3. List expected phenotype, especially if there are any animal welfare concerns.
   4. Describe any special care or monitoring procedures.
   5. Describe other procedures used to minimize pain, distress, or discomfort.
H. Animal use in other protocols: If animals are to be used on more than one protocol, then this should be scientifically justified.

5.8 ANIMAL CARE, HOUSING, AND TRANSPORTATION

A. Husbandry: Many protocols refer to standard husbandry SOPs. If standard SOPs are being followed, then a simple acknowledgment of that fact is normally sufficient since these SOPs are reviewed by the IACUC. For USDA-regulated species, the housing, husbandry, and transportation must be in accordance with 9 CFR Part 3 Standards, which exist for each regulated species.
   1. Standard versus nonstandard checklist.
   2. Nonstandard/specialized requirements: Should provide justification for each nonstandard item with the frequency and duration of time that the animal will

be exposed to the nonstandard husbandry condition and any anticipated consequences. The person responsible for the nonstandard husbandry item should also be identified.

    a. Caging: Type of cage (e.g., wire bottom with justification), cage change interval, ventilated or static, autowater versus water bottle or pouch, other.

    b. Food: Name of specialized/medicated diet, how the food is stored, its expiration, and who is responsible for feeding.

    c. Water: If medicated, give compound and concentration, and identify who is responsible for changing water bottles.

    d. Other environmental parameters (light cycles and intensity, temperature, humidity, etc.).

B. Housing: Important not only for planning purposes, but also for regulatory compliance given all of the strict requirements for animal housing and physical plant.

  1. Location

    a. Primary housing location (building, room number).

    b. Secondary housing location (greater than 12 hours USDA/24 hours PHS) outside of the core vivarium; it is also important to identify activities associated with these areas and who is responsible.

    c. All other areas where animals are used for all of the procedures described in the protocol, such as surgery (survival and nonsurvival), hazardous agent, behavioral, and other nonsurgical procedures. Maximum duration of animal use in these areas.

  2. Management: Any PI-managed areas and personnel should be identified with specific roles and responsibilities for animal care, monitoring, and oversight.

  3. Social housing: For nonhuman primates (NHPs), there needs to be an environmental enhancement plan that includes specific provisions to address the social needs of NHPs of species known to exist in social groups in nature (9 CFR §3.81(a)). Social housing should be the default for social laboratory species (NRC 2011). Justification should be given for individually housed animals and limited to the minimum period necessary (AAALAC 2014). If individually housed, animals should be provided with environmental enrichment.

  4. Environmental enrichment: Environmental enrichment is part of the institution's behavior management program and should facilitate and promote the expression of species-specific behavior and psychological well-being (AAALAC 2013, NRC 2011).

    a. Provide scientific justification if no environmental enrichment will be used.

    b. Provide time frame for lack of enrichment.

D. Transportation: Procedures should be identified for all animals to be transported outside of the central vivarium. Questions to be addressed include:

  1. Will animals be transported outside the central vivarium?

  2. Who will be responsible for their transport? Are they qualified and trained?

  3. Where will the animals be transported?

  4. How will the animals be transported? What equipment will be used? Will transport involve the use of a private vehicle?

  5. How long will it take to transport the animals?

  6. Will transport occur through any public or patient areas? What means will be used during transport to minimize exposure to nonresearch personnel?

5.9 ANIMAL PROCEDURES/EXPERIMENTAL DESIGN

A. Checklist of major procedures: Most of the protocols reviewed by the author have developed modular approaches to their protocol form, in which major- or high-risk/monitoring procedures are described separately in appendices; in the case of electronic systems, these sections are only visible if the associated procedure is part of the protocol. Having a simple checklist at the beginning of this section (or potentially identified earlier in the protocol form, such as with the protocol purpose in the administration section above) will provide a procedural roadmap for both the PI and the reviewer.

B. Provide a clear, concise, complete, and sequential description of all animal use procedures. Details of any of the procedures checked above are covered in their respective sections, but they should be listed here for clarity. Examples include

1. The animal acclimation and identification method (if different from above).
2. The type and number of experimental groups and control groups. These can be grouped into pain categories.
   a. How long animals are in each group.
   b. Detailed procedures in each group if not covered elsewhere; otherwise list.
   c. Description of anticipated or established clinical signs of disease, illness, lesions, behavioral abnormalities, and so on.
   d. Anticipated or established morbidity/mortality with each group if applicable.
   e. Signs used to assess pain, distress, or discomfort.
   f. Humane end points for each group.
      i. Describe the anticipated clinical signs that may develop in the model (e.g., tumors, percentage body-weight loss/gain, inability to eat or drink, behavioral abnormalities, and signs of toxicity).
      ii. What are the proposed study/early euthanasia criteria with regard to above clinical signs, and what treatment or action will be initiated for each (e.g., humanely euthanize, contact veterinary staff)?
         1. Provide scientific justification for any unrelieved pain/distress or if using death as an end point.
   g. Unanticipated outcomes:
      i. Does the PI want to be notified before treatment is initiated or animal is euthanized? Supply emergency contact information.
3. Method of restraint:
   a. Chemical
   b. Physical (prolonged restraint addressed in physical restraint section)
4. Agent administration (details of anesthesia, hazardous chemicals, and non-pharmaceutical agents addressed in other sections).
5. Blood, fluid, tissue collection (see Appendix D: Guidelines for Blood Sample Withdrawal). Any exceptions to these guidelines need to be scientifically justified, and any safeguards to prevent adverse effects must be described.
   a. Method of collection
   b. Frequency
   c. Volume of a single blood withdrawal
   d. Volume of total blood withdrawn per day and week
6. Antibody Production. If using ascites production to produce antibodies, provide a justification for not using an *in vitro* system.
   a. Will antibody production occur at an off-site vendor (NIH 2014a)?

7. Tumor Passage: Provide details on care for animals injected with cells producing solid tumors:
   a. Frequency with which animals will be observed and tumor(s) measured/monitored for ulceration, body weights taken, and body-conditioning scores performed
   b. Maximum size of tumor(s) and anticipated impact on health and well-being of animals
   c. Supportive care that will be provided; humane end points

5.10 ANIMAL-RELATED PROCEDURES

A. Hazardous Agents

Animal experiments involving hazards deserve special consideration. Many institutions choose to have a separate committee, such as the Institutional Biosafety Committee (IBC), Radiation Safety Committee (RSC), Stem Cell Research Oversight Committee (SCRO), or Environmental Health and Safety (EHS) office review and approve these procedures separately. A checkbox is helpful to identify which hazard type will be used with animals, such as chemical/nanomaterial, biohazardous, biological, or radiation.

1. Chemical/nanomaterials: This section is used to document use of hazardous substances (chemicals including nanomaterials) in animals.
   a. Personnel information
   b. Agent name, location where hazard administered, and housing location after administration
   c. Hazard class: examples include carcinogen, mutagen, toxicity level, and other
   d. Species, route of administration, maximum concentration and dose, volume administered, and frequency
   e. Effect of agent on animal well-being
   f. Period of time from the end of animal exposure to study termination
   g. Route of excretion, hazardous metabolites, half-life if known, and decontamination procedures
   h. Engineering controls and personal protective equipment (PPE)
   i. Waste disposal arrangements
   j. Transportation/shipping methods

2. Biohazardous: This section is used to document the use of biohazardous substances (biological) in animals.
   a. Type of biohazardous agent: for example, human/NHP cells, tissues or fluids; stem cells (see Section 10B); active virus/bacteria/prion; attenuated virus/bacteria; recombinant DNA (NIH 2009)
   b. Personnel information
   c. Risk group level and biosafety level
   d. Agent name, location where hazard administered, and housing location after administration
   e. Species, route of administration, maximum concentration and dose, volume administered, and frequency
   f. Effect of agent on animal well-being
   g. Period of time from the end of animal exposure to study termination

      h. Route of transmission, period of infectivity, decontamination procedures, and whether the agent has zoonotic/biosecurity implications

      i.   Engineering controls and PPE

      j.   Waste disposal arrangements

      k. Transportation/shipping methods

3. Radiation: Does the research involve *in vivo* use of radioisotopes or the use of irradiators or radiation-generating machines?

      a. Check all that apply: Radioisotopes, irradiators, x-ray, MRI, PET, CT scan, fluoroscopy, laser, other

          i.   Use of human patient medical equipment/patient areas

          ii. Scheduling

          iii. Decontamination procedures

          iv. Hospital infection control panel approval

      b. Radioisotope name, route of administration, dosage/curies

      c. Location where administered, housing location after exposure

      d. Species information

      e. Effect of agent on animal well-being

      f.   Period of time from the end of animal exposure to study termination

      g. Route of excretion, half-life if known, decontamination procedures

      h. Engineering controls and PPE

      i.   Waste disposal arrangements

      j.   Transportation/shipping methods

B. Biological Material/Animal Products for Use in Animals

1. Human stem cells and other cells of human origin

      a. Cell type, route of administration, concentration, special handling and use, biosafety/SCRO panel approval if applicable

      b. Precautions to prevent pregnancies in animals given human embryonic stem cells (hESCs)

      c. NIH/state-specific restrictions

      d. Pathogen profile of donor for cells of human origin

2. Cells/tissues of rodent origin

      a. Screening biological materials for rodent pathogens

C. Use of Non-Pharmaceutical-Grade Compounds

Animal Care Policy No. 3 (USDA 2014), the Guide, and the NIH-OLAW all offer guidance on the use of non-pharmaceutical-grade compounds in live animals (NIH 2014e). In some cases, the use of non-pharmaceutical-grade compounds may be described in the chemical use hazard section.

1. Will any non-pharmaceutical-grade compounds be used in live animals?

2. If yes, provide scientific justification for its use. Address availability of pharmaceutical-grade compounds.

3. Describe efforts in considering the following: grade, purity, sterility, acid–base balance, pyrogenicity, osmolality, stability, site and route of administration, compatibility of components, side effects and adverse reactions, storage, and pharmacokinetics.

D. Surgery

A checklist indicating the type or classification of surgical procedure(s) is helpful at the beginning of this section: these can include survival major, survival minor, non-survival, multiple minor survival, multiple major survival, and vendor-conducted surgery.

1. Basic information for surgical procedures (excluding vendor-conducted):
    a. Title and name of personnel involved (Note: detailed training and quali-
        fications should be listed previously in the Personnel section. If not, they
        should be described here).
    b. Location(s) of where procedure is to be performed.
    c. Preoperative procedures if applicable, such as withholding of food or
        water prior to surgery and duration, preoperative physical exam, or blood
        or chemistry profile.
    d. Detailed description of surgical procedures to be performed, includ-
        ing instrument sterilization method; aseptic techniques and methods
        used, including surgeon preparation (for survival); surgical incision/site
        preparation; anticipated time to perform procedure; preoperative anes-
        thetics, analgesics, and sedatives given; supportive care given during
        procedure (e.g., intravenous (IV) fluids, mechanical ventilation, oph-
        thalmic ointment, temperature control); parameters monitored includ-
        ing ranges, if known, during anesthesia (vital signs such as respiration
        rate, temperature, mucous membrane color, saturated oxygen, heart
        rate, blood pressure) and identification of actions taken if parameter is
        outside of range; and method used to assure adequate anesthetic level
        (e.g., toe pinch).
2. Survival procedures:
    a. Identification if minor or major survival surgery.
    b. Location where animal will be recovered.
    c. Housing of animal during recovery.
    d. Personnel involved in recovery.
    e. What are provisions for after-hours, weekend, and holiday care?
    f. Description of expected condition of animal after full recovery from
        anesthesia.
    g. How will animals be monitored? What clinical signs and parameters will
        be used to determine pain, distress, or discomfort?
    h. Description of potential postoperative complications and how they will be
        managed.
    i. What postoperative care will be given after the procedure?
        A. Supportive care (e.g., temperature control, IV fluids)
        B. Postoperative analgesia and sedation: name of agent, dose, route, fre-
            quency, expected time frame of effect of drug
    j. What humane end points will be used to prevent continued pain or
        distress?
3. Multiple survival surgeries:
    a. Description of all survival surgeries performed on the single animal.
    b. What is the scientific justification for multiple survival surgeries?
    c. What is the estimated time between the survival surgeries?
4. Vendor-conducted survival surgery:
    a. Name of vendor
    b. Description of surgery
    c. Number of animals required for study
    d. Acclimation period after arrival and prior to use
E. Anesthesia, Analgesia, Tranquilization, Sedation
    1. Identify species and procedure.

2. Name of agent, dose (recommend use of ranges whenever possible), route (recommend multiple routes whenever possible), frequency.
   a. If gas anesthesia:
      i. Location of use: EHS or some equivalent office should assess and approve of all areas where gas anesthesia is being used.
      ii. Delivery method.
      iii. Scavenging method.
      iv. Personnel and verification of training.

F. Physical Restraint

The Guide considers prolonged physical restraint as deserving special consideration and that it should be avoided unless it is scientifically justified (NRC 2011).

1. Describe procedure(s) requiring prolonged restraint.
2. Describe method and restraint device used to restrain the animal.
3. Describe the duration and frequency of prolonged restraint (should be minimum necessary to reach scientific objectives) and how often animals are observed.
4. Describe location(s) where prolonged restraint and associated procedures will be conducted.
5. Describe the veterinary care plan for animal care and support during the restraint.
6. Describe procedures used to train and acclimate animals to the restraint device.
7. Describe alternatives that were considered.
8. Describe criteria used to remove animals from the study if they fail to adapt.
9. Assurance that veterinary care will be provided if lesions or illnesses are observed, and that the purpose and duration of the restraint has been communicated to all personnel involved in the study.

G. Food/Fluid Regulation

The Guide considers food and fluid regulation as deserving of special consideration (NRC 2011).

1. Describe the nature, extent, and frequency of food and water regulation and how this determination was made.
2. What are the potential adverse consequences of the regulation on the animal's health and well-being?
3. What methods and signs will be used in assessing the animal's health and well-being and how often? (Note: The Guide states that "Body weights should be recorded at least weekly and more often for animals requiring greater restrictions.") (NRC 2011)
4. What criteria will be used to remove the animal from the study?
5. Justify the use of food and water regulation.
6. What alternative methods were considered, for example, positive reinforcement?

H. Behavioral Testing

1. Animal subjects information:
   a. Species, age, weight, sex, number.
2. Name of behavioral test.
3. Describe any equipment and it use as part of the test.
4. Describe the behavioral test.
5. Are there any potential adverse effects (e.g., pain, distress, or discomfort) associated with the test?

6. What signs will be used to determine if the animal is experiencing any pain, distress, or discomfort?
7. What humane end points will be used to end the experiment?
8. How often will the animal be monitored?
9. Personnel information.

I. Canine Opportunity for Exercise
 1. Will there be any exceptions or restrictions to the institution's program for the opportunity to exercise?
    a. If yes, provide scientific justification for the exception or restriction.
    b. Describe the extent and duration of the exception.

J. Psychological Well-Being of NHPs
 1. Will there be any exceptions or restrictions to the institution's program for environmental enhancement to promote psychological well-being of NHPs?
    a. If yes, provide scientific justification for the exception or restriction.
    b. Describe the extent and duration of the exception.

K. Field Studies/Investigations
 Field investigations involving wildlife are challenging. The AWRs define a *field study* as "a study conducted on free-living wild animals in their natural habitat" and exempt such studies from IACUC review (USDA 2013). However, if the field research involves an invasive procedure or harms or materially alters the behavior of an animal under study, it is excluded from this exemption and must be reviewed by the IACUC. The PHS Policy, on the other hand, has no such exemption, and all PHS-funded activities must be conducted in accordance with the Guide. The Guide refers to field research as *field investigations*, which are defined as studies that "may involve the observation or use of nondomesticated vertebrate species under field conditions" (NRC 2011). If the activity is USDA exempt and non-PHS-funded, the institution should consider following taxon-specific guidelines. You can find an example of a detailed protocol form, developed by the Ornithological Council and the American Society of Mammologists, on the OLAW website: http://grants.nih.gov/grants/olaw/20140320_SampleWildlifeProtocolB.docx.
 1. Provide animal subjects information if not previously identified in 'Animal Subjects' section.
 2. Describe location(s) where field study will take place.
 3. Describe how animals will be observed and all nonphysical interactions. Will these observations and interactions materially alter their behavior?
 4. Describe precautions taken to ensure the health and safety of personnel working in the field and handling animals.
 5. Will animals be captured? If yes, describe:
    a. Method of capture and handling
    b. Equipment used in capture
       i. Detailed description of equipment and its use
       ii. How often the equipment is checked if left unattended
       iii. Maximum potential time for animal in capture device
    c. All procedures conducted on the animal after capture
    d. Maximum length of time for capture and procedures
    e. Transportation of animals:
       i. Justification for transportation of animals
       ii. Method of transport and procedures used to ensure animal welfare

      iii. Length of time for transport

      iv. Final destination

   f. Disposition of animal after all procedures are completed

6. Describe procedures used to minimize injury or mortality.
7. Is there a potential to capture nontarget species? If so, please describe which species if possible.
8. Describe procedures used to minimize take of nontarget species.
9. Are permits (local, regional, state, federal, national, international, the Convention on International Trade in Endangered Species of Wild Flora and Fauna [CITES]) required for the observation, capture, or any of the procedures conducted on the animal?

   a. If yes, provide the following information for each authorization:

      i. Agency name

      ii. Agency contact information

      iii. Permit or authorization number

      iv. Approval date

   b. Attach a copy of the permit or authorization.

   c. If authorization is still pending, attach a copy of the permit application.

10. Will animals be brought back to the institution? If yes, describe.

5.11 EUTHANASIA/FINAL DISPOSITION

A. Indicate final disposition of animal, such as euthanasia, transfer to other protocol, adoption, release of animal (such as in a field study).

1. Indicate or describe method of euthanasia:

   a. Standard, preapproved method. A list can be provided for PI to check from.

   b. If nonstandard, is this method recommended by the American Veterinary Medical Association (AVMA) Guidelines for the Euthanasia of Animals?

      i. Acceptable: see Appendices 1 and 2 of the AVMA Guidelines 2013, p. 99–101.

      ii. Acceptable with conditions: see Appendices 1 and 2 of AVMA Guidelines 2013, p 99–101.

      A. Justification for using acceptable with conditions.

      B. How will conditions be met? For example, if using CO_2 euthanasia, what secondary method will be used to ensure death?

   c. If not recommended by the AVMA Guidelines for the Euthanasia of Animals, provide scientific justification as to why such methods must be used.

   d. How will death of animal be ensured?

2. Will fluid or tissues be collected during or following euthanasia?
3. What is the final disposition of carcass?
4. Will there be sharing of tissues, fluids, or carcasses?

5.12 PAIN AND DISTRESS CATEGORIES

Many institutions choose to address USDA's pain and distress classifications, which are used for annual reporting (9 CFR §2.36 (a)(5–8); Appendix G).

5.12.1 USDA Classifications and Examples

Classification B: Animals being bred, conditioned, or held for use in teaching, testing, experiments, research, or surgery, but not yet used for such purposes.

Examples:

- Breeding colonies of any animal species that are handled in accordance with IACUC approval, the Guide, and other applicable regulations. Breeding colony includes parents and offspring. (Note: The USDA does not require listing of non-regulated rats, mice, and birds.)
- Newly acquired animals that are handled in accordance with IACUC approval and applicable regulations.
- Animals held under proper captive conditions or wild animals that are being observed.

Classification C: No pain or distress to animals, and no use of pain-relieving drugs.

Examples:

- Procedures performed correctly by trained personnel such as the administration of electrolytes/fluids, administration of oral medication, blood collection from a common peripheral vein per standard veterinary practice (dog cephalic, cat jugular) or catheterization of same, standard radiography, parenteral injections of nonirritating substances.
- Manual restraint that is no longer than would be required for a simple exam; short period of chair restraint for an adapted NHP.

Classification D: Pain or distress to animals for which appropriate anesthetic, analgesic, or tranquilizing drugs are used.

Examples:

- Surgical procedures conducted by trained personnel in accordance with standard veterinary practice, such as biopsies, gonadectomy, exposure of blood vessels, chronic catheter implantation, and laparotomy or laparoscopy.
- Blood collection by more invasive routes, such as intracardiac or periorbital collection from species without a true orbital sinus (e.g., guinea pigs).
- Administration of drugs, chemicals, toxins, or organisms that would be expected to produce pain or distress but which will be alleviated by analgesics, anesthetics, tranquilizers, or supportive care.

Classification E: Pain/distress to animals for which the use of appropriate anesthetic, analgesic, or tranquilizing drugs are withheld due to adverse effects on procedures, results, or interpretations.

Examples:

- Procedures producing pain or distress unrelieved by analgesics, such as toxicity studies, microbial virulence testing, radiation sickness, and research on stress, shock, or pain.

- Surgical and postsurgical sequella from invasion of body cavities, orthopedic procedures, dentistry, or other hard- or soft-tissue damage that produces unrelieved pain or distress.
- Negative conditioning via electric shocks that would cause pain in humans.
- Regulatory/mandatory testing, such as leptospirosis vaccine potency testing using hamsters.

5.12.2 Note Regarding Classification E

An explanation of the procedures producing pain or distress in these animals and the justification for not using appropriate anesthetic, analgesic, or tranquilizing drugs must be provided. This information is required to be reported to the USDA, will be available from the USDA under the Freedom of Information Act (FOIA), and may be publicly available through the Internet via the USDA's website.

The required information for the Column E explanation is:

1. Registration number.
2. Number of animals used in the study.
3. Species (common name) of animals used in the study.
4. Explanation of the procedure producing pain and/or distress.
5. The scientific justification why pain and/or distress could not be relieved. State methods or means that pain and/or distress relief would interfere with test results.
6. Federal regulations that require the procedure. Cite the agency, the code of Federal Regulations (CFR), title number, and the specific section number.

In addition to the requirements, the author recommends the following description of measures and procedures used to minimize and evaluate pain and distress.

- Nonpharmacological procedures used to minimize pain and distress
- Signs used to assess pain and distress and how often they will be monitored and by whom
- Humane end points used to remove or euthanize animals from the study

Studies involving death as an end point must be well documented and justified.

5.13 ASSURANCES

In the author's review of various protocols, most of them have a list of assurances or certifications. Here are a couple of examples:

A. From the author's institution:
  1. I agree to abide by the University of Oregon policies for the care and use of animals; the provisions of the Guide for the Care and Use of Laboratory Animals; and all federal, state, and local laws and regulations governing the use of animals in research.

I understand that emergency veterinary care will be administered to animals showing evidence of pain or illness, in addition to routine veterinary care as prescribed for individual species in the Standard Operating Procedures.

2. I declare that all experiments involving live animals will be performed under my supervision or that of another qualified biomedical scientist listed on this protocol.

3. I certify that all personnel having direct animal contact, including myself, have been trained in humane and scientifically acceptable procedures in animal handling, administration of anesthetics, analgesics, and euthanasia to be used in this project. I assure that personnel will be allowed adequate time to attend training sessions.

4. I understand that personnel with live animal contact are required to participate in the Occupational Health and Safety Program.

5. I further declare that the information provided in the accompanying protocol is accurate to the best of my knowledge. Any proposed revisions to the animal care and use data will be promptly forwarded in writing to the IACUC for approval, including changes in personnel and location.

6. I am aware that any deviation from an approved protocol or violations of pertinent policies, guidelines, or laws could result in immediate suspension of this project.

B. From the NIH-OLAW sample protocol form:

1. I certify that I have attended the institutionally required investigator training course. Year of Course Attendance: _____ Location: _____

2. I certify that I have determined that the research proposed herein is not unnecessarily duplicative of previously reported research.

3. I certify that all individuals working on this proposal who are at risk are participating in the institution's Occupational Health and Safety Program.

4. I certify that the individuals listed in Section A are authorized to conduct procedures involving animals under this proposal, have attended the institutionally required investigator training course, and received training in: the biology, handling, and care of this species; aseptic surgical methods and techniques (if necessary); the concept, availability, and use of research or testing methods that limit the use of animals or minimize distress; the proper use of anesthetics, analgesics, and tranquilizers (if necessary); and procedures for reporting animal welfare concerns.

5. For all USDA Classification D and E proposals (see section H.1.): I certify that I have reviewed the pertinent scientific literature and the sources and/or databases as noted in Section H.2. and have found no valid alternative to any procedures described herein which may cause more than momentary pain or distress, whether it is relieved or not.

6. I certify that I will obtain approval from the IACUC before initiating any significant changes in this study.

7. I certify that I will notify the IACUC regarding any unexpected study results that impact the animals. Any unanticipated pain or distress, morbidity, or mortality will be reported to the attending veterinarian and the IACUC.

8. I certify that I am familiar with and will comply with all pertinent institutional, state, and federal rules and policies.

PI Name: _____ Signature: _____ Date: _____

REFERENCES

AAALAC International (Association for Assessment and Accreditation of Laboratory Animal Care, International). 2014. Position statements: Social housing. AAALAC, Frederick, MD.

AAALAC International (Association for Assessment and Accreditation of Laboratory Animal Care, International). 2013. Accreditation 4. Environmental enrichment. AAALAC, Frederick, MD.

HHS (U.S. Department of Health and Human Services). 2009. *Biosafety in Microbiological and Biomedical Laboratories*, 5th edn. U.S. Department of Health and Human Services, CDC/NIH, U.S. Government Printing Office, Washington, DC.

HHS (U.S. Department of Health and Human Services). 2013. Public health service grant application PHS 398. Office of Laboratory Animal Welfare, NIH, Bethesda, MD. http://www.grants.nih.gov/grants/funding/phs398/phs398.pdf.

NIH (National Institutes of Health). 1985. U.S. government principles for the utilization and care of vertebrate animals used in testing, research, and training. http://www.grants.nih.gov/grants/olaw/references/phspol.htm#USGovPrinciples.

NIH (National Institutes of Health). 2002. Public Health Service policy on humane care and use of laboratory animals. Office for Protection from Research Risks, NIH, Bethesda, MD.

NIH (National Institutes of Health). 2009. NIH guidelines for research involving recombinant DNA molecules. *Federal Register* 74 FR 48275. Office of Laboratory Animal Welfare, NIH, Bethesda, MD.

NIH (National Institutes of Health). 2010. NOT-OD-10-027: Instructions for completion and peer review of the vertebrate animal section (VAS) in NIH grant applications and cooperative agreements. Office of Laboratory Animal Welfare, NIH, Bethesda, MD. http://grants.nih.gov/grants/guide/notice-files/NOT-OD-10-027.html.

NIH (National Institutes of Health). 2011. Animal study proposal. Office of Laboratory Animal Welfare, NIH, Bethesda, MD. http://grants.nih.gov/grants/olaw/sampledoc/animal_study_prop.htm.

NIH (National Institutes of Health). 2012a. NIH Grants Policy Statement Part II. NIH, Bethesda, MD. http://grants.nih.gov/grants/policy/nihgps_2012/nihgps_ch15.htm#_Toc271265264.

NIH (National Institutes of Health). 2012b. Worksheet for review of the vertebrate animal section (VAS). Office of Laboratory Animal Welfare, NIH, Bethesda, MD, January 18. http://grants.nih.gov/grants/olaw/vaschecklist.pdf.

NIH (National Institutes of Health). 2014a. Frequently asked questions: PHS policy on humane care and use of laboratory animals. Office of Laboratory Animal Welfare, NIH, Bethesda, MD. http://www.grants.nih.gov/grants/olaw/faqs.htm.

NIH (National Institutes of Health). 2014b. Frequently asked questions: PHS policy on humane care and use of laboratory animals: Does the PHS policy apply to the production of custom antibodies or to the purchase of surgically modified animals? Office of Laboratory Animal Welfare, NIH, Bethesda, MD. http://grants.nih.gov/grants/olaw/faqs.htm#App_2.

NIH (National Institutes of Health). 2014c. Frequently asked questions: PHS policy on humane care and use of laboratory animals: Is the IACUC required to review the grant application? Office of Laboratory Animal Welfare, NIH, Bethesda, MD. http://grants.nih.gov/grants/olaw/faqs.htm#proto_10.

NIH (National Institutes of Health). 2014d. Frequently asked questions: PHS policy on humane care and use of laboratory animals: Is the IACUC responsible for judging the scientific merit of proposals? Office of Laboratory Animal Welfare, NIH, Bethesda, MD. http://grants.nih.gov/grants/olaw/faqs.htm#proto_12http://www.ncbi.nlm.nih.gov/pubmed/.

NIH (National Institutes of Health). 2014e. Frequently asked questions: PHS policy on humane care and use of laboratory animals: What is considered a significant change to a project that would require IACUC review? Office of Laboratory Animal Welfare, NIH, Bethesda, MD. http://grants.nih.gov/grants/olaw/faqs.htm#proto_9.

NIH (National Institutes of Health). 2014f. Frequently asked questions: PHS policy on humane care and use of laboratory animals: When institutions collaborate, or when the performance site is not the awardee institution, which IACUC is responsible for review of the research activity? Office of Laboratory Animal Welfare, NIH, Bethesda, MD. http://grants.nih.gov/grants/olaw/faqs.htm#proto_8.

NIH (National Institutes of Health). 2014g. How to write an application involving research animals: NIAID research funding. Office of Laboratory Animal Welfare, NIH, Bethesda, MD. http://www.niaid.nih.gov/researchfunding/sci/animal/pages/anitutorial.aspx.

NIH (National Institutes of Health). 2014h. NIH grants policy statement (2013) Part I. Office of Laboratory Animal Welfare, NIH, Bethesda, MD. http://grants.nih.gov/grants/policy/nihgps_2013/nihgps_ch1.htm.

NRC (National Research Council). 2011. *Guide for the Care and Use of Laboratory Animals*, 8th edn. Washington, DC: National Academies Press.

USDA (U.S. Department of Agriculture). 2014. USDA-APHIS-animal care policy manual. USDA, Washington, DC. http://www.aphis.usda.gov/animal_welfare/policy.php.

USDA (U.S. Department of Agriculture). 2013. *Animal Welfare Act and Animal Welfare Regulations* (Animal Care Blue Book). Code of Federal Regulations (CFR), Title 9, Chapter 1, Subchapter A, Parts 1–4.

U.S. DHHS (U.S. Department of Health and Human Services). 2013. Public health service grant application PHS 398. Office of Laboratory Animal Welfare, NIH, Bethesda, MD. http://www.grants/funding/phs398/phs398.pdf

Semiannual Program Evaluation, Facility Inspections, and Postapproval Monitoring
All Part of the Same Thing

Deborah A. Frolicher

CONTENTS

Oversight, accuracy, and efficiency are integral to the scientific process, and this is also true for the Institutional Animal Care and Use Committee (IACUC) regulatory component of the scientific process. As the complexity of scientific research has increased over the last several decades, many in biomedical research believe there has been a concomitant increase in the regulations, policies, and standards governing the use of animals in research. It is vital that institutions meet minimum requirements, but it is by strengthening existing standards and enhancing oversight that institutions can ensure that the required components of their animal care programs effectively and efficiently balance humane care and use of animals with the scientific method. Institutional officials (IOs) and IACUCs are charged with providing the necessary program oversights.

Semiannual program evaluations, facility inspections, and postapproval monitoring (PAM) provide an institution the opportunity to assess the effectiveness of its animal care program and its compliance with the program and to recommend enhancements to the program. The conduct of evaluations, inspections, and monitoring should compare an institution's program against veterinary, management, and oversight best practices. Taken together, semiannual program evaluations, facility inspections, and PAM can provide the qualitative and quantitative evidence essential to confirm that the care and use of animals are happening as they should. The formulation of policies and procedures for conducting evaluations and inspections will increase the IACUC's long-term efficiency by reducing the need to discuss issues every time they arise and will contribute to the consistency of committee decisions, enhancing fair treatment for all investigators.

6.1 EVALUATIONS, INSPECTIONS, AND POSTAPPROVAL MONITORING

The first step in this process is to clearly communicate requirements and expectations so that the complexities of an institution's Animal Care and Use Program (ACUP) are apparent to interested parties, such as investigative staff, regulatory oversight bodies and the public sector. One component of clear communication is word choice, and the place to start a discussion on semiannual program evaluations, facility inspections, and PAM is with clear definitions of terms. For instance, is there a difference between the terms *evaluation* and *inspection*? Although there are differences in the definitions of these two terms, those most applicable to this topic may be that an *evaluation* is a process used to examine a system or system component to determine the extent to which specified properties are present; and an *inspection* is an official examination or careful scrutiny of an act or process. So although these terms may be used interchangeably, consistent terminology and precise descriptions reduce misconceptions and ensure that those individuals or entities with a stake in the success of your institution's ACUP are on the same page. For example, facility inspection and PAM may imply policing and enforcement actions; but these terms, if well defined and coupled with processes that are well conducted, will act in conjunction with semiannual program evaluations to assist an institution with ensuring that the program and facilities adequately support the research, testing, and teaching objectives of the institution. For the purposes of this review, the following terms are defined:

- Semiannual program evaluation: A review of all components of the entire ACUP that occurs every six months or twice a year at six-month intervals
- Facility inspection: Visual examination of an institution's animal housing and support areas

- PAM: Mechanisms, either formal or informal, by which animal research activities are assessed for compliance against approved protocols and regulatory requirements (Note: As indicated in Table 6.1, the term *postapproval monitoring* is not to be interpreted as the regulatory requirement for "continuing IACUC oversight" (NIH 2006) or "continuing reviews" (9 CFR 2.31 (d)(5); USDA 2013).)

Other terms that may be used include semiannual program review, semiannual inspections, semiannual assessment, facility evaluation, readiness rounds, protocol facilitation, protocol compliance, protocol assessment, and protocol reviews, to name only a few. No matter the terminology used, the important idea is to ensure that all interested parties understand which terms are used at their institution and that they know the function and intent of these processes at their institutions. Training and dissemination of information by the IACUC, veterinarians, facility supervisors, and other key individuals will help ensure that all involved know what is expected.

6.2 REGULATORY REQUIREMENTS

Table 6.1 provides the regulatory citations for the components of oversight. The Animal Welfare Act Regulations (AWRs) require that reviews be conducted using the Animal Welfare Regulations Title 9, Chapter I, subchapter A: Animal Welfare as a basis for these evaluations (USDA 2013). The Public Health Service (PHS) Policy on Humane Care and Use of Laboratory Animals (the PHS Policy) (NIH 2002) requires that institutions base their program of animal care and use on the Guide for the Care and Use of Laboratory Animals (the Guide) (NRC 2011) and that they comply with applicable U.S. Department of Agriculture (USDA) regulations. It notes that when the Guide and USDA differ, the requirement for compliance with the USDA regulations is absolute. The Department of Defense (DOD) (DOD 2005, 2010) and the Department of Veterans Affairs (VA) (VA 2011) have similar requirements and list the Guide (NRC 2011) as well as the AWRs as a basis for evaluation. For those institutions conducting biomedical research with agricultural animals, it is expected that the Federation of Animal Science Societies Guide to the Care and Use of Agricultural Animals in Research and Teaching (the Ag Guide) (FASS 2010) be used to determine oversight expectations.

6.3 PROGRAM COMPONENTS

The next step after determining what oversight requirements are applicable at your institution is to define your ACUP and its components. Several documents can assist with this task. Required program components include an IO, who shows support for the program and the IACUC; an IACUC, with a willingness to serve and take its responsibility seriously; training programs; and IACUC policies and procedures. As defined in the Guide, the ACUP is the segment of an institution's overall organization comprised of "the policies, procedures, standards, organizational structure, staffing, facilities, and practices put into place by an institution to achieve the humane care and

Table 6.1 Regulatory Requirements for Oversight

	USDA/AWA/AWRs	PHS	DOD	VA
Semiannual program evaluation	2.31(c)(1) "review, at least once every six months, the research facility's program for humane care and use of animals"[a]	IV.B.1 "review at least once every six months the institution's program for human care and use of animals"[b]	AR 40-33 "perform semiannual reviews of animal care and use programs and facilities"[c]	1200.07(8.f.1) "the designated VA IACUC must perform a self-assessment review of the program of animal care and use, and an inspection of the animal facilities and husbandry practices at least every 6 months"[d]
Facility inspection	2.31(c)(2) "inspect, at least once every six months, all of the research facility's animal facilities, including animal study areas"[a]	IV.B.2 "inspect at least once every six months all of the institution's animal facilities (including satellite facilities)"[b]	DOD 3216.01 "all DOD institutions using or housing animals for RDT&E or training for more than 12 hours shall conduct a program review, including a facility inspection, at least semiannually using DOD Form 2856"[c]	1200.07(8.f.1.a) "review must include all facilities and investigator areas where laboratory animals purchased with local VA funds are used in procedures, or housed longer than 12 hours."[d]
Postapproval monitoring	No specific citation however 2.31 (d)(5) infers continued review "the IACUC shall conduct continuing reviews of activities covered by this subchapter at appropriate intervals as determined by the IACUC, but not less than annually"[a]	No specific citation however IV.C.5 infers continued review "the IACUC shall conduct continuing review of each previously approved, ongoing activity covered by this Policy at appropriate intervals as determined by the IACUC, including a complete review at least once every three years"[b]	No specific citation however AR 40-33 states "Perform other duties as listed in Title 9, Code of Federal Regulations" (see USDA requirement)[c]	No specific citation however 1200.07(8.f.1.b) states "as part of the Program review, the IACUC must randomly review IACUC records representing at least 5 percent of the total active projects"[d]

Source: [a]USDA (U.S. Department of Agriculture). 2013. Animal Welfare Act and Animal Welfare Regulations: Animal Care Blue Book. Code of Federal Regulations (CFR), Title 9, Chapter 1, Subchapter A, Parts 1–4; [b]NIH (National Institutes of Health). 2002. Public Health Service Policy on Humane Care and Use of Laboratory Animals. NIH, Bethesda, MD: Office of Laboratory Animal Welfare; [c]DOD (Department of Defense). 2010. DOD Instruction 3216.01. Use of animals in DOD programs. Washington, DC: DOD; [d]VA, VHA (Department of Veterans Affairs, Veterans Health Administration). 2011. *VHA Handbook 1200.07*, Use of Animals in Research. Washington, DC: Department of Veterans Affairs.

use of animals in the laboratory and throughout the institution" (NRC 2011). Basically, it is the institution's responsibility to establish and maintain a program that meets all the physical, procedural, medical, and human resources standards required to ensure that animals are cared for and used in ways judged to be scientifically, technically, and humanely appropriate. A well-defined, well-described program formalizes the best practices at your institution and provides an education and evaluation tool.

As a starting point, chapter headings and subheadings within the Guide and the Ag Guide, as well as the AWRs, can be used to outline the components of your ACUP. For example, the chapter headings within the Guide can be used to define four key components of a program; namely, (1) ACUP, (2) environment, housing, and management, (3) veterinary care, and (4) physical plant. Similar components can also be found in the AWRs, including (1) IACUC, (2) attending veterinarian, and (3) species-specific standards in regard to housing, husbandry, feeding, watering, and transportation. For those facilities receiving PHS funding, the institution's Assurance document describes the specifics of the ACUP and presents this information in an outline format that can be easily adapted for use in the evaluation of the program. The Office of Laboratory Animal Welfare (OLAW) website also provides several resources that can be used to help describe and define the ACUP. For those institutions working with USDA-covered species, but not funded by PHS or accredited by the Association for Assessment and Accreditation of Laboratory Animal Care (AAALAC) International, the AWRs can be used to outline the standards for each species maintained in regard to housing, husbandry, feeding/watering, and transportation. Finally, for institutions accredited by AAALAC International, the program description serves as a complete description of the ACUP.

Once the major components of a program have been determined, core requirements within each of those sections should be developed. Input from various participants of the program, such as IACUC members, veterinarians, facility support staff, investigative staff, and administrative staff, is invaluable when defining a program and its components, because it provides a baseline level of knowledge across the many aspects of the ACUP. These core requirements should be specific to the institution and be revised as necessary to address changes within the research program. As an example, within the Guide the chapter on the ACUP is further divided into regulations, policies, and principles; program management; program oversight; and disaster planning and emergency preparedness. McEntee and Sandgren (2007) and Sandgren (2005) provide useful information for defining an ACUP and offer an example of a program review worksheet that can be modified to develop a similar tool at your institution.

6.4 PROGRAM EVALUATION, FACILITY INSPECTION, AND POSTAPPROVAL MONITORING PROCEDURES

6.4.1 Participants Invited/Interviewed

The list of individuals invited to participate in a program evaluation, facility inspection, or PAM process is as varied as the types of institutions that undertake

Table 6.2 Regulatory Requirements for Conducting Program Evaluations and Facility Inspections

Oversight Activity	PHS	USDA	DOD	VA
Semiannual program evaluation	IACUC members or *ad hoc* consultants (IV.B.1)	IACUC subcommittee of at least two committee members (2.31.c.3)	IACUC (40-33; 4.f.3)	At least three IACUC members (including the veterinarian) (1200.07 8.f(1)5
Facility inspection	IACUC members or *ad hoc* consultants (IV.B.2)	IACUC subcommittee of at least two committee members (2.31.c.3)	IACUC (40-33; 4.f.3)	At least three IACUC members (including the veterinarian) (1200.07 8.f(1)5

these procedures. Consideration for the inclusion of individuals from the IACUC, the research staff, the animal care staff, the environmental health and safety program, the occupational medicine provider, the physical plant staff, and the administration staff will aid in ensuring an effective review of an institution's ACUP. Assignments to evaluate the various components of an ACUP can be made based on individual areas of expertise. For example, the occupational medicine provider might not be necessary for a facility inspection, or as part of a PAM process, but his or her input is invaluable when assessing the implementation and management of an institution's occupational health and safety program. Further, the knowledge and expertise of the veterinarian or a well-qualified IACUC administrator can be crucial to assisting the IACUC in formulating defensible conclusions when interpreting the regulations. Provided each individual's role is clearly defined, discussion and review with this large a group can still be effective in determining the health of your ACUP. Be sure to consider possible conflicts of interest when assigning individuals to attend facility inspections or conduct PAM; you must be sure they are not charged with inspecting areas for which they are responsible.

Except for the specific USDA regulation requiring an IACUC subcommittee of at least two members to conduct program evaluations and inspections, regulations and guidance do not state who must conduct evaluations and inspections. However, they do emphasize the responsibility of the IACUC in overseeing and evaluating these activities. Table 6.2 summarizes the federal oversight requirements specific to the conduct of program evaluations and facility inspections.

The following are considerations when assigning individuals to conduct program evaluations, facility inspections, or PAM:

- No individual IACUC member may be prevented from attending a program evaluation review or a facility inspection (9 CFR §2.31 (c)(3), USDA 2013).
- Regardless of the process in place for PAM and continuing review, the IACUC should be informed about the findings of such a review process.

- Husbandry staff are excellent escorts when conducting facility inspections due to their familiarity with the facilities and the work processes involved. Their guidance can make the inspection process more efficient.
- Assigning one or more of the program components to members of the IACUC or the IACUC staff for evaluation and presentation at an IACUC-convened meeting on a periodic basis can provide a snapshot of the program and ease the semiannual evaluation process.

6.4.2 Training

Once individuals have been appointed to evaluation, inspection, or monitoring assignments there are tools that can be provided to assist in training and educating these individuals, specific to their assignment. Facility inspections are physical and visual assessments of the buildings and environment where animals are housed and the equipment used. Since individual IACUC members may not be familiar with the specifics of the housing of each species maintained at an institution, it is recommended that facility inspection teams include animal care staff or veterinarians, or both, with knowledge of the specific species whose housing facilities are being inspected. Wake Forest University Health Services and the U.S. Department of Health and Human Services (DHHS) developed an online IACUC Member's Guide to Animal Facility Inspections available at http://ori.hhs.gov/education/products/IACUC/start.html# (WFSM 2014). This web-based teaching tool is useful not only for the novice but also for veterans of the facility inspection process. The course is broken into three parts: virtual tours, resources, and a quiz. In the virtual tour section, one can select the specific type of area to be inspected using the panoramic image provided. Clicking on numbered boxes provides specific information about the item being viewed. The quiz, if taken online, will indicate when an answer is correct but does not prevent an individual from guessing more than once on the same question. Therefore, if the quiz is to be used by your institution to document training, it is suggested that the quiz be converted into a format that allows only one guess per question. If your institution subscribes to the Collaborative Institutional Training Initiative Program (www.citiprogram.org), the Essentials for IACUC Members course offers modules that cover topics on facility inspections and identifying, documenting, and correcting deficiencies, which may be useful for training purposes. For institutions with zebra fish or other aquatic species, the Institute for Laboratory Animal Research's *ILAR Journal* (Sanders 2012) devoted an entire issue to zebra fish health and husbandry, and the article by Koerber and Kalishman (2009) may be useful when training IACUC members prior to inspection of aquatic facilities.

Training in the conduct of program evaluations and PAM is more institution specific and probably best developed by the institution with guidance available from sources such as OLAW, AAALAC International, USDA, and the Guide. Attendance at national and local meetings sponsored by Public Responsibility in Medicine and Research (PRIM&R), OLAW, and Scientists Center for Animal Welfare, as well as participation in IACUC 101, 201, 301, or Essentials of IACUC Administration classes, are also helpful when developing components of an institutional training program on facility inspections, semiannual program evaluation, and PAM. The best advice to give individuals conducting inspections or evaluations is to ask questions, be nosy: open drawers, open cabinets, open refrigerators. These simple instructions can be most helpful in educating personnel as to their responsibilities and roles in evaluating an institution's ACUP.

6.4.3 Tools to Assist in Evaluations, Inspections, and Reviews

IACUCs use a variety of standards, documents, and guidelines to assist in their evaluation of the ACUP. Many documents maintained as part of routine IACUC record keeping can be useful when conducting semiannual evaluations, facility inspections, or PAM. At the very least, copies of previous inspection/evaluation reports should be provided to ensure that previously recognized deficiencies have been corrected or that a recurrence of a particular deficiency is not indicative of a systemic program shortcoming. Copies of approved protocols should be used when conducting PAM. Use of performance standards can be helpful in establishing specific components of an appropriate ACUP, but care should be taken to ensure that the flexibility inherent in performance standards do not allow for a divergence in opinion as to what is considered appropriate. Copies of institutional policies, guidelines, standard operating practices, and preventive maintenance records are useful and can be reviewed during the semiannual program evaluation for accuracy in their descriptions and completion of required maintenance. A review of IACUC minutes may also highlight controversial animal protocols/procedures that may benefit from additional evaluation. The institution's PHS Assurance document and, if applicable, the AAALAC International program description should also be reviewed to ensure that any changes within the program have been properly communicated to the regulatory or accreditation oversight bodies. Institutions may also want to consider referencing the USDA Animal Care Inspection Guide, available for download from the Animal Welfare section of the Animal and Plant Health Inspection Service (APHIS) website, as a tool to facilitate and improve the quality and uniformity of inspections and program evaluations. Not only does this document provide information on inspection procedures, it also provides insight into what is expected with regard to the review of IACUC responsibilities, functions, and activities. The OLAW website provides sample checklists (http://grants. nih.gov/grants/olaw/sampledoc/cheklist.htm) that may be used when evaluating the program and conducting facility inspections. Use of checklists, although easy for quick reporting of problems, can sometimes lead to complacency, and the influence of individual biases, leading to either overreporting or underreporting. For example, some IACUC members may believe that investigator training is all that is necessary for research personnel, where other members may believe training conducted by the veterinary staff is necessary. This may lead to one member indicating that research staff training is acceptable and another indicating a minor deficiency. As stated in Section 6.1, this is just another example illustrating the need for clear communication of terminology and education to ensure that all involved in these processes know what is expected. Finally, other records that may be assessed during facility inspections or during PAM include principal investigator–managed standard operating practices, surgical and postsurgical records, controlled substances logs, Drug Enforcement Administration records, and quality assurance procedures. AAALAC International's *Connection* publication (AAALAC 2005) notes that the best approach to conducting effective evaluations may be to use a combination of these tools and vary them each time to avoid complacency, encouraging "fresh, critical thinking that makes sure the right questions get asked—and answered."

6.4.4 Facilities to Be Inspected

The PHS Policy (NIH 2002) states that the IACUC must "inspect at least once every six months all of the institution's animal facilities (including satellite facilities) using the Guide as a basis for evaluation." Section 2143 (b)(3) of the AWA broadens this requirement to indicate "inspect at least semiannually all animal study areas and animal facilities" (USDA 2013). Both of these regulatory documents then provide further definitions for facilities, satellite facilities, and study areas as follows:

- Research facility: According to §2132 (e), "The term 'research facility' means any school (except an elementary or secondary school), institution, organization, or person that uses or intends to use live animals in research, tests, or experiments, and that (1) purchases or transports live animals in commerce, or (2) receives funds under a grant, award, loan, or contract from a department, agency, or instrumentality of the United States for the purpose of carrying out research, tests, or experiments: Provided, that the Secretary may exempt, by regulation, any such school, institution, organization, or person that does not use or intend to use live dogs or cats, except those schools, institutions, organizations, or persons, which use substantial numbers (as determined by the Secretary) of live animals the principal function of which schools, institutions, organizations, or persons, is biomedical research or testing, when in the judgment of the Secretary, any such exemption does not vitiate the purpose of this chapter."
- Federal research facility: Defined in §2132 (o) (USDA 2013) as "each department, agency, or instrumentality of the United States which uses live animals for research or experimentation."
- Satellite facility: Any building, room, area, enclosure, or other containment outside of a core facility or centrally designated or managed area in which animals are housed for more than 24 h (PHS definition).
- Study area: Any building, room, area, enclosure, or other containment outside of a core facility or centrally designated or managed area in which animals are housed for more than 12 h (AWRs definition).

The list of areas requiring inspection is as varied as are institutions. Institutions may find the broad terms defined in this section confusing, depending on the diversity of species being maintained and the types of research conducted. Limiting the use of laboratories and areas outside the centralized animal facilities minimizes the number of inspection sites. Special considerations may be required for institutions with several satellite facilities (sometimes located geographically distant from the main facilities); for institutions with facilities with practical impediments, such as germfree or biohazard containment facilities or facilities for agricultural use; and for institutions involved in field studies.

As mentioned previously, there are many resources that can assist an institution in developing a list of areas and items requiring inspection. The OLAW website provides a broad listing of five physical facility areas that require visual examination. These are terrestrial animal housing and support; aquatic animal housing and support; cage wash facilities; aseptic surgery; and procedure areas, nonsurvival surgeries, laboratories, and rodent surgeries. Within each of these areas, consideration should be given to cleanliness, maintenance, and orderliness. Macroenvironment (defined as facility maintenance; heating, ventilation, and air-conditioning [HVAC]; electrical system; noise/vibration; light; temperature; humidity; and food/bedding storage) as well as microenvironment (identification, primary enclosures, density, biosecurity, and record keeping) need to be evaluated.

Animal rooms, cage wash areas, and procedure rooms should be maintained and evaluated separate from personnel areas, with rooms identified by use and conformance to the standards relative to their use. For example, feed storage areas and feed handling procedures should ensure proper feed rotation and storage procedures to provide palatable, uncontaminated diets that meet each species' specific nutritional requirements. Procedures should be in place to minimize contamination by potential disease vectors (insects and other vermin) and ensure use within the shelf life recommended by the manufacturer. Housekeeping and cleaning supplies should be stored separately from food supplies. Walls, doors, ceilings, and floors should be clean and well maintained, with surfaces constructed of impervious, smooth, sanitizable materials that are also suitable to enable adequate footing for terrestrial animals. HVAC systems and lighting systems should be evaluated for their ability to maintain and control environmental parameters, such as room temperature, humidity, and air exchanges. Although not all members of an inspection team will know the suggested ranges for these parameters, any inspection team member can evaluate the comfort level within animal facilities and request confirmation of acceptability from care staff more familiar with the ranges recommended by the Guide and the AWRs.

Other physical plant areas that require confirmation of adequacy include water quality, vermin control, sentinel programs, availability and use of personnel protective equipment, loading docks, receiving areas, and transportation vehicles. These assessments can be made by requesting documentation from responsible entities. For example, water quality can be assessed by reviewing the local water supplier's quality control documentation. Vermin control can be assessed not only by visually inspecting for signs of vermin infestation but by reviewing or requesting an evaluation of the program from the entity responsible for placement of vermin control devices.

Finally, periodic review of institution policies and procedures will ensure that current practices correlate with written descriptions. It is left to the IACUC to determine which standard operating procedures (SOPs), policies, and procedures are elements of the ACUP and to develop a method of reviewing these as part of the program review. There is no requirement that these be reviewed semiannually; however, it is suggested that the IACUC have an SOP in place for reviewing SOPs, policies, and procedures (NABR 2013). For example, are procedures in place for facility security and access restrictions as well as fire alarm and emergency preparedness? What are the procedures in place for reporting ill/injured/abnormal animals, and are facility and investigative staff familiar with these procedures?

For institutions conducting field studies, semiannual IACUC inspections of the field location are not required by the AWRs as long as the study falls under the AWRs' definition of a *field study*. As defined in 9 CFR 1.1, (USDA 2013) a field study is "any study conducted on free-living wild animals in their natural habitat, which does not involve an invasive procedure, and which does not harm or materially alter the behavior of the animals under study." Research conducted in the field on wildlife that does not fit the AWRs' definition of a field study requires IACUC oversight (USDA 2013). IACUCs should be aware of circumstances under which field studies or field investigations are conducted so that they can consider the risks to personnel and the impact on study subjects. The IACUC review may be accomplished by reviewing written descriptions, photographs, or videos that document specified aspects of the study site. The IACUC should also ensure that appropriate permits are in place by consulting with local, state, and/or federal fish and wildlife offices. In the case of marine mammals, the IACUC should consult with the National Oceanic and Atmospheric Administration and similar local and state-level agencies. If the study will take place outside of the United States, international laws and permit requirements may apply.

Other areas that may require special consideration include containment areas and facilities where agricultural animals are used in research or teaching. For these two specific areas, guidance can be obtained by reviewing the Biosafety in Microbiological and Biomedical Laboratories (BMBL) (HHS 2009) and the Ag Guide (FASS 2010). The BMBL and the Ag Guide provide guidance on practice standards as well as authoritative references on the safe handling and containment of hazardous agents and the use of agricultural animals in biomedical research, respectively.

Regardless of the number and type of facilities inspected at your institution, remember that well-designed, well-constructed, and properly maintained facilities are important elements of a quality research program and ACUP.

6.4.5 Scheduling

As stated in both the PHS Policy and the AWRs, program evaluations and facility inspections must be conducted at least once every six months or semiannually. The most recent edition of the Guide (NRC 2011) suggests these procedures be conducted "at least annually or more often as required (e.g., by the AWA and PHS Policy)." For PHS-assured or USDA-covered institutions that conduct inspections on a monthly rolling basis, it is important to ensure that each facility is checked at least once every six months.

6.4.6 Documentation and Follow-Up

Once evaluations and inspections are concluded, it is necessary to develop reports describing the conduct of these activities and submission requirements associated with their conduct. Table 6.3, taken from the Institutional Animal Care and Use Committee Guidebook (NIH/ARENA 2002), provides an overview of the documentation and submission requirements for semiannual reports, including facility inspections.

Reports should include appropriate detail and be reviewed by the IACUC for accuracy, specificity, and use of an unbiased tone. The report must describe findings and categorize these as either significant or minor. As defined by the PHS Policy, a significant deficiency is one that is or may be a threat to animal health or safety (NIH 2002). The report must also provide a reasonable and specific plan and schedule

Table 6.3   Documentation and Submission Requirements of Semiannual Reports and Facility Inspections

	PHS	USDA
Timetable	Every six months; an AAALAC report may fulfill these requirements	Every six months; an AAALAC report may fulfill these requirements
Submit to	IO	IO
Submitted by	IACUC, as committee action	IACUC, signed by a majority of members
Form used	Not specified (OLAW sample report: http://grants.nih.gov/grants/olaw/sampledoc/ioreport.htm)	Not specified
Contents	Describe adherence to Guide and PHS Policy and departures from Guide and PHS Policy	Describe adherence to AWRs and departures from AWRs
	State reasons for departures; identify significant and minor deficiencies; include plan/schedule to correct deficiencies; include minority views	State reasons for departures; identify significant and minor deficiencies; include plan/schedule to correct deficiencies; include minority views
	Approved by IACUC	Reviewed and signed by majority of IACUC members
	Maintained by institution	Maintained by research facility
	Available to OLAW upon request	Available to APHIS and funding agency upon request
	Other: Identify facilities accredited by AAALAC	Other: Report failure to adhere to plan/schedule through IO to APHIS and funding agency within 15 business days
		9 CFR Part 2, Subpart C 2.31 (c) (3)

Source: PHS Policy IV.B.3, IV.E.1.d & IV.F.4, OER NIH Notice OD-00-007, Release date December 21, 1999

for correcting each noted deficiency. Specific for USDA-covered institutions, it should be noted that failure to adhere to a stated correction schedule for a significant deficiency must be reported within 15 business days to prevent noncompliance. Departures, deviations, and exceptions to stated regulatory requirements must also be described within the semiannual report, in addition to any minority reviews submitted by IACUC members. Consideration should be given to including both recommendations for improvement and praise for positive aspects and improvements to the program. Finalized reports can be used as a tool to track trends and assist in suggestions for improvements to the program.

When documenting evaluation activities, IACUCs should consider coding facilities and their locations, since these documents may be obtained through the Freedom of Information Act process. In addition, the IACUC, in conjunction with institutional administration, should determine the process for precise, candid reporting to both the institution and required outside entities. Semiannual reports require review by the IACUC and—specific for USDA-covered entities—signature by a majority of the IACUC members to indicate that that they were provided the opportunity to review the final document and its findings. Any IACUC member may file a minority view when he or she is not in agreement with the majority of the membership about a specific issue and wants this noted in the IACUC meeting minutes.

Once the report has been approved by the IACUC and submitted and signed by the IO, ascertain that a mechanism is in place for notifying responsible parties, tracking remediation of deficiencies, and promptly reporting any issues of noncompliance. OLAW provides guidance on documenting departures from the Guide (Departures from the Guide: http://grants.nih.gov/grants/olaw/departures.htm) and reporting noncompliance (Reporting Noncompliance: http://grants.nih.gov/grants/olaw/reporting_noncompliance.htm) on its website.

6.4.7 Postapproval Monitoring (PAM)

The utilization of PAM programs by IACUCs to assess the use of live vertebrate animals after approval has received increased attention in the laboratory animal community. As stated previously, there are no specific federally mandated requirements for a PAM program, with the exception of the VA programs where the IACUC must randomly review at least 5% of the total active projects with a minimum of five protocols as part of the semiannual self-assessment review of the ACUP (VA 2011). However, there are many references within regulatory documents for continual monitoring of animal activities. The AWRs require the IACUC to conduct semiannual reviews of animal facilities and animal study areas to ascertain that the control of pain and suffering in experimental animals occurs as described in IACUC-approved protocols, and this can be accomplished by review of the procedure and the condition of experimental animals via a PAM program. The Guide stresses the use of PAM to facilitate ongoing protocol assessment and regulatory compliance (NRC 2011). AAALAC International's program description requests a description of the mechanisms used to review ongoing studies. This lack of regulatory requirement intensifies the need for each institution to develop a specific mechanism by which animal research activities are monitored for compliance with the protocols approved by the IACUC. PAM should not replace federally mandated IACUC responsibilities, but an efficient PAM process can provide significant additional information to strengthen the institution's confidence that its research program is meeting both the letter and the spirit of federal, institutional, and accreditation mandates.

A PAM program may or may not rely directly on the IACUC, but it should be self-auditing, collegial, and nonconfrontational. An ideal program should create a positive and open environment. Processes should be clearly defined, consistent, and applicable to all users. This will ensure operational integrity. Banks and Norton (2008) describe three types of PAM and outline advantages and disadvantages to each model. When performed by attentive and observant individuals, PAM can extend the IACUC's oversight, management, training, and communication resources. PAM programs can also build bridges, encourage partnerships, enhance education, and ensure animal well-being. An effective PAM program involves knowledgeable individuals who can, on behalf of the IACUC, monitor procedures and personnel and provide IACUC-mandated training or retraining of investigative staff. Further, an efficient PAM process can provide significant additional information that enables an institution to be confident that it is meeting both the letter and the spirit of the federal regulations developed to ensure humane animal care.

The PAM program can be used as one mechanism to provide continuing review of animal research activities after IACUC approval to ensure activities are being conducted in accordance and in congruence with approved procedures. PAM typically takes place independently from semiannual inspections, program reviews, and the daily monitoring of animals. PAM personnel should be excellent communicators and be able to maintain a professional demeanor in challenging circumstances. Their knowledge of laboratory animal care, invasive procedures, and regulations enables them to harmonize the pursuit of scientific research with adherence to regulations. An institution's PAM can be supplemented by animal procurement software that prevents the institution from ordering species that are not approved or exceeding the animal numbers specified in the protocol. More and more software tools that can facilitate the collection, management, and tracking of PAM results, as well as semiannual inspection information, are becoming available.

PAM processes can be conducted either formally or informally. Formal processes usually consist of a series of ongoing observations and reviews that provide firsthand observation and monitoring of procedures and personnel. As described by Collins (2008), formal PAM processes generally include reviews of specific documents, such as medical records; pre-, peri-, and postoperative procedure records; on-site interviews with research personnel; and audits of animal activities, such as nonsurgical procedures, noninvasive imaging, and behavior assessments, to name a few. The advantages of this type of process include prompt identification of concerns and efficient resolutions. However, formal programs generally require specific funding and the use of qualified personnel. On the other hand, informal processes are generally conducted in conjunction with semiannual program evaluations, together with required periodic protocol reviews, as part of daily husbandry and veterinary reviews, or at the time of animal welfare concern investigations. These informal processes can be a practical alternative to a formalized program, especially if there is a strong institutional commitment to compliance, and if costs are a concern. Smaller institutions, or those with an actively engaged IACUC, may also make an informal process work. Regardless of the type of process used, the PAM program should facilitate research in accordance with appropriate performance standards in the care and use of laboratory animals that are based on regulations (the AWA, the PHS Policy, and the Guide) and the professional judgment of the IACUC.

Record keeping of PAM processes should identify which protocols, operating practices, or activities were monitored. To further support the efficacy of PAM processes, attempts should also be made to collect evidence of good performance and to issue recognition post audit for items such as attention to detail and professional manner. Findings should be presented to the IACUC for review, with any additional concerns discussed and addressed. As stated by Collins (2008), if an IACUC decides to use PAM to evaluate an institution's programs or facilities, the committee must maintain responsibility for evaluating and disseminating the resulting report. In review, the goal of a PAM program should be to find deficiencies when they are small and easily correctable, thereby averting costly compliance concerns that may result in protocol suspension or closure. A PAM program should not be implemented only as a consequence of a noncompliant event or an accusation. As stated by Plante and James (2008), "implementing a formal PAM process for the sole purpose of identifying protocol deviations—without a subsequent reassessment of the adequacy of the program component(s) that should have prevented noncompliance in the first place—creates just another time-consuming and expensive process that falls short of its full potential and funnels monetary and personnel resources away from other program components that could benefit from them." Further, the Essentials of IACUC Administration class, offered by PRIM&R, recommends that an institution's PAM program be SMART—that is, specific, measurable, attainable, realistic, and timely.

6.5 FINAL THOUGHTS

In closing, it should be understood that any processes used to conduct semiannual program reviews, facility inspections, and PAM serve the IACUC in many ways, including

- Focusing education efforts to address repeat noncompliant findings
- Trending observations for further evaluation
- Expanding the training program to address specific negative trends

Regular inspection and assessment of your institution's ACUP serve to ensure that the program is adhering to the highest standards for humane handling, care, and treatment of research animals. Individuals involved in the oversight of ACUPs should strive to be upbeat and helpful. Employees at all levels must believe that the institution is committed to high standards of care. These attributes, combined with a willingness to lend a hand as a problem solver, will go a long way toward achieving and maintaining a strong, compliant, and effective ACUP. Goal setting after inspections/evaluations should include agreements about the metrics of performance that will be used to measure success and will help everyone understand whether the program is meeting set standards.

In spite of the best efforts of individuals dedicated to the humane care of laboratory animals, human error, equipment malfunctions, and accidents will occur. Ensuring that your IACUC is aware of these incidents will enable an evaluation of whether they are isolated incidents or an indication of a broader problem. An effective program evaluation protects both the individual investigator and the institution while inspiring confidence among the general public that animal research is being performed in an ethical manner. Institutions should be careful to avoid excessive self-imposed regulations and to assure all concerned that evaluation and inspection processes are not intended to slow or impede research but to support and establish a foundation for a strong ACUP. Plante and James (2008) describe the use of program oversight enhancements to coordinate the myriad processes, procedures, and personnel that are integral to a persuasive and sustainable culture of responsibility and dedication to compliance. Semiannual inspections and evaluations, along with other PAM program components, provide the qualitative and quantitative evidence that everything is happening as it should.

REFERENCES

AAALAC International (Association for Assessment and Accreditation of Laboratory Animal Care International). 2005. Preparing for the semiannual review. *Connection*, Fall issue, pp. 1–7. Rockville, MD: AAALAC International. http://www.aaalac.org/publications/newsletter.cfm.

Banks, R. E. and J. N. Norton. 2008. A sample postapproval monitoring program in academia. *ILAR Journal* 49 (4):402–418.

Collins, J. G. 2008. Postapproval monitoring and the institutional animal care and use committee (IACUC). *ILAR Journal* 49 (4):388–392.

DOD (Department of Defense). 2005. The care and use of laboratory animals in DOD programs. Washington, DC: Departments of the Army, Navy, Air Force, Defense Advanced Research Projects Agency, and the Uniformed Services, University of the Health Sciences.

DOD (Department of Defense). 2010. DOD Instruction 3216.01. Use of animals in DOD programs. Washington, DC: Departments of the Army, Navy, Air Force, Defense Advanced Research Projects Agency, and the Uniformed Services, University of the Health Sciences.

FASS (Federation of Animal Science Societies). 2010. Guide for the care and use of agricultural animals in agricultural research and teaching. Champaign, IL: FASS.

HHS (U.S. Department of Health and Human Services). 2009. *Biosafety in Microbiological and Biomedical Laboratories*. 5th edn. Washington, DC: US Government Printing Office.

Koerber, A. S. and J. Kalishman. 2009. Preparing for a semiannual IACUC inspection of a satellite zebrafish (*Danio rerio*) facility. *Journal of the American Association for Laboratory Animal Science* 48 (1):65.

McEntee, H. I. and E. P. Sandgren. 2007. A tool for semiannual review of the institutional animal care and use program. *Lab Animal* 36 (9):36–40.

NABR (National Association for Biomedical Research). 2014. NABR webinars: Q&A with the USDA (July 9, 2013). http://www.nabr.org/Webinars.aspx.

NIH (National Institutes of Health). 2002. Public Health Service policy on humane care and use of laboratory animals. Bethesda, MD: Office of Laboratory Animal Welfare, U.S. Department of Health and Human Services, NIH.

NIH (National Institutes of Health). 2014. Frequently asked questions: PHS policy on humane care and use of laboratory animals: Is post approval monitoring required? NIH, Bethesda, MD: Office of Laboratory Animal Welfare. http://grants.nih.gov/grants/olaw/faqs.htm#instresp_6.

NIH/ARENA (National Institutes of Health/Applied Research Ethics National Association). 2002. *Institutional Animal Care and Use Committee Guidebook*. 2nd edn. Bethesda, MD: Office of Laboratory Animal Welfare.

NRC (National Research Council). 2011. *Guide for the Care and Use of Laboratory Animals*. 8th edn. Washington, DC: National Academies Press.

Plante, A. and M. L. James. 2008. Program oversight enhancements (POE): The big PAM. *ILAR Journal* 49 (4):419–425.

Sanders, G. E. 2012. Zebrafish housing, husbandry, health, and care: IACUC considerations. *ILAR Journal* 53 (2):205–207.

Sandgren, E. P. 2005. Defining the animal care and use program. *Lab Animal* 34:41–4.

USDA (U.S. Department of Agriculture). 2013. *Animal Welfare Act and Animal Welfare Regulations* (Animal Care Blue Book). Code of Federal Regulations (CFR), Title 9, Chapter 1, Subchapter A, Parts 1–4.

VA, VHA (Department of Veterans Affairs, Veterans Health Administration). 2011. Use of animals in research, *VHA Handbook 1200.07*. Washington, DC: Department of Veterans Affairs.

WFSM (Wake Forest School of Medicine). 2014. Laboratory animal training and oversight. Winston-Salem, NC: WFSM. http://ori.hhs.gov/education/products/IACUC/about_afi.html.

CHAPTER 7

IACUC Oversight of Training and Qualification in Animal Care and Use

Nicole Duffee

CONTENTS

7.1 REGULATORY REQUIREMENTS FOR TRAINING AND QUALIFICATION

Two pillars of humane care and use of research animals are the training and qualification of personnel to perform this work. The *Guide for the Care and Use of Laboratory Animals* (the Guide) (NRC 2011) states, "all personnel involved with the care and use of animals must be adequately educated, trained, and/or qualified in basic principles of laboratory animal science to help ensure high-quality science and animal well-being." The Guide stresses that training is for all researchers—that is, principal investigators, study directors, research technicians, postdoctoral fellows, students, and visiting scientists. The Animal Welfare Regulations (AWRs) 9 CFR §2.32 (USDA 2013a) likewise require institutions to ensure all scientists, research technicians, animal technicians, and other personnel involved in animal care, treatment, and use are qualified to perform their duties. The Public Health Service (PHS) Policy on Humane Care and Use of Laboratory Animals (NIH 2002) has similar language and requires a description of the training program in the institution's Animal Welfare Assurance. Other mandates may also be relevant, such as the American Veterinary Medical Association Guidelines for the Euthanasia of Animals, 2013 Edition (AVMA 2013), the Guide for the Care and Use of Agricultural Animals in Research (FASS 2010), Good Laboratory Practice regulations (FDA 1997), the Department of Defense (DOD 2010), and Biosafety in Microbiological and Biomedical Laboratories (HHS 2009). If the regulatory mandates of other countries are applicable, additional resources should be sought on national requirements for training, as described by van Zutphen (2007), Bayne et al. (2011), and Guillen (2012). Per all mandates, the institution has the overarching responsibility for ensuring personnel training and qualification via a training program. The Institutional Animal Care and Use Committee (IACUC) assumes this responsibility on behalf of the institution and thereby has the function of overseeing the training program.

The training program must focus on humane methods of animal maintenance and experimentation (see 9 CFR §2.32 for guidance on these methods). Furthermore, personnel qualifications to perform the work on animals must be reviewed with sufficient frequency. The AWRs specify minimum requirements for training in animal husbandry, animal handling and care, periprocedural care, aseptic technique in surgery and other procedures, alternatives to limit the use of animals or minimize their distress, medications to prevent or alleviate pain and distress, and reporting methods for deficiencies in animal care and treatment, as well as for services available to provide information on biomethodologies, animal alternatives, avoidance of unnecessary duplication of animal use in research, and the intent and requirements of the Animal Welfare Act (AWA). Of these listed, the greatest challenge is teaching the fundamentals of aseptic surgery due to the procedural complexities and the rigors of maintaining asepsis. Hèon et al. (2006) described a model for developing a comprehensive training program for both rodent and large animal surgery. Training on species-specific biomethodologies typically includes ethics of animal care and use, humane methods of euthanasia, occupational health and safety considerations, and biosafety practices and equipment (Pritt and Duffee 2007), according to the nature of the research program. Personnel should be trained on guidelines and standard operating procedures relevant to their work. Moreover, scientists should be trained on the preparation of animal protocols, how important issues in animal care and use are to be addressed, and how to interact effectively with the IACUC.

The development of an institution's training curriculum can be aided by the example outlines and content recommendations documented by the National Research Council (NRC 1991), Anderson (2007), and Medina et al. (2007). Sample training program descriptions and training content on institutional websites may be browsed from links on the IACUC home page IACUC Central, formerly IACUC.org (AALAS 2014b).

Many institutions require repeat training (retraining, as distinguished from continuing education) for core content, such as regulatory mandates or safety topics. Many institutions require personnel to periodically repeat a course or sometimes a shortened version in a planned activity scheduled annually or when a protocol is renewed. Besides aiming to refresh knowledge, retraining is an opportunity to convey updated information on mandates, policies, and practices. Retraining may also be needed when compliance issues are identified, such as during postapproval monitoring visits or other inspections, or when animal care staff observe a problem in the animals. In these circumstances, communication among all individuals involved is important in order to customize the retraining with a precise determination of the content to be delivered.

7.2 VALUE IN TRAINING

Training provides valuable support to a research program, though the return on investment is not easy to measure. Mountains of evidence have shown that pain, stress, and distress in animals alter the physiological state of many body systems, which affect the quality of the animals as research subjects, thus undermining the integrity of data collected in research studies (Whiting 2011). For example, poor tissue handling in surgery can exacerbate the pain and discomfort associated with wound healing during postoperative recovery. Animals that are stressed or in pain have increases in blood levels of stress hormones. They are metabolically compromised and make substandard research models.

When poor practices are frequent, the institution faces liabilities of regulatory citations and financial penalties through discoveries made during regulatory inspections. Its public reputation can be damaged if onlookers broadcast embarrassing reports and video footage to the news media. Furthermore, inadequate training may increase the risk of injuries or exposures to infectious agents in personnel. The training program counters these liabilities with the goals of advancing a culture of animal welfare and developing competence in all personnel working with animals, so that the animals are handled humanely, pain and discomfort are minimized, and the animals' physiological state is sound for research. This can be aptly summarized: Good animal care is good science (Bennett 1994).

An institutional training program that effectively prepares personnel to work appropriately and humanely with animals is an important component of the good animal care supporting the research mission of the institution. Training, inclusive of continuing education, is also the cornerstone of an efficient and productive workforce in the animal facility. Training facilitates professionalism among the staff and promotes high-quality husbandry practices. Training improves morale, and higher job satisfaction in animal technicians translates to better employee retention and customer service (Huerkamp 2006). Lockworth et al. (2011) described a reorganization of staff that was grounded on a new training program aimed at empowering animal technicians to aid in veterinary case management. The outcomes were a more efficient use of staff resources, more consistent animal care, and improved animal health. Overall, resources invested in an effective training program yield humane and responsible care of laboratory animals, which are vital to biomedical research.

7.3 PERSONNEL TRAINING AND QUALIFICATION

7.3.1 Training for the Institutional Official

The chief institutional official (CIO or IO) has duties to appoint the IACUC and act upon the committee's recommendations on the program and facility. Therefore, training the IO on these responsibilities is helpful, although it is not specified in the regulatory mandates. In the limited time an IO may have available for such training, orientation to the animal research issues can begin with the U.S. Government Principles for the Utilization and Care of Vertebrate Animals Used in Testing, Research, and Training (NIH 1985). The IO needs a brief overview of the regulatory mandates and agencies; the roles of the IO and the IACUC; the requirements for the IACUC, attending veterinarian (AV), and scientists; the requirements for inspections, filings, and assurances; the value of facility accreditation and staff certifications; and the potential consequences of deficiencies and citations. Greene et al. (2007) offered recommendations on training and continuing education for the IO and the IACUC.

7.3.2 Training for IACUC Members

The AWA (USDA 2013b) and the PHS Policy (NIH 2002) require the IACUC to be qualified through the experience and expertise of its members to oversee/assess the institution's Animal Care and Use Program (ACUP), facilities, and procedures. This includes, at a minimum, an understanding of the applicable mandates, protocol review, and facility inspections. Ideally, IACUC members and administrative staff should be trained on the responsibilities and functions related to oversight of the ACUP. Skills in the IACUC process may be developed through participation in related online courses, webinars, workshops, and conferences. An abundance of IACUC training opportunities is available from the National Institutes of Health (NIH) Office of Laboratory Animal Welfare, Public Responsibility in Medicine and Research (PRIM&R), the Scientists Center for Animal Welfare (SCAW), the National Association for Biomedical Research, and the American Association for Laboratory Animal Science (AALAS). IACUCs often devote a portion of a meeting to training, which should be documented as such in the minutes. Nonscientist and nonaffiliated IACUC members benefit from additional training to orient them to the field of animal research (Mondschein 2007).

7.3.3 Training for Veterinarians and Animal Care Staff

All individuals whose duties affect the health or well-being of the animals must be qualified to work humanely with each species. Although personnel are generally neither hired nor supervised by the IACUC, the IACUC must ensure that the animal research program is run by qualified and competent staff. According to the Guide, the AV who oversees the veterinary care program "is certified or has training or experience in laboratory animal science and medicine or is otherwise qualified in the care of the species being used." The AWRs further define the AV as

> a person who has graduated from a veterinary school accredited by the American Veterinary Medical Association's Council on Education, or has a certificate issued by the American Veterinary Medical Association's Education Commission for Foreign Veterinary Graduates, or has received equivalent formal education as determined by the Administrator; has received training and/or experience in the care and management of the species being attended; and who has direct or delegated authority for activities involving animals at a facility subject to the jurisdiction of the Secretary. (USDA 2013a)

Likewise, the clinical veterinarians must be trained and experienced in laboratory animal medicine and science. Veterinarians may be qualified as diplomats of a college of laboratory animal medicine (United States or other nation), or they may acquire the necessary training in nondiplomat specialization programs or through mentoring on the job.

Animal care personnel must also be appropriately qualified according to their job functions. Although their duties are typically learned on the job by following a mentor, they need training services, which, at a minimum, should educate them on institutional policies, occupational health and safety, facility operations, and animal care standards. Foshay and Tinkey (2007) discussed testing strategies for evaluation of training effectiveness for animal technicians. Administrative support personnel need training to carry out duties related to their role in the animal research program, such as animal procurement and record keeping.

All personnel involved in the oversight or operation of the animal research program should be engaged in and encouraged to obtain professional certifications relevant to their roles and duties. For the professional development of technical and managerial staff, most institutions provide some training support in certification programs from AALAS. This may entail providing classes and instructional materials. AALAS offers three levels of certification for technicians—assistant laboratory animal technician, laboratory animal technician, and laboratory animal technologist—and one for supervisors and managers (certified manager of animal resources). Surgical technicians should aim for professional recognition as a surgical research anesthetist and either surgical research technician or surgical research specialist, conferred by the Academy of Surgical Research. For IACUC staff, PRIM&R offers the credential of certified professional IACUC administrator. Veterinarians and veterinary technicians typically have state professional licensing that is maintained with continuing education credits. Opportunities and support for meeting the certification and licensure requirements for continuing education are important for maintaining professional stature, which enhances the institution's record of staff qualifications. This may involve participating in membership organizations, workshops, or conferences. Doing so expands knowledge of the field and promotes career development as laboratory animal professionals. As the laboratory animal field evolves, new certifications may emerge in the future and should be embraced for elevating the professional status of staff.

7.3.4 Training for Research Staff

The responsibility for the oversight of qualifications and training in animal care and use extends to researchers and educators through an institutional training program (Conarello and Shepherd 2007). The researcher training program aims to instill compliance with animal welfare mandates, develop technical skills, and promote a culture of adherence to animal welfare standards. Two training goals dominate: regulatory standards and humane procedures. Communicating about the animal research mandates leads to an understanding of the institution's policies and guidelines, which emanate from these mandates. A best practice in developing a training program is to take input from scientific staff, perhaps with the involvement of a focus group. The IACUC is responsible for evaluating the effectiveness of the training program for animal users. A framework for assessing proficiency and competency in animal procedures, described by Clifford et al. (2013), may be helpful for this purpose. The postapproval monitoring program, too, can be a source of information to help assess training effectiveness when retraining needs are identified. A high frequency of these occurrences can reveal strategic weaknesses in the training program that may be addressed by changes in training methods or through other forms of communication.

7.4 STAFFING A TRAINING PROGRAM

The emphasis of regulatory and accrediting authorities on personnel competence in animal care and use procedures necessitates that a training program be properly organized and staffed. Training personnel are often recruited from the program's veterinary or husbandry staff, but other individuals, such as laboratory managers, may become trainers as well. Depending on the size and complexity of the program, it may be run by a coordinator, manager, or director (Kennedy 2002, Conarello and Shepherd 2007, Pritt and Duffee 2007). The training program staff may report to the animal facility management, a compliance office, or the IACUC administration. Trainers may be dedicated to wholly supporting the program or may balance training with other duties. Research staff may be identified as auxiliary trainers for specific techniques. Some programs are outsourced to an external organization. A common example is when the husbandry staff are employed by a contract service organization that also provides the training services for all personnel. Contract workers or companies may be hired to provide training in such areas as surgical skills or AALAS certification preparation, or to produce online courses built to the specifications of the institution.

The training program should have a process to qualify trainers, expand their skills, and verify training proficiency. Verification of trainer proficiency may involve observing training sessions and providing constructive feedback on teaching methods. Ideally, trainees should have the opportunity to give their feedback on the session, such as through a satisfaction survey. Continuing education and communication among the training staff help ensure they maintain technical and training standards in line with institutional policies. Effective training requires knowledge and skills in adult education, which are not typically acquired on the job as individuals ascend the career ladder from technician to trainer (Dobrovolny et al. 2007). Train-the-trainer workshops help individuals learn how to teach specific techniques and may impart general teaching skills. To support this career step, some trainers may take general education courses and even earn a degree in that field. Trainers should participate in professional associations, such as AALAS and the Laboratory Animal Welfare Training Exchange. Networking with other trainers can benefit the institution through exposure to new resources and approaches on training.

7.5 TYPE OF TRAINING METHODS

The type of training methods used depends on the nature of the audience, the geographic relationship among facility sites, available technologies, and the expertise of trainers.

Face-to-face training is effective for building a relationship between a new hire and senior staff. Face-to-face training introduces researchers to animal facility personnel and identifies who they can turn to for future assistance or additional training. Orientation sessions convey the requirements for using the animal facility and induct the recipient into a culture of animal welfare and compliance. When training takes place through conversation among few individuals, the trainer may verify lesson comprehension through discussion. In larger groups, as is often the case for researchers, face-to-face training takes the form of a lecture, in which policies and standards can be effectively communicated; verifying lesson comprehension is best accomplished by incorporating a quiz.

More and more, topics on regulatory and policy matters are presented in virtual learning modules (see Section 7.9) instead of face-to-face. This allows trainer sessions to focus on personal interactions for facility orientation, procedure demonstrations, and relationship building between researchers and animal facility personnel. Hands-on training is best for teaching correct and humane methods of animal procedures and for helping the recipient develop skills and acquire confidence. Formal on-site workshops may be arranged to teach a group. Media resources (see Section 7.9)

can be a valuable adjunct to hands-on training by preparing the recipient with preliminary information, reinforcing technical steps during a presentation, and reviewing critical points afterwards.

7.6 TRAINING PROTOCOL

The use of animals for training falls under the scope of research training/
teaching covered in the AWA, the PHS Policy, and the Guide. All animals covered
under regulatory mandates must be assigned to an animal protocol that is reviewed
and approved by the IACUC. A training protocol is most practical when it is struc-
tured to cover procedures commonly taught, possible animal species used, and
likely individuals teaching hands-on techniques (Conarello and Shepherd 2007).
In this way, hands-on training involving animals will be automatically covered
by one protocol. Before training on a new procedure, trainers should consult the
training protocol to verify that the proposed animal use is included. Additional
training procedures should be reviewed and approved beforehand as a protocol
amendment.

7.7 DOCUMENTATION OF TRAINING

Training and qualifications applicable to the animal research program must be
documented per the Guide. There are no requirements for type of data or record
format, but it is generally expected that records of training activities and individuals' training histories be maintained and be reasonably accessible (Pritt et al. 2004).
Although the AWRs do not specifically require documentation of training, records
are valuable for proving that training took place on specific procedures when ques-
tioned by an inspector or site visitor (Slauter 1999). If applicable to the research
program, Good Laboratory Practice regulations make specific requirements on documentation integrity, archiving, storage, security, and retention (FDA 1997).

Training documentation systems may be paper files, computerized databases, or
a hybrid of technologies. Ideally, the training documentation system can yield tabu-
lated information to aid preparation of reports on the training program, such as for
semiannual reports and Association for Assessment and Accreditation of Laboratory
Animal Care International program descriptions. Simple check-off lists and paper
records of attendance may be sufficient for some institutions. For others, computerized systems are needed to manage the training program data. Learning management
systems (LMSs) have been developed that automatically document the completion
of online courses and exams. This training documentation can be combined from
multiple sources (course delivery systems) into one database so administrative personnel can see all records in one place. For example, transcript data from animal
welfare compliance courses may be downloaded from one system and merged with
data on human resource courses from a second system. Some LMSs also allow the
manual input of data from nonvirtual training events, such as face-to-face sessions,

so that documentation of multiple types of training can be maintained together in one location. Integrating training data on an LMS typically involves a high degree of customization. Although complex and costly to develop and maintain, a good LMS makes it easy to access training records on demand.

The data to be included in training documentation should address the questions of when, what, how, and who. Records should specify the date when training occurred, what the training topic was (at the minimum, a title), how the training was delivered (type of training), who the trainer was, and who received the training. Exam scores may be included. For animal procedure training, the degree of detail documented for the topic should match how the training need is specified. For instance, if an individual is to receive training on tail vein injection in the rat, the session's learning objectives should include that procedure. A training documentation system may link session titles with lists of procedures taught, like lesson objectives. This allows a session title in an individual's record to be related to qualifications for particular procedures. To go on with this example, if a session entitled "rat handling and blood collection techniques" is documented to include tail vein injection, then the individual who completes this training can be recognized for learning this procedure and meeting the training requirement. The number and species of animals used in training are not necessary for documentation but, if tracked, may be useful as another metric of the training program. The period of time for maintaining training records will depend on institutional policies and applicable regulatory mandates, for example, Good Laboratory Practice regulations.

7.8 DISSEMINATING INFORMATION ABOUT THE TRAINING PROGRAM

Information on the training program should be disseminated throughout the institution, so anyone can learn about the training requirements, services, and resources. An intranet website is the first place where people commonly seek out this information. A website alone is insufficient, however, to adequately inform the community about the program, because visiting the site takes initiative. Communication is more effective when people are contacted, and various media can be helpful to this end. Newsletters (print or electronic) can announce training events, highlight current issues, give updates on animal care and use, and disseminate news about the animal facility. A LISTSERV can be used for specific interest groups, such as a department or facility users.

7.9 EXTERNAL RESOURCES FOR RESEARCHER TRAINING

Abundant media resources, available free or commercially, are valuable to enhance training programs. Some items are best used as adjuncts—for example, to accompany a procedure demonstration. Others may be used entirely on their own to replace a face-to-face session with virtual training, as in introducing animal welfare concepts or regulatory requirements of animal research. A sampling of resources is presented below, and individuals operating a training program may consider how best to use them and for which audiences. Readers are reminded that a list of this kind is out of date once published. Hence, the resources in this section should be seen as a starting point for exploring current resources beyond those listed here.

7.9.1 Regulatory Mandates and Bioethics

Online learning is frequently used to orient researchers to regulatory requirements and bioethics. The AALAS Learning Library (AALAS 2014a) and the Collaborative Institutional Training Initiative Program (CITI 2014) summarize these requirements in similar courses: "Working with the IACUC" and other introductory courses relating regulatory issues to specific species (amphibian, cat, dog, ferret, gerbil, goat, guinea pig, hamster, mouse, nonhuman primate, rabbit, rat, sheep, and swine). The AALAS Learning Library also has in-depth courses on key mandates for animal research.

7.9.2 Common Animal Procedures

Books and digital media provide step-by-step demonstrations of common procedures, such as physical restraint, blood sampling, and compound administration. A select listing of these resources is as follows: A select listing of these resources is as follows: mouse, rat, rabbit, minipig (AALAS 2012–2014), mouse and rat with video clips on DVD (Bogdanske et al. 2014), and mouse and rat vascular catheterization (Liu and Heiser 2007).

The University of Newcastle offers a collection of tutorials on a website called Assessing the Health and Welfare of Laboratory Animals (AHWLA 2014). One tutorial teaches basic animal handling and procedures for gerbil, hamster, mouse, rat, guinea pig, rabbit, and ferret.

A video article presenting a tutorial on restraint and compound administration in mice and rats (Machholz et al. 2012) can be found in the *Journal of Visualized Experiments* (JoVE.com), a scientific video journal.

Online courses in biomethodologies are available on the AALAS Learning Library for dog, ferret, mouse, poultry, rat, *Xenopus*, and zebrafish.

7.9.3 Recognition of Animal Pain and Distress

Pritchett-Corning (2011) produced a handbook that portrays clinical signs of illness in rodents and rabbits.

The University of Newcastle (AHWLA 2014) offers two tutorials: Basic Assessment of Laboratory Animal Health and Welfare, and Recognizing Post-Operative Pain in Animals.

The AALAS Learning Library has two courses on pain alleviation: Pain Management in Laboratory Animals, and Post-Procedure Care of Mice and Rats in Research. Additionally, signs of pain and distress are incorporated in its species-specific courses.

7.9.4 Anesthesia and Surgical Technique

The NIH has three online video tutorials originally published as a CD: General Training in Survival Rodent Surgery, Simple Suture Patterns for Rodent Surgery, and Special Considerations for Aseptic Surgery in a Transgenic Mouse Facility. Baran et al. (2009, 2010) described the application of electronic learning and multimedia to surgical training.

JoVE.com offers how-to information on many surgical techniques. Its veterinary advisory board reviews JoVE articles that involve live animal work to ensure that proper welfare and sterility standards are observed. Principles of Rodent Surgery for the New Surgeon is a video article presented by Pritchett-Corning et al. (2011).

7.9.5 Occupational Health and Safety and Biosafety

The AALAS Learning Library offers courses on occupational health and safety in animal research, laboratory animal allergy, ergonomics for animal technicians, and animal biosafety. Information on zoonoses is included in all species-specific courses.

7.10 CONCLUSION

By shaping attitudes and behaviors about animal care and use in research, a training program enhances compliance with regulatory mandates and supports the institution's research mission. The IACUC has a responsibility to ensure that effective training is provided to all personnel whose work contributes in various ways to animal care and use. There is great flexibility in how a program can be configured to achieve best results. Customer input on the training program is valuable to mold the training to meet the needs often known best by those doing the work. Customer satisfaction feedback is vital for improving the training experience. Trainers should be encouraged to develop their teaching skills, which should be evaluated in performance reviews. Summaries of information and data about the training program should be prepared periodically for the IACUC's review. Through carrying out its oversight responsibility, the IACUC ensures the training program achieves a high quality of service to the institution, its personnel, and the animals.

REFERENCES

AALAS (American Association for Laboratory Animal Science). 2014a. AALAS Learning Library. AALAS. https://www.aalaslearninglibrary.org/Pages/Courses/Tracks. aspx?intLibraryID=10.

AALAS (American Association for Laboratory Animal Science). 2014b. IACUC central: Institutional animal care & use training programs. Memphis, TN: AALAS. https://www. aalas.org/iacuc/resources/iacuc-resources/training-program-webpages.

AALAS (American Association for Laboratory Animal Science). 2012–2014. *Techniques Training Series: Mouse* (2012), *Rat* (2013), *Minipig* (2013), *Rabbit* (in press). Memphis, TN: AALAS.

AHWLA (Assessing the Health Welfare of Laboratory Animals). 2014. BVA Animal Welfare Foundation. Practical animal handling: Tutorial guide. http://www.ahwla.org.uk/site/ tutorials/BVA/BVA01-Title.html.

Anderson, L. C. 2007. Institutional and IACUC responsibilities for animal care and use education and training programs. *ILAR Journal* 48 (2):90–95.

AVMA (American Veterinary Medical Association). 2013. *Guidelines for the Euthanasia of Animals*. Schaumburg, IL: AVMA.

Baran, S. W., E. J. Johnson, and J. Kehler. 2009. An introduction to electronic learning and its use to address challenges in surgical training. *Lab Animal* 38 (6):202–210.

Baran, S. W., E. J. Johnson, J. Kehler, and F. C. Hankenson. 2010. Development and implementation of multimedia content for an electronic learning course on rodent surgery. *Journal of the American Association for Laboratory Animal Science* 49 (3):307–311.

Baran, S. W., E. J. Johnson, M. A. Stephens, and J. Kehler. 2009. Development of electronic learning courses for surgical training of animal research personnel. *Lab Animal* 38 (9):295–304.

Bayne, K., D. Bayvel, J. M. Clark, G. Demers, C. Joubert, T. M. Kurosawa, E. Rivera, et al. 2011. Harmonizing veterinary training and qualifications in laboratory animal medicine: A global perspective. *ILAR Journal* 52 (3):393–403.

Bennett, B. T., M. J. Brown, and J. C. Schofield. 1994. *Essentials for Animal Research: A Primer for Research Personnel*. Beltsville, MD: U.S. Department of Agriculture, National Agricultural Library. http://www.nal.usda.gov/awic/pubs/noawicpubs/essentia.htm.

Bogdanske, J. J., S. Hubbard-Van Stelle, M. R. Riley and B. M. Schiffman. 2014. *Laboratory Mouse and Laboratory Rat Procedural Techniques*. Boca Raton, FL: CRC Press.

Clifford, P., N. Melfi, J. Bogdanske, E. J. Johnson, J. Kehler, and S. W. Baran. 2013. Assessment of proficiency and competency in laboratory animal biomethodologies. *Journal of the American Association for Laboratory Animal Science* 52 (6):711–716.

CITI (Collaborative Institutional Training Intiative) Program. 2014. CITI program. https:// www.citiprogram.org/.

Conarello, S. L. and M. J. Shepherd. 2007. Training strategies for research investigators and technicians. *ILAR Journal* 48 (2):120–130.

Dobrovolny, J., J. Stevens, and L. V. Medina. 2007. Training in the laboratory animal science community: Strategies to support adult learning. *ILAR Journal* 48 (2):75–89.

DOD (Department of Defense). 2010. DOD instruction 3216.01. Use of animals in DOD programs. http://www.dtic.mil/whs/directives/corres/pdf/321601p.pdf.

FASS (Federation of Animal Science Societies). 2010. *Guide for the Care and Use of Agricultural Animals in Agricultural Research and Teaching*, 3rd edn. FASS, Champaign, IL.

FDA (Food and Drug Administration). 1997. Good laboratory practice for nonclinical laboratory studies. Department of Health and Human Services, Code of Federal Regulations 21:272–285.

Foshay, W. R. and P. T. Tinkey. 2007. Evaluating the effectiveness of training strategies: Performance goals and testing. *ILAR Journal* 48 (2):156–162.

Greene, M. E., M. E. Pitts, and M. L. James. 2007. Training strategies for institutional animal care and use committee (IACUC) members and the institutional official (IO). *ILAR Journal* 48 (2):131–142.

Guillen, J. 2012. FELASA guidelines and recommendations. *Journal of the American Association for Laboratory Animal Science* 51 (3):311–321.

Hèon, H., N. Rousseau, J. Montgomery, G. Beauregard, and M. Choiniere. 2006. Establishment of an operating room committee and a training program to improve aseptic techniques for rodent and large animal surgery. *Journal of the American Association for Laboratory Animal Science* 45 (6):58–62.

HHS (U.S. Department of Health and Human Services). 2009. *Biosafety in Microbiological and Biomedical Laboratories*. 5th edn. Washington, DC: U.S. Government Printing Office.

Huerkamp, M. J. 2006. Job dynamics of veterinary professionals in an academic research institution. I. Retention and turnover of veterinary technicians. *Journal of the American Association for Laboratory Animal Science* 45 (5):16–25.

Kennedy, B. W. 2002. Creating a training coordinator position. *Lab Animal* 31 (6):34–38.

Liu, J. H. K. and A. Heiser. 2007. *Rat Jugular Vein and Carotid Artery Catheterization for Acute Survival Studies: A Practical Guide*. New York, NY: Springer.

Lockworth, C. R., S. L. Craig, J. Liu, and P. T. Tinkey. 2011. Training veterinary care technicians and husbandry staff improves animal care. *Journal of the American Association for Laboratory Animal Science* 50 (1):84–93.

Machholz, E., G. Mulder, C. Ruiz, B. F. Corning, and K. R. Pritchett-Corning. 2012. Manual restraint and common compound administration routes in mice and rats. *J Vis Exp* (67):e2771.

Medina, L. V., K. Hrapkiewicz, M. Tear, and L. C. Anderson. 2007. Fundamental training for individuals involved in the care and use of laboratory animals: A review and update of the 1991 NRC Core Training Module. *ILAR Journal* 48 (2):96–108.

Mondschein, S. G. 2007. A current perspective on the role and needs of IACUC unaffiliated members. *Lab Animal* 36:21–26.

NIH (National Institutes of Health). 1985. U.S. government principles for the utilization and care of vertebrate animals used in testing, research and training. Bethesda, MD: NIH. http://grants.nih.gov/grants/olaw/references/phspol.htm#USGovPrinciples.

NIH (National Institutes of Health). 2002. Public Health Service policy on humane care and use of laboratory animals. Bethesda, MD: Office of Laboratory Animal Welfare, NIH.

NRC (National Research Council). 1991. *Education and Training in the Care and Use of Laboratory Animals: A Guide for Developing Institutional Programs*. Washington, DC: National Academy Press.

NRC (National Research Council). 2011. *Guide for the Care and Use of Laboratory Animals*. 8th edn. Washington, DC: National Academies Press.

Pritchett-Corning, K. R. 2011. *Handbook of Clinical Signs in Rodents and Rabbits*. Wilmington, MA: Charles River Laboratories.

Pritchett-Corning, K. R., G. B. Mulder, and Y. Luo. 2011. Principles of rodent surgery for the new surgeon. *Journal of Visualized Experiments* (47), e2586.

Pritt, S. and N. Duffee. 2007. Training strategies for animal care technicians and veterinary technical staff. *ILAR Journal* 48 (2):109–119.

Pritt, S., P. Samalonis, and L. Bindley. 2004. Creating a comprehensive training documentation program. *RESOURCE* 33 (4).

Slauter, E. 1999. AWIC bulletin: When the USDA veterinary medical officer looks at your training program. *AWIC Bulletin* 10:1–2.

USDA (U.S. Department of Agriculture). 2013a. *Animal Welfare Act and Animal Welfare Regulations* (Animal Care Blue Book). Code of Federal Regulations (CFR), Title 9, Chapter 1, Subchapter A, Parts 1–4.

USDA (U.S. Department of Agriculture). 2013b. Animal Welfare Act of 1966 intended to regulate the transport, sale and handling of dogs, cats, guinea pigs, nonhuman primates, hamsters and rabbits intended to use for research or other purposes. P.L. 89-544, pp. 2131–2156.

van Zutphen, B. 2007. Education and training for the care and use of laboratory animals: An overview of current practices. *ILAR Journal* 48 (2):72–74.

Whiting, T. 2011. Understanding animal welfare: The science in its cultural context. Review. *Canadian Veterinary Journal* 52 (6):662.

CHAPTER 8

Navigating the Search for Alternatives

Mary W. Wood and Michael Kreger

CONTENTS

The Animal Welfare Act (AWA, Laboratory Animal Welfare Act, P.L. 89-544; USDA 2013a) was signed into law by President Lyndon Johnson in 1966 and is recognized in the United States as the minimally acceptable standard for laboratory animal treatment and care. The U.S. Department of Agriculture's (USDA) Animal and Plant Health Inspection Service (APHIS) oversees the AWA, while the House and Senate Agriculture Committees have primary legislative jurisdiction.

Since its passage, the AWA has continued to evolve, illustrated by its several significant amendments over the years, most recently in 2008. It was the 1985 amendments, however, that remain arguably most significant for animals used in research, teaching, and testing. Called the Improved Standards for Laboratory Animals Act and tucked within the Food Security Act of 1985 (P.L. 99-198), these amendments strengthen standards for laboratory animal care, increase the enforcement of the AWA, provide for the dissemination of information to reduce unintended duplication of animal experiments, and mandate training for personnel who handle animals. Notably, the 1985 amendments require each research facility covered by the AWA, including federal facilities, to appoint a committee to assess animal care, treatment, and practices in experimental research (USDA 2013b).

The 1985 amendments defined and established the requirement for an oversight body called the Institutional Animal Care and Use Committee (IACUC). One of the IACUC's many roles is to verify consideration of the availability of alternatives; the principal investigator (PI) must convince the IACUC that they have considered alternatives to any procedures that may cause more than momentary or slight pain or distress to the animals, and that they have determined that the proposed animal studies are not unnecessarily duplicative. The IACUC evaluates these requirements, in part, by reviewing the provided written narrative of the methods used and sources consulted to determine the availability of alternatives, including refinements, reductions, and replacements. If the IACUC is unsatisfied with the alternatives search or the explanatory narrative on the protocol form, they will return the protocol to the PI for revision.

While literature searches have been used to address alternatives concerns since 1985, questions remain; the related regulations and compliance are still an area of confusion. Many are uncertain what a search of the alternatives literature looks like and are unclear about what is required by law and, especially, what the benefits may be.

The APHIS has the responsibility for interpretation and clarification of the AWA, both for the inspectors and the inspected. The APHIS Animal Care Inspection Guide (APHIS 2013) provides insight into what the USDA inspectors are expecting, and the APHIS Animal Care Policies (APHIS 2011) provide guidance for compliance for the IACUC and the PIs. In particular, Animal Care Policy #12 addresses the search for literature on alternatives and explains what is meant in the AWA by a "written narrative for alternatives to painful procedures" (APHIS 2011). While there are many complicated ways to design and execute a search, this chapter will provide a good starting point, as well as tips for the researcher and information specialist; we will outline the legislative background and describe how the alternatives search can best be performed.

8.1 DEFINING ALTERNATIVES

The Principles of Humane Experimental Technique was first published in 1959 (Russell and Burch 1959). It was written by two British researchers, William Russell and Rex Burch, who were the first to advocate the three Rs in animal research: replacement, reduction, and refinement. The book and the subject were fairly well ignored for about 25 years, after which time the book was rediscovered. It has since become the basis for and the source of the common language used in the discussion of alternatives in biomedical research, legislation, and regulations.

Replacement refers to the replacement of animals with nonanimal models or techniques or a species phylogenetically lower. Reduction means reducing the number of animals used; it can also refer to the minimization of any unintentionally duplicative experiments. Reductions in the number of animals used can be brought about by using no more animals than necessary to accomplish the purpose of the test, by combining tests in such a way that fewer animals are needed, and by retrieving information that allows any unintentional duplication of earlier work to be avoided. A thorough literature search of articles similar to the proposed study may help determine appropriate animal numbers while also verifying unnecessary duplication. Refinement is a technique or procedure to reduce pain and distress. Refinement offers the best opportunity for immediate implementation and is the least often considered. Proper use of analgesics and anesthetics; knowledge of the test species' physiology and behaviors; modifications in restraint, handling, and blood collection techniques; and proper training of personnel all constitute refinements (Wood 2000). The 1989 Final Rules, called the preamble to the AWA 1985 amendment, specifically references the three Rs, and states that the PI must consider not just alternatives, but all three Rs (NAL 2014b).

8.2 LEGISLATION

The AWA emphasizes the importance of minimizing pain and distress, stating "that the principal investigator consider alternatives to any procedure likely to produce pain or distress in an experimental animal" (USDA NAL 2014b).

Title 9 of the Code of Federal Regulations (9CFR) codifies the regulation and delineates how the consideration of alternatives should be made. The "IACUC shall determine that ... the principal investigator has considered alternatives to procedures that may cause more than momentary or slight pain or distress to the animals, and has provided a written narrative description of the methods and sources ... used to determine that alternatives were not available" (USDA NAL 2014b).

The *Federal Register* provides a rationale for making alternatives consideration a written requirement and suggests databases that can be searched to document whether or not alternatives are available:

The principal investigator must provide a written narrative of the sources, such as Biological Abstracts, Index Medicus, the Current Research Information Service

(CRIS), and the AWIC that is operated by the NAL. We believe that in fulfilling this requirement committee members will discuss these efforts with the principal investigator in reviewing the proposed activity. We also believe that considerations of alternatives will be discussed during committee meetings where proposed activities are presented for approval, and made part of the meeting minutes. (USDA NAL 2014b)

The legislation mandates that the investigator provide a written narrative demonstrating to the IACUC that alternatives to potentially painful or stressful procedures were considered in the experimental design. A thorough search of the literature is suggested as the best way to demonstrate a good faith effort. IACUC members, as well as the USDA Animal Care (AC) inspector, should be able to follow the provided search strategy, the list of databases searched, and the keywords used to verify that the investigator has reliably determined whether or not alternatives exist. The literature search provides a consistent, transparent way to evaluate if a replacement, refinement, or reduction is possible (Kreger 1998).

8.2.1 USDA Policy 12

USDA-APHIS Animal Care Policy #12 interprets and clarifies what the inspectors consider to be an adequate consideration of alternatives. It paraphrases the legal statements from 9CFR, specifically noting that

> When a database search is the primary means of meeting this requirement, the narrative should include: the name(s) of the databases searched (due to the variation in subject coverage and sources used, one database is seldom adequate); the date the search was performed; the time period covered by the search; and the search strategy (including scientifically relevant terminology) used.
> Regardless of the alternatives source(s) used, the written narrative should include adequate information for the IACUC to assess that a reasonable and good faith effort was made to determine the availability of alternatives or alternative methods. If a database search or other source identifies a bona fide alternative method (one that could be used to accomplish the goals of the animal use proposal), the IACUC may and should ask the PI to explain why an alternative that had been found was not used. The IACUC, in fact, can withhold approval of the study proposal if the Committee is not satisfied with the procedures the PI plans to use in his study. (USDA NAL 2014b)

8.3 RESEARCH BENEFITS OF PERFORMING AN ALTERNATIVES SEARCH

Beyond the legal mandate in the AWA, there are other benefits to an alternatives search. The Public Health Service (PHS), the U.S. Government Principles for the Utilization and Care of Vertebrate Animals Used in Testing, Research, and Training (NIH 2002), the PHS Policy on Humane Care and Use of Laboratory Animals (PHS 2002), and the *Guide for the Care and Use of Laboratory Animals* (the Guide) (NRC 2011) all require consideration of alternatives when awarding project funding.

Such laws and policies extend to all vertebrates, including those beyond the scope of the AWA. Additionally, complying with the AWA and the Guide is required in order for an institution to become accredited by the Association for Assessment and Accreditation of Laboratory Animal Care International (AAALAC International) (AAALAC International 2014). There may also be an economic benefit if the animal sample size can be reduced or a nonanimal alternative is found. Finally, and notably, an alternatives search takes the researcher beyond the journals in her/his area of expertise to a world of literature about advances in procedures and methods, and to areas that encourage collaboration and discovery, and that improve the well-being of the study animals.

8.4 COMPLIANCE: THE SEARCH FOR ALTERNATIVES

The search begins with the researcher describing the protocol. As the search strategy is drafted, the field widens to cover not just the specifics of the protocol but also methods that can reduce, refine, or replace animal use. This effort is followed by database selection, which involves choosing databases relevant to the researcher's area of interest, as well as other databases that may address specific questions or procedures. For example, databases might include, in addition to medical databases, a computer technology database that gives computer simulations of a particular procedure. The search is run and then evaluated by reviewing a list of citations or abstracts and retrieving relevant articles. Finally, the search must be documented, and a narrative is written describing whether any identified alternatives can or cannot be used. This is probably the broadest step of all in that it should cover all three Rs.

8.4.1 How to Conduct a Literature Search for Alternatives

The aim of any comprehensive information search is to collect all essential documents. The efficacy and utility of the search are directly affected by how one searches (appropriate search terms, expertise, and training) and where (scientific databases, indexes, and online sources) (Roi 2013).

8.4.1.1 Search Strategy

There is no single correct method for designing a search strategy. Searching is an iterative process, and any strategy will require modification and rethinking as the search is performed; the results of one inquiry often generate another not previously considered. Librarians often approach a search by making use of subject headings, category codes, and thesauri unique to and provided by individual databases; however, because databases differ by design, the search in each database may be different. Identifying concepts, gathering synonyms, and searching by keywords is an approach that works effectively across databases and is a good practice when doing a multidatabase search. The unique considerations of the alternatives search can be readily integrated into this search strategy approach.

Legislation specifically mentions searching for alternatives to painful procedures, requiring a search of the entire area of study. The procedure may appear in
title, abstract, or descriptor fields, but more often it is in the methods section within
the article. To consider and evaluate possible alternatives to a potentially painful procedure may require keyword searching and reading specific sections from articles.

Searching for appropriate animal numbers is also part of the alternatives search.
A comprehensive alternatives search will retrieve citations that cover studies similar
to the one proposed, with animal numbers, again, often noted in the materials and
methods sections. Together with a biostatistician consult, this information facilitates
the determination of and justification for the proposed number.

In toxicology testing, the search is easily run if the type of compound is known.
If the test compound is unknown, or if certain tests are required by other federal
agencies, it is important to remember that *alternatives* means more than simply
searching for a replacement technique. The investigator can search for a method that
uses fewer animals or where mortality is not the end point, or search for techniques
that minimize pain or distress by using analgesics.

8.4.1.2 Key Term Selection

Searches often begin with a semantic search query, asking a question in the hope
that the articles retrieved will provide the answer. This type of preliminary search
of citations similar to the area of research will allow consideration of refinements
to the proposed methods, but it can also be useful in identifying additional relevant
keywords and concepts. Making use of these specific key terms used in the published
literature may allow the retrieval of unexpected results. Effective searching is dependent on appropriate search terms; the relevant synonyms and concepts identified
should be integrated into the evolving search strategy.

8.4.2 Where to Search

Once the topic is clear and the search strategy outlined, with keywords and
synonyms as well as specific questions and concerns, deciding what information
resources to search is essential. There is no right or wrong number of databases to
select when running an alternatives search. However, it is important to recognize
that no single database reviews all the literature in all research fields. Databases do
overlap somewhat in the journals they index and the subject areas they cover, but
they also complement each other. Testing a new medical device, for example, might
involve searching biomedical, engineering, and even computer sciences databases.
The objectives of the search are to demonstrate whether alternatives are available and,
if so, their possible utility. A thorough search always requires more than one database.

Bibliographic databases provide the foundation for a good search for alternatives. With the exception of some historic literature, online databases have virtually
replaced printed journal indexes. Usually, bibliographic databases are collections of
article citations, with or without abstracts, from hundreds of subject-related journals.
It is important to recognize, when selecting databases, what kinds of publications are

indexed in each. Some include journal articles only, whereas others also include conference proceedings, audiovisuals, book chapters, and reports. Each citation includes the title, author, year of publication, publisher, and keyword descriptors. These, plus abstracts, are usually prepared by the authors or may be specially written by the database producer.

8.4.2.1 Evidence-Based, Systematic Review

Different databases require different approaches to searching, as well as an understanding of what is covered and how it is indexed. For example, Medline and PubMed have an extensive medical subject headings structure called MeSH; many databases, including AGRICOLA, CAB, and Embase, also have a controlled vocabulary thesaurus. Knowing about these tools and how to use them allows the search to be more complete and the results more reliable, as not all publications are equal in their authority and scientific reliability. Database selection may be the first authority filter: PubMed indexes more selectively than Google Scholar, Google Scholar does not index using a thesaurus, and Cochrane Database of Systematic Reviews includes only systematically assessed reviews (Cochrane Collaboration 2014). It is incumbent on the researcher to evaluate the material uncovered and determine if the information therein is valid and useful. Considering the evidence and evaluating the studies on which a publication is based are part of the search process.

Evidence-based decision making necessitates identification of the best available evidence and its application, together with the researcher's expertise, to the proposed study. There are guidelines and definitions to help the scientist determine the level of evidence in each piece. Scientists in the Netherlands have identified steps to assist scientists in performing a comprehensive literature search, while considering the scientific quality of the search results. Of primary importance is identification of all potentially relevant studies, immediately followed by their evaluation, which involves assessing the quality of the evidence based on study design (Leenaars 2012, Hooijmans 2013).

8.4.2.2 Database Selection

Most researchers and librarians are well acquainted with literature databases such as Medline and PubMed, Embase, AGRICOLA, CAB, and BIOSIS. Although they are not typically considered as databases on alternatives, they index the results of millions of peer-reviewed biomedical studies and technical papers. Consequently, these authoritative databases, and other similar resources, should be the databases of choice when conducting an initial literature review (Smith 2005).

The single most determinate factor in database selection is availability. At academic research institutions, there are often many excellent and relevant databases from which to choose, depending on the question; however, due to subscription costs, it is a limited, select list of database options. Private research facilities may subscribe to an online database service that, while expensive, allows access to essentially every possible database. Others may rely solely on resources that are freely available. In any scenario, selecting those databases most relevant to your search topic is very important.

Sometimes you may not know about a database that may be of interest. Sometimes there are questions that need to be answered that may be in publications outside of your research area and perhaps indexed in databases other than those with which you are familiar. Identifying both databases that may be relevant and databases to which you have access will depend on your facility and library. If you have an information professional available to you, we strongly suggest you make use of their expertise and insight. Another option is to contact the information specialists at the Animal Welfare Information Center (AWIC). While they will not know your particular library, they will know how to advise you on database options and selection.

8.4.2.3 Bibliographic Databases

National libraries index and organize vast amounts of information into various databases, which are then available free of charge. The National Library of Medicine (NLM) lists nearly 300 publicly available databases and resources (NIH 2014a). Of those, the most heavily used and recognizable are Medline and PubMed. They are two resources in the NLM's enormous biomedical and genomic information collection called the National Center for Biotechnology Information (NCBI), and they primarily index human clinical medicine journals; they do not index nonjournal publications like reports, audiovisuals, or conference proceedings (NCBI 2014). Other resources in NCBI include PubChem, BioSystems, BLAST, GenBank, Gene, and PubMed Central (PMC). Of significant value in pharmaceutical and toxicology studies is the NLM collection of resources that make up the Toxicology Data Network (TOXNET). These and other NLM databases (e.g., ClinicalTrials and AIDSInfo) cover human and laboratory animal medicine and research, making up the "world's largest biomedical library" (NIH 2014a).

The National Agricultural Library (NAL) produces the AGRICOLA database, which indexes journals dealing with alternatives, laboratory animal care and use, and veterinary medicine, as well as many other related conference proceedings, reports, audiovisuals, and newsletters (NAL 2014a). Because AWIC is part of NAL, AGRICOLA covers the recent alternatives literature particularly well.

While the databases Medline and PubMed are often used interchangeably, there is a slight difference between them. Started in the 1960s, Medline is the NLM journal citation database and provides references to biomedical and life sciences journal articles. PubMed has been available since 1996 and includes the entire Medline database plus in-process citations, ahead-of-print citations, citations to out-of-scope articles, and citations to a few other articles meeting special criteria. Both databases are exceptional resources, including biomedical and clinical research, veterinary medicine and science, and laboratory animal science. MeSH includes related subject headings such as *animal welfare*, *laboratory animal science*, *animal testing alternatives*, *animal use alternatives*, *animal experimentation*, *research design*, and *animal models* (Smith 2005).

TOXNET includes databases on toxicology, hazardous chemicals, and environmental health. It provides extensive coverage of alternative testing techniques, offering access to 14 different toxicology-related databases, including the Hazardous Substances Data Bank (HSBD), the Integrated Risk Information System (IRIS), the Genetic Toxicology Data Bank (GeneTox), the comprehensive Toxicology Literature Online (Toxline), and the Developmental and Reproductive Toxicology database (DART). The 14 databases can be searched individually or together. The site also serves as a gateway to other NLM toxicology resources.

AWIC was established in 1986 by the U.S. Federal Government as an information center within NAL; its purpose is to assist scientists in finding alternatives to painful procedures performed on animals (NAL 2014a). In the past, AWIC produced an array of bibliographies focusing on laboratory, farm, and exhibit animals. The bibliographies cover topics on husbandry, handling, alternatives, and database searching, as well as issues of concern to animal care committees such as food and water regulation, caging, animal numbers, and humane end points. AWIC continues to provide an extensive selection of links to databases, guidelines, and regulatory information. The information specialists are available for assistance with literature searching.

Beyond the databases provided by the national libraries are valuable and unique bibliographic databases produced by various organizations. CAB Abstracts is produced by the CABI organization and provides extensive coverage of the world's veterinary and laboratory-animal medicine and science literature. Searching both the CAB and AGRICOLA databases will address the veterinary, animal science, and laboratory animal literature, with a particular focus on large animal and welfare topics. CAB indexes appropriate citations with the terms *animal welfare* or *animal testing alternatives*. AGRICOLA also uses the terms *animal use alternatives, alternative toxicity testing, end points, animal use reduction, animal use refinement,* and *animal use replacement,* as well as the broad category *laboratory and experimental animals*. CAB Abstracts uses the term *laboratory animal science* to allow users to focus on that specific body of literature. Searchable subjects covered by both databases include analgesics and anesthetics, animal behavior, and animal husbandry, in addition to basic research (Smith 2005).

Embase is a powerful biomedical and pharmacological database produced by Elsevier and, if possible, should be included in a database search. Many researchers regularly search PubMed or Medline, but relatively few realize that Embase covers the same subject areas with very little citation overlap, and it includes citations and abstracts from conference proceedings as well as journal articles. It offers a European perspective and is arguably the database of choice for finding drug-related research information. Access to Embase is not universal, however, due to cost. While international information specialists and the experienced AWIC staff recommend searching Embase as frequently as Medline, that is not always an option in practical terms.

BIOSIS Previews is another highly recommended multidisciplinary database that covers biomedical research, biological research, veterinary science, pharmacology, and other life-science topics. It is useful for finding information on alternative techniques because of its broad coverage of the life sciences, and the interdisciplinary nature of the database allows scientists to find information on models and techniques that may fall outside the journals that they normally read. It is an extraordinarily well-indexed database, and its useful thesaurus terms include *animal care, animal husbandry, models and simulations, laboratory techniques,* and *methods and techniques.* BIOSIS indexes books, reports, and conference proceedings as well as journal articles and is worth searching for general natural-history information on behavior and animal welfare studies.

Each of these literature databases is useful for locating information on replacement, reduction, and refinement techniques. Because the number of animals used in a study is partially dependent upon the variability in the response of the animals, reviewing literature from similar research may assist researchers in determining the appropriate numbers of animals required. If invasive procedures are to be performed on animals, researchers should also review the appropriate veterinary literature to ensure that less invasive techniques are not available and that, for potentially painful procedures, the best analgesic and general care protocols are used. Similarly, for studies that may involve the use of large numbers of animals, the general biomedical and veterinary literature should be reviewed to determine if alternative methods or techniques could be used instead (Smith 2005). This type of information can be obtained from these large multidisciplinary databases.

8.4.2.4 Alternative Databases

In addition to the numerous bibliographic databases, there are many valuable but less well-known specialized databases, which often address animal welfare or specific aspects of the three Rs. Information centers with a mandate to assist scientists in locating information on the three Rs have been established in several countries. Internationally, guidelines for the care and use of animals in research have been produced by scientific organizations and regulatory bodies. Researchers should be experts on the scientific literature in their field; they may not, however, have the same familiarity with the literature addressing replacement, reduction, and refinement. Finding unfamiliar information from unknown resources is a particular challenge to complying with the required search for alternatives. Identifying these useful resources and evaluating the publications for relevant and new ideas can offer new possibilities for a proposal; considering also the relevant specialized alternatives databases or resources will ensure adequate and compliant consideration.

Reliable and authoritative databases and resources on alternatives are often produced by government or academic entities. The U.S. government supports several alternatives-focused resources that are worth checking, including a resource offered by the NLM Specialized Information Services named ALTBIB (Resources for Alternatives to the Use of Live Vertebrates in Biomedical Research and Testing). ALTBIB provides access to information on refined animal testing methods and testing strategies and offers related preformulated searches of PubMed. Another U.S. government site is produced by the Interagency Coordinating Committee on the Validation of Alternative Methods (ICCVAM). Under the auspices of the National Toxicology Program Interagency Center for the Evaluation of Alternative Toxicological Methods, ICCVAM is relevant to any regulatory and research agencies requiring alternatives information in toxicological and safety testing. Finally, AWIC is an essential piece of the puzzle and is worth mentioning again here. In addition to creating resources and providing education and support in the search for alternatives, the site offers suggestions and lists of additional resources to consider. The examples noted on the AWIC Sample Literature Searches for Alternatives site are instructive and enlightening (NAL 2014a).

Altweb, produced by the Johns Hopkins Center for Alternatives to Animal Testing (CAAT), is a good example of an academia-based alternatives resource. It serves as a collaborative project with industry, government, and humane organizations and contains science-based alternatives news, education resources, and scientific and regulatory information. Conference proceedings (e.g., monoclonal antibody production), full-text articles, and links to other sites are included.

Internationally, there are government, regulatory, academic, and privately funded sites of authoritative scientific information. Norecopa is the Norwegian Consensus Platform for Replacement, Reduction and Refinement of animal experiments, representing government, research, industry, and animal welfare. It supports a variety of websites and resources, a highlight being the NORINA database, which features information on alternatives to, or supplements for, the use of animals in teaching and training protocols.

The National Centre for the Replacement, Refinement and Reduction of Animals in Research (NC3Rs) was formed in 2005, funded by the British government in support of research into the three Rs. NC3Rs produces information resources and guidelines on humane techniques and organizes conferences and symposia on initiatives relating to the three Rs. Of particular relevance here are the microsites, notably the Blood Sampling Microsite, the Information Portal, and the Guidelines and Factsheets. NC3Rs developed the related Animal Research: Reporting of *In Vivo* Experiments guidelines (ARRIVE), which are intended to improve the reporting of animal experiments and are endorsed by several journal publishers (NC3Rs 2014).

The Fund for the Replacement of Animals in Medical Experiments (FRAME) is a privately funded U.K. organization dedicated to the development of new and valid methods that will replace the need for laboratory animals in medical and scientific research, education, and testing. As part of that effort, they publish *Alternatives to Laboratory Animals (ATLA)*, an international peer-reviewed scientific journal. Additionally, the group's web pages on Information Resources and Guide to Searching for Alternatives are worth noting.

The Canadian Council on Animal Care (CCAC) oversees the ethical use of animals in science in Canada. While not exactly the same, U.S. and Canadian regulations are similar enough to make the resources at the CCAC website extremely useful, in particular the 3Rs Microsite, the 3Rs Search Guide, and the Alternatives Test Methods Table.

8.4.2.5 *Use of Google as a Search Engine*

Google may be an essential tool in information dissemination, but it is not appropriate for searching research literature. When there is a known title, Google offers a very quick verification tool, and, if there is some obscure citation, Google is sometimes the only place to verify and correct it, allowing further searching and access. But it is not designed to provide reliable information or identify authoritative publications from a general subject search inquiry. Google Scholar, however, offers a focused search option, and it can be quite useful, keeping in mind that verification and evaluation of each resource is required. There is no indexing, so the searching is limited to keywords, but its breadth and reach is quite extraordinary. It allows you to search across disciplines and sources, including articles, theses, books, and abstracts from academic publishers, professional societies, online repositories, and universities. It may uncover otherwise unfindable manuscripts, conference proceedings, and society publications. While it cannot be relied on to be the sole database searched for alternatives, it can be one of a few.

8.4.2.6 Other Methods and Sources

There may be situations where databases are insufficient. There are certainly particular fields of study and, more likely, particular questions that cannot be adequately addressed in the databases and websites noted previously. In these situations, Google may be viewed as a supplemental resource, offering assistance in retrieving very current information that is otherwise very difficult to uncover. Conference abstracts and proceedings, colloquia presentations and discussion, and even current and ephemeral conversations appearing in alternative Internet-based resources, including blog and twitter posts, may be searched using special limits in Google. Other scholarly bibliographic tools available with the emerging technology include resources such as Mendeley, CiteULike, Zotero, ResearchGate, Academic.edu, and Lanyrd.com. Unique possibilities emerge with the now available relational searching, online tracking of scholarly discussion and activity, and scholarly social networks. Like an expert consultation or an esoteric conference presentation, sometimes additional and perhaps even as-yet undefined approaches may be necessary to fully consider a topic or a question in a comprehensive manner.

8.4.2.7 Tools Available to Assist with Search

Tools exist to help with managing information, such as Endnote, Mendeley, and Zotero. While each offers something unique, all organize publications and other informational resources, facilitating repeat access as well as future composition. Another exceedingly useful tool for the researcher is the freely available My NCBI, available from the PubMed page. Perhaps more relevant to the issue at hand, My NCBI offers several features that help with searching and with compliance. My NCBI allows the searcher to save searches and to create automatic alerts, to use a filter to modify and narrow search results, and to retain recent search activity for six months. This last function can be used to very accurately reflect in the protocol exactly what search strategies were used, using a simple copy and paste. Additionally, My NCBI accounts sync with eRA Commons accounts, facilitating National Institutes of Health (NIH) public access policy compliance and managing other NIH funding requirements.

8.4.3 Evaluating Search Results

After the searches are run, the PI must review the information and determine whether or not alternatives are available. Often, full-text articles are required in order to determine the usability and possible efficacy of an alternative. Large academic or pharmaceutical research facilities will have access to many of the articles online or perhaps on the shelf in the library but certainly not all. Smaller institutions often do not have that luxury. In either case, if material is needed and not readily available, efforts should be made to obtain the full text. A Google search of the title is recommended in case the article has been deposited in PMC or another open repository. Contacting the author remains a practical way of obtaining a copy. Interlibrary loan is an option; if the library is part of a consortium, exchanges can be very quick and are the preferred method.

The literature search coupled with findings from other sources used (e.g., websites, conferences attended, personal training, and experience) will help the PI reach a decision regarding any possible replacements, reductions, or refinements to the proposal. An alternative may be as simple as a way to house the animals that is more comfortable or an analgesic given to relieve pain caused by an adjuvant. The bottom line is that the researcher must use the search to assure the IACUC members that the proposed study plan is the most humane way to meet the objectives of the study.

8.4.4 Documenting Results

USDA AC Policy #12 specifically states that

When a database search is the primary means of meeting this requirement, the narrative should include:

1. the name(s) of the databases searched (due to the variation in subject coverage and sources used, one database is seldom adequate);
2. the date the search was performed;
3. the time period covered by the search; and
4. the search strategy (including scientifically relevant terminology) used. (APHIS 2011)

After all of the searching is complete, the material evaluated, and the proposal modified as needed, record keeping is necessary in order to comply. The requirements listed in Policy #12 are fairly straightforward, asking for the names of the databases searched and the date the search was performed. If searched on multiple days, the most recent date will suffice. The time period covered by the search is requested. This can be trickier than it appears, as it is not always apparent what dates the specific database covers. If given the option, search at least the most recent ten years. For PubMed, the default search is from 1966 to the present, while for BIOSIS, it is from 1926 to the present. It would be reasonable and is acceptable to note *all years through the present*. Given this information, together with the date searched, the IACUC can be assured that a reasonable search of the available literature was made.

The narrative also requires the search strategy used, including the scientifically relevant terminology. This effort may be facilitated when searching NLM databases, as My NCBI retains a query history, providing a record of the search strategy and search date. This information can be copied and pasted into the protocol or saved as an attachment. Most other databases also have at least a temporary search history, which may be copied and pasted. Regardless of the sources used, Policy #12 notes that "the written narrative should include adequate information for the IACUC to assess that a reasonable and good faith effort was made to determine the availability of alternatives or alternative methods" (APHIS 2011).

Any other methods used to supplement the literature search, such as websites, consultations with experts, or conferences attended, should be included as such on the protocol form. As suggested previously, some research questions may require information not found in traditional bibliographic databases. In those cases, sufficient documentation should be provided to assure the IACUC of the value and validity of the source.

8.5 CONSULTING WITH INFORMATION SCIENTISTS

Seeking assistance from a librarian or information specialist regarding search strategies and database selection can minimize time and effort while increasing the value of the search results. Many literature searches are typically run during the study design period, which helps verify unnecessary duplication and provides background information on the topic of interest. Such searches can easily be tailored to address alternatives, and with some search guidance, researchers can improve the relevancy of the search results, and can find that the alternatives search can be a tool for improving the quality of research.

8.6 AVAILABLE TRAINING

Meeting the Information Requirements of the AWA: A Workshop is offered multiple times each year by AWIC at NAL in Beltsville, Maryland. The workshop is invaluable for anyone interested in maximizing their efforts in the search for alternatives or learning how to meet the requirements of the AWA. The AWIC information specialists also present at conferences and, when invited, will offer the workshop at remote sites or by webinar. Their guidance is available over the phone, and valuable tools and resources may be found on the AWIC website.

Other training resources include the 2013 re-edition of the European Union Reference Library for alternatives to animal testing (EURL ECVAM) *Search Guide: Good Search Practice on Animal Alternatives*. This European Commission Joint Research Centre publication is available free online from the EU Bookshop and contains extensive data sheets on information resources, basic principles of data retrieval procedures, and a table of organizations including their strengths and features (Roi 2013).

Additional useful guides that discuss this type of search and the evaluation of the results are available and are listed in the references and suggested readings.

8.7 CONCLUSION

The literature search shows a good faith effort on the part of the researcher to demonstrate that the research is as humane as possible. Alternatives may be found that can lead to adoption of experimental methods that are less painful, use fewer animals, and make better scientific and economic sense. If alternatives are not found, the search demonstrates that there is no other way and no more humane way to do the research than what is proposed.

REFERENCES

AAALAC International (Association for Assessment and Accreditation of Laboratory Animal Care International). 2014. http://aaalac.org. Accessed December 2, 2013.

APHIS (Animal and Plant Health Inspection Service. Animal Care). 2011. USDA-APHIS-animal care policy manual. APHIS, USDA. http://www.aphis.usda.gov/animal_welfare/policy.php.

Cochrane Collaboration. 2014. Cochrane database of systematic reviews. Cochrane Library. University Medical Centre Freiburg. http://www.thecochranelibrary.com/view/0/index.html.

Kreger, M. 1998. Why conduct literature searches for alternatives. *ASLAP Newsletter* 30(3):19–23.

Leenaars, M., C. R. Hooijmans, N. van Veggel, G. ter Riet, L. Leeflang, L. Hooft, G. J. van der Wilt, A. Tillema and M. Ritskes-Hoitinga. 2012. A step-by-step guide to systematically identify all relevant animal studies. *Laboratory Animals* 46(1): 24–31.

NAL (National Agricultural Library). 2014a. Animal Welfare Information Center home page. U.S. Department of Agriculture. http://awic.nal.usda.gov/.

NAL (National Agricultural Library). 2014b. Legislative history of the Animal Welfare Act. U.S. Department of Agriculture. Animal Welfare Information Center. http://awic.nal.usda.gov/legislative-history-animal-welfare-act-table-contents.

NCBI (National Center for Biotechnology Information). 2014. National Center for Biotechnology Information (NCBI) home page. Bethesda, MD: National Library of Medicine. http://www.ncbi.nlm.nih.gov/.

NC3Rs (National Centre for the Replacement, Refinement and Reduction of Animals in Research). 2014. NC3Rs home page. http://www.nc3rs.org.uk/.

NIH (National Institutes of Health). 2014. U.S. National Library of Medicine home page. NIH, Bethesda, MD. http://www.nlm.nih.gov/.

NIH. OER. OLAW (National Institutes of Health. Office of Extramural Research. Office of Laboratory Animal Welfare). 2014a. OLAW. Office of laboratory animal welfare. http://grants.nih.gov/grants/olaw/olaw.htm.

NRC (National Research Council). 2011. *Guide for the Care and Use of Laboratory Animals*, 8th edn. Washington, DC: National Academies Press.

Roi, A. J. and B. Grune. 2013. *The EURL ECVAM Search Guide: Good Search Practice on Animal Alternatives*. Luxembourg: Publications Office of the European Union.

Russell, W. M. S. and R. L. Burch. 1959. *The Principles of Humane Experimental Technique*. London: Methuen.

Smith, A. J. and T. Allen. 2005. The use of databases, information centers and guidelines when planning research that may involve animals. *Animal Welfare* 14(4):347–359.

USDA (U.S. Department of Agriculture). 2013a. Animal Welfare Act of 1966 intended to regulate the transport, sale and handling of dogs, cats, guinea pigs, nonhuman primates, hamsters and rabbits intended to use for research or other purposes. *Public Law* 89 (544):2131–2156.

USDA (U.S. Department of Agriculture). 2013b. *Animal Welfare Inspection Guide*, 1st edn. Washington, DC: USDA. http://www.aphis.usda.gov/animal_welfare/downloads/ Inspection%20Guide%20-%20November%202013.pdf.

Wood, M. W. and L. A. Hart. 2000. Searching for the 3Rs: Facilitating compliance in the bibliographic search for alternatives. In *8th ICML Conference Proceedings*. http://web. archive.org/web/20010522084641/www.icml.org/monday/icahis3/wood.htm.

SUGGESTED READINGS

Chilov, M., K. Matsoukas, N. Ispahany, T. Y. Allen, J. W. Lustbader. 2007. Using MeSH to search for alternatives to the use of animals in research. *Medical Reference Services Quarterly* 26(3):55–74.

Crawford, R. L. and T. Allen. 2008. Databases for biomedical animal resources. In *Sourcebook of Models for Biomedical Research*, ed. P. M. Conn, 49–54. Totowa, NJ: Humana Press.

Grune, B., M. Fallon, C. Howard, V. Hudson, J. A. Kulpa-Eddy. 2004. Report and recommendations of the international workshop retrieval approaches for information on alternative methods to animal experiments. *Altex* 3:115–127.

Hakkinen, P. and D. K. Green. 2002. Alternatives to animal testing: Information resources via the Internet and world wide web. *Toxicology* 173(1):3–11.

Hooijmans, C. R. and M. Ritskes-Hoitinga. 2013. Progress in using systematic reviews of animal studies to improve translational research. *PLoS Medicine* 10(7).

Hooijmans, C. R., M. Leenaars and M. Ritskes-Hoitinga. 2010. A gold standard publication checklist to improve the quality of animal studies, to fully integrate the three Rs, and to make systematic reviews more feasible. *Alternatives to Laboratory Animals* 38(2):167–182.

Kilkenny, C., W. J. Browne, I. C. Cuthill, M. Emerson, D. G. Altman. 2010. Improving bioscience research reporting: The ARRIVE guidelines for reporting animal research. *PLoS Biology* 8(6):e1000412.

Nesdill, D. and K. M. Adams. 2011. Literature search strategies to comply with institutional animal care and use committee review requirements. *Journal of Veterinary Medical Education* 38(2):150–156.

NHMRC (National Health Medical Research Council). 2000. *How to Use the Evidence: Assessment and Application of Scientific Evidence*. Canberra: National Health and Medical Research Council, Canberra.

NIH (National Institutes of Health). 2002. Public Health Service policy on humane care and use of laboratory animals. Bethesda, MD: Office of Laboratory Animal Welfare, U.S. Department of Health and Human Services, NIH. http://grants.nih.gov/grants/olaw/references/phspolicylabanimals.pdf. Accessed December 31, 2013.

OACU (Office of Animal Care and Use). 1999. Using animals in intramural research: Guidelines for investigators and guidelines for animal users. U.S. Department of Health and Human Services, NIH. http://oacu.od.nih.gov/training/pi.htm.

Smith, C. P. 1991. AWIC tips for searching for alternatives to animal research and testing. *Animal Welfare Information Center Newsletter* 2(1): 3–5.

OTA (U.S. Congress, Office of Technology Assessment). 1986. *Alternatives to Animal Use in Research, Testing, and Education*. Washington, DC: U.S. Government Printing Office. http://www.princeton.edu/~ota/disk2/1986/8601_n.html.

Vries, R., M. Leenaars, J. Tra, et al. 2013. The potential of tissue engineering for developing alternatives to animal experiments: A systematic review. *Journal of Tissue Engineering and Regenerative Medicine*. Published electronically April 3, 2013. doi: 10.1002/term.1703.

Wood, M. W. 2008. Bibliographic searching tools on disease models to locate alternatives for animals in research. In *Sourcebook of Models for Biomedical Research*, ed. P. M. Conn, 35–41. Totowa, NJ: Humana Press.

Wood, M. W. and L. A. Hart. 2011. Selecting appropriate animal models and strains: Making the best use of research, information and outreach. *AATEX* 14(Special Issue):303–306.

CHAPTER 9

The Relationship between the IACUC and Principal Investigators

Bill Yates

CONTENTS

The challenges of a scientific career have never been more daunting than they are today. It is difficult to obtain the funding necessary for running a laboratory, so scientists need to spend an increasing amount of time writing grants. The competitive funding environment also places a premium on scientific achievement, as only the most productive scientists are likely to be successful in securing grants. At the same time, the regulatory burden on scientists is increasing. The Federal Demonstration Project has estimated that over 40% of an investigator's time is spent in addressing regulatory burden, leaving less than 60% of their effort for scholarly pursuits (Haywood and Greene 2008). It is no wonder that some scientists have developed an adversarial relationship with the offices in their institution that handle regulatory affairs, as they do not believe those offices understand the challenges that scientists face or attempt to reduce their regulatory burden.

The goal of this chapter is to provide suggestions to investigators on how best to cope with the administrative responsibilities associated with the care and use of laboratory animals. These strategies include becoming acquainted with the relevant regulations, developing a proactive relationship with the Institutional Animal Care and Use Committee (IACUC), writing effective animal use protocols, rapidly addressing noncompliance with animal use regulations, reducing the likelihood that violations of animal care and use regulations will occur in the future, and conducting outreach to minimize the administrative burden.

9.1 THE FIRST STEP: UNDERSTANDING THE REGULATORY FRAMEWORK

In order to work effectively with an IACUC, investigators must first understand the IACUC's mission and the rationale for the IACUC's actions. The IACUC and the administrative officials that support the committee, including the institutional official (IO), have a legal obligation to assure that the institution complies with the Animal Welfare Act (AWA) and Regulations (AWRs) and the Public Health Service (PHS) Policy on Humane Care and Use of Laboratory Animals (PHS Policy) if the institution receives funding from the PHS (NIH 2002). Compliance with the PHS Policy requires that the institution must adhere to the Guide for the Care and Use of Laboratory Animals (the Guide) (NRC 2011), which was extensively revised in 2011. Failure to comply with the AWA and AWRs can result in fines for the institution as well as potential prosecution in federal court (Cohen 2006). Findings from inspection reports for facilities that use animals for research, teaching, and testing are available to the public on the U.S. Department of Agriculture (USDA) Animal and Plant Health Inspection Service (APHIS) website. Noncompliance with PHS Policy can result in withdrawal of grant funds (NIH 2002). Thus, to protect an institution, the IACUC must assure full compliance with the laws and regulations administered through both the PHS and the USDA.

To provide a regulatory framework, most IACUCs generate local rules and policies that are based on regulations promulgated by state and local governments (e.g., the AWA and AWRs) or funding agencies (e.g., the PHS Policy on Humane Care and Use of Laboratory Animals). In addition, past noncompliant actions of investigators may lead to local policies that exceed the letter of the law. For example, an institution with several citations from the USDA related to a particular problem may generate new policies to limit the potential for the problem to reoccur.

As a first step in working effectively with an IACUC, investigators should become familiar with the regulations that govern their work. The AWA and AWRs as well as the Guide are long and complex documents, although a synopsis of the AWA is available on the USDA website. In addition, the Guide (NRC 2011) is well indexed and is available on OLAW's website so that investigators can readily find pertinent information in the publication. Investigators are encouraged to obtain copies of these documents and to bookmark their IACUC's website so they can have easy access to pertinent information when writing animal use protocols or designing new studies. Many institutions offer seminars related to the care and use of laboratory animals, and investigators are encouraged to take advantage of these opportunities. If an investigator has limited time and seeks a condensed education regarding animal welfare regulations, they are encouraged to attend a national meeting that focuses on this topic. Organizations such as the Scientist's Center for Animal Welfare (SCAW; http://www.scaw.com) (SCAW 2014) and Public Responsibility in Medicine and Research (PRIM&R; www. primr.org) (PRIM&R 2014) offer annual conferences that can provide extensive training to an investigator within a few days. It is well worth the effort to attend such a meeting.

9.2 WRITING IACUC PROTOCOLS

The most important interaction between an investigator and their IACUC occurs when an investigator submits an animal use protocol (NIH 2002). A fundamental tenet of animal care and use regulations in the United States is the prospective review of all procedures to be performed on vertebrate animals. Failure to follow the procedures outlined in the IACUC-approved protocol or the performance of procedures that are not specified in the protocol are common causes of citations by the USDA to institutions (USDA 2014). Furthermore, the polices of the NIH require reporting of protocol deviations to the Office of Laboratory Animal Welfare (OLAW) (NIH 2002). The NIH does not permit the charging of procedures that were not approved by the IACUC to grants awarded by the agency (Brown 2012). Such circumstances always are problematic for an institution to deal with, since institutional funds must be diverted to cover the costs of the unapproved work.

The information required in an IACUC protocol is specified in the AWA and AWRs, PHS Policy, and the Guide. Although all institutions must abide by the same standards, the ways in which those standards are addressed in a protocol can vary. For example, the AWA mandates that planning of studies entailing procedures that may cause more than momentary or slight pain or distress include a consultation with the attending veterinarian (AV) or his or her designee (Cohen 2006). To address this mandate, some programs require investigators to schedule a face-to-face meeting with a veterinarian before a protocol is submitted. In other programs, a completed protocol must be sent to a veterinarian for preview, and the investigator must address comments from the veterinarian before the protocol is routed to the IACUC reviewers. A third common strategy is for the veterinary review to occur concurrently with the consideration of the protocol by IACUC members. Thus, to avoid frustration, investigators should schedule a meeting with the IACUC office director or IACUC chair soon after relocating to a new institution to become familiar with the processes used at that institution to consider animal care and use protocols. An IACUC typically collaborates with other regulatory offices (such as the radiation safety office and the biosafety office) when completing protocol reviews. Investigators should also learn about the dynamics of such interactions and whether applications to other offices should precede or accompany an IACUC protocol submission. Taking some time to understand the processes used by an institution's IACUC in managing the review of a protocol is well worth the effort.

A common mistake of principal investigators (PIs) is to delegate the writing of a protocol to a technician or junior laboratory member without proper oversight of the protocol preparation. Although a senior technician in a laboratory can contribute significantly to the planning of a study, they may not understand the scientific nuances of contemplated experiments, and thus could exclude crucial animal manipulations from the protocol. This may lead to the submission of an incomplete protocol to the IACUC, which raises concerns on the part of IACUC reviewers that could easily have been averted if the PI had thoroughly proofread and corrected the protocol. Considerable time for both IACUC reviewers and laboratory staff members can be saved when a senior investigator is actively involved in IACUC protocol preparation. Such oversight can also prevent the omission of animal manipulations from the protocol and findings of noncompliance related to performance of unapproved procedures.

As part of protocol review, an IACUC can require modifications prior to the approval of a study. The modifications should be weighed very deliberately and investigators should challenge any modifications that would prevent a study from being completed successfully. For example, the IACUC may approve studies that include pain and distress for animals provided that adequate justification is provided (Brown and Gipson 2012). Concerns on the part of IACUC reviewers often stem from an inadequately prepared protocol and are best addressed by providing the necessary information to the reviewers. If an investigator reaches an impasse in addressing IACUC concerns during protocol review, they should speak to the IACUC chair about strategies to overcome the impasse. It is typically possible to find a solution that meets the needs of the investigator while addressing the IACUC's concerns. However, under no circumstances should an investigator include the IACUC's suggestions in the protocol if they intend to perform different procedures in the laboratory. For instance, if an investigator believes that administration of an analgesic would interfere with a study, they should not include analgesic administration in the protocol "to get it past the IACUC," while planning to withhold analgesia during experiments. As noted above, deviation from the procedures outlined in a protocol is serious noncompliance that may lead to sanctions for the investigator and must be reported by the institution.

Although the information provided to the IACUC in protocols should be relatively detailed, it must not be so prescriptive that a deviation from the protocol is likely. The most effective protocols provide contingencies, such as alternate methods for euthanizing an animal. It is always helpful to anticipate potential problems in a study and to include strategies for addressing these problems in the protocol.

By its nature, scientific investigation is fluid, and corrections in strategies are often needed. New scientific strategies often entail the ordering of new reagents and supplies as well as the modification of existing IACUC protocols. Investigators should include in their planning sufficient time for the IACUC to process the protocol modification request and should also be aware of the average protocol-processing time for their IACUC office.

9.3 MAINTAINING CONGRUENCY BETWEEN
GRANTS AND IACUC PROTOCOLS

The NIH grants policy (NIH 2014a), as well as the policies of many other agencies that fund research grants, requires that an IACUC must assure that all the manipulations of animals proposed in a grant are addressed in approved IACUC protocols. For NIH grants, the congruency check usually occurs during the "just in time" period following the grant review and prior to the release of funding (NIH 2010). IACUCs address this mandate in a variety of ways, and investigators who submit research grants should become familiar with this mechanism. It is also worth noting that IACUC protocols must be considered *de novo* by the IACUC every three years, whereas a NIH grant can be funded for a period of up to five years. With rare exceptions (NIH 2014b), the NIH grants policy requires grantees to include all manipulations of animals in their protocols, even if that phase of the research will not start until year four or five of their PHS-funded grant. Although investigators frequently challenge this requirement, IACUCs at PHS-assured institutions must require this information in order to be in compliance with the NIH grants policy.

9.4 SEMIANNUAL INSPECTIONS: SCRUTINY OF AN
INVESTIGATOR'S RESEARCH PROGRAM BY THE IACUC

Nobody appreciates someone looking over their shoulder, but both the AWA and the Guide require that an IACUC maintain oversight of the Animal Care and Use Program (ACUP) that extends beyond the prospective review of animal care and use protocols (Dale 2008). For example, IACUCs are required to conduct semiannual inspections of areas where animals are housed or used in experiments, identify deviations in research practices from established guidelines, and formulate corrective actions for those deviations (USDA 2013, NIH 2002). IACUCs are also required to conduct a continuous review of animal research activities under 9 CFR §2.31 (d)(5). Many IACUCs fulfill this requirement by establishing additional procedures for postapproval monitoring (PAM) of studies (Dale 2008). Investigators must understand that continuous monitoring (such as through a PAM program) is expected and should make use of the opportunity to improve their procedures for animal care and use. During continuous monitoring, investigators have a prime opportunity to discuss their experimental problems with IACUC members and to develop strategies to improve experimental practices. Although investigators should never be confrontational with IACUC and administrative staff members during these sessions, they should feel comfortable in asking about the rationale for policies implemented by the IACUC and in suggesting improvements in the implementation of the policies. Continuous monitoring should be considered an opportunity for the education of investigators and their staff members as well as of the IACUC members participating in the sessions. If conducted appropriately, both the productivity of the investigator's laboratory and the implementation of IACUC policies will be improved.

An IACUC is also compelled to investigate concerns regarding the care and use of laboratory animals (9 CFR §2.31(c)(4); USDA 2013, NIH 2002). Such concerns often arise from animal facility staff members who note unanticipated animal morbidity or mortality as well as deviations from regulations, policies, or guidelines. Concerns may also arise from members of an investigator's own laboratory. It is natural to consider the raising of such concerns, particularly by a member of an investigator's own laboratory, as a betrayal. Under AWRs 9 CFR §2.32(c)(4), an institution is required to train those involved in animal activities on the methods whereby deficiencies in animal care and treatment are reported, with a provision that such a person or committee member cannot be discriminated against or be subject to reprisal as a result. The U.S. Department of Labor enforces protection against whistleblowers as well (USDL 2014). When the IACUC initiates an investigation related to a concern, the best strategy for an investigator to follow is to provide the IACUC with all of the information that is requested and to answer in good faith any questions that are raised. If the concern is credible, an investigator will likely minimize sanctions by acknowledging the validity of the concern. Sometimes whistleblower concerns are not credible and stem from the motivations of a disgruntled employee. An investigator should remain confident that if they cooperate fully in the ongoing investigation, they will be vindicated from false charges.

9.5 SOMETHING WENT WRONG: WHAT SHOULD I DO, AND HOW DO I PREVENT NONCOMPLIANCE IN THE FUTURE?

Nobody is perfect, and in spite of an investigator's diligence in running an exemplary research program, at some point a member of their laboratory will inevitably violate animal care and use regulations, policies, or guidelines. Such lapses may be unintentional and the result of a careless mistake or inattention. In addition, even when complying fully with the protocols approved by an IACUC, unexpected animal morbidity or mortality may occur. In such cases, the best strategy is to report the violation or animal welfare issues to the IACUC and to work proactively with the IACUC in formulating a corrective action plan. Even if the problem was serious, the IACUC's concerns will almost certainly be mitigated if the problem was reported and addressed by the investigator. This is especially true when an unanticipated event has compromised animal welfare. In such cases, rapid consultation with a veterinarian to minimize animal pain and distress is the only ethical path that an investigator can take. Experimental animals can be very expensive, and research problems diminish the productivity of a laboratory. Rapid mitigation of noncompliance or unanticipated problems will allow research productivity to continue unabated.

Investigators should also create an environment in their laboratory where all members are comfortable in communicating their concerns and mistakes so that problems are not covered up and allowed to become serious. It is additionally important to provide assistance to new laboratory members, who are most likely to make mistakes. Taking extra time to assure that new laboratory workers are well trained is worth the effort, as poorly trained individuals make mistakes that result in the loss of valuable time and resources.

The laboratory should foster collaboration, and not competition, between members. It is often helpful for laboratory members to work in teams in order to diminish the potential for omitting critical steps in procedures or failing to record a manipulation in an experimental record. At many institutions, undergraduate students have a desire to participate in laboratory research. Introducing undergraduate students to the laboratory environment is essential to assure that there is a stable scientific workforce in the future. A good assignment for such students is to manage record keeping for the more senior laboratory members and to perform cross-checks to assure that approved protocols are followed. By assigning appropriate tasks to undergraduate student volunteers, a PI can increase laboratory productivity while diminishing the risk of noncompliance.

Setting expectations that are too high is a recipe for disaster, since overworked individuals have a tendency to take shortcuts that lead to noncompliance with approved protocols. Investigators need to bear in mind that such noncompliance will cause serious problems with the IACUC and regulatory agencies, and that these problems have a considerable impact on productivity. Investigators should focus on long-term success and not short-term accomplishments by encouraging laboratory members to work carefully and diligently and by taking the time to double-check their work.

9.6 ESTABLISHING A POSITIVE RELATIONSHIP WITH THE IACUC

Some investigators mistakenly believe that the membership of their institution's IACUC is limited to veterinarians and administrators who have never worked in a laboratory. Although the AWRs only require a veterinarian and a nonaffiliated member to represent public concerns (9 CFR §2.31(b)(3)), many IACUCs have scientists as members to fulfill the PHS Policy. Rather than complaining about the policies formulated by an IACUC, it is a better strategy to become a member of the IACUC and help to shape institutional policies related to the use of animals. Most effective IACUCs include membership of stakeholders from a variety of departments to assure that none of its decisions will have adverse effects on scientific achievement. An investigator should learn if their department has a representative on the IACUC, and if it does, should communicate their concerns to that individual, who can then report them at an IACUC meeting. If an investigator's department is not represented on the IACUC, they should consider volunteering to serve on this important committee. There is no better way for an investigator to remain familiar with animal welfare regulation, and learn effective strategies for managing a compliant laboratory than to serve as an IACUC member. If an investigator is interested in serving on the IACUC, they should discuss this interest with the IACUC chair, IACUC office director, AV, or IO.

Even if an investigator does not have the opportunity to become a member of their institution's IACUC, they have the ability to influence the committee and should take advantage of this opportunity. Most importantly, if an investigator believes that an IACUC policy could be implemented in a better fashion, they should communicate their concern to the IACUC chair or ask to speak to the IACUC members at the next convened meeting. It is possible that the IACUC was not aware of all of the implications of the policy when it was formulated and may be willing to modify the policy on the basis of concerns. If an investigator believes that the IACUC is not functioning as well as it could, then their specific concerns should be relayed to the IACUC chair or IO.

A weakness of some IACUCs is that decisions and policies are not communicated effectively to the research community. Investigators should attempt to work proactively with the IACUC in assuring that a two-way dialogue is maintained. However, any feedback from investigators to the IACUC should be constructive and not provided in a combative fashion. Most IACUCs attempt to implement governmental mandates and the requirements of granting agencies in the fashion that is least onerous to investigators. Accordingly, investigators should learn about the rationale for any new policies or decisions before offering criticism.

9.7 REDUCING REGULATORY BURDEN BY ESTABLISHING A CULTURE OF COMPLIANCE

In most laboratories, students, technicians, and postdoctoral associates perform the majority of the manipulations on animals, and thus it is essential to assure that all laboratory members are committed to compliance with IACUC policies. Failure to faithfully follow the protocols approved by the IACUC is one of the most common problems in a laboratory, and to avoid this problem, all laboratory members must be familiar with the protocols relevant to their work. Copies of IACUC protocols should be readily available in the areas where animal manipulations occur so they can be easily referenced. It is often helpful to circulate protocols to all laboratory members as they are being written in order to assure that no animal manipulations are excluded from the protocol. The protocols should be reviewed periodically at laboratory meetings to assure that laboratory members understand which manipulations of animals have been approved. All laboratory members should also have access to the IACUC's policies, and those relevant to ongoing work in the laboratory should be discussed during laboratory meetings, particularly after those policies have been revised by the IACUC. Taking these steps will generate a culture of compliance in the laboratory.

Mentorship regarding animal care and use regulations should be provided for all new laboratory members. To facilitate such mentorship, it is useful to appoint a local expert in animal care and use regulations. Some investigators hire a laboratory manager whose primary role is to remain acquainted with the policies generated by the IACUC and other regulatory committees at the institution and to assure that they are implemented properly in the laboratory. Such an individual can also take charge of mandatory laboratory record keeping as well as training of new laboratory members. Since students and postdoctoral associates tend to remain in a laboratory for a limited time, it is often best to designate a senior laboratory technician as the laboratory manager. A seasoned laboratory manager can relieve a considerable portion of an investigator's administrative burden; thus, these individuals are highly valuable.

Many IACUCs have implemented policies and requirements that exceed those prescribed by the government or funding agencies. Often, the IACUC is compelled to take measures that pose a burden to all investigators due to continuing noncompliance with existing policies. The old adage "one rotten apple spoils the barrel" certainly applies to the research environment, since onerous regulatory burden often stems from the egregious actions of a minority of investigators. For instance, NIH was pressured by Congress to implement burdensome conflict-of-interest regulations due to the inappropriate relationships of a few scientists with industry (Lo and Field 2009). Thus, equally as important as maintaining a compliant laboratory is reminding your colleagues about the importance of compliance. Institutional leaders should also strive to establish a culture of compliance, which balances rewards for compliant investigators with sanctions for noncompliance. By exerting peer pressure on their colleagues, investigators can go a long way toward eliminating the occurrences of noncompliance that lead to regulatory burden.

9.8 EFFECTS OF ADVOCACY GROUPS

A major goal of the animal rights movement is to reduce or eliminate the use of animals in biomedical research. Successful actions of animal advocacy groups have resulted in increased regulations, which have led to increased research costs (Ludmerer 2005). It is the author's opinion that legislators may receive a false perspective about animal research from these advocacy groups and as a result may enact burdensome new laws and regulations that do little to improve animal welfare. Investigators are encouraged to become more vigilant and aware of the concerns and petitions raised by these groups and to exercise their ability to exert political influence on local, state, or federal policy makers as well. Many professional societies distribute alerts to their members when state or local governments are considering laws that are in opposition to animal research. Investigators should pay close attention to such alerts and contact their representatives to provide a balanced perspective about the potential impacts of the new law.

One of the most effective tools used by activists who strive to eliminate animal use in biomedical research is to publicize noncompliance with animal use regulations, particularly when the noncompliance has affected animal welfare. Since the USDA lists violations of the AWA and AWRs on its website, such violations are public information. Animal rights groups can gain access to reports made by an institution to OLAW through provisions of the Freedom of Information Act (FOIA). At public institutions, IACUC records such as noncompliance notices to investigators or findings from semiannual inspections may be obtained through the provisions of state laws on open records. When publicized by animal rights groups, such reports and records provide a negative perspective about animal research to members of the public, including legislators. In light of this, it is in the research community's best interest to ensure full compliance with animal welfare regulations at all times.

9.9 SUMMARY

This chapter has provided commonsense steps that investigators can take to maximize their productivity by effectively managing the ACUP in their laboratory. These steps include becoming familiar with the laws, regulations, and policies that govern animal use and fostering a laboratory environment where all members are dedicated to regulatory compliance. Protocols submitted for IACUC review must be thorough and accurate, while at the same time not so prescriptive that they will likely result in noncompliance at some point. Investigators should treat an IACUC-approved protocol as if it were a contract with their institution, as violations have very serious repercussions. Investigators should work toward establishing a two-way dialogue with their IACUC and consider the IACUC to be a partner in their research program. Finally, investigators must always bear in mind the high price of noncompliance with animal care regulations, which often includes additional regulatory burden. Animal rights groups publicize instances of noncompliance in an attempt to undermine animal research and to convince legislators that further restrictions on animal research are needed. Any short-term time savings achieved by circumventing animal use regulations or conducting procedures that are not approved will eventually be erased by the sanctions and additional regulatory burden that follow the discovery of these activities by the IACUC or regulatory agencies.

REFERENCES

Brown, P. 2012. OLAW online seminar: Grants policy and congruence. Office of Laboratory Animal Welfare, NIH, Bethesda, MD.

Brown, P. and C. Gipson. 2012. Response to protocol review scenario: A word from OLAW and USDA. *Lab Animal* 41:220.

Cohen, H. 2006. The Animal Welfare Act. *Journal of Animal Law* 12:13–26.

Dale, W. E. 2008. Postapproval monitoring and the role of the compliance office. *ILAR Journal* 49 (4):393–401.

Haywood, J. R. and M. Greene. 2008. Avoiding an overzealous approach: A perspective on regulatory burden. *ILAR Journal* 49 (4):426–434.

Lo, B. and M. J. Field. 2009. *Conflict of Interest in Medical Research, Education, and Practice*. Washington, DC: National Academies Press.

Ludmerer, K. M. 2005. *Time to Heal: American Medical Education from the Turn of the Century to the Era of Managed Care*. New York: Oxford University Press.

NIH (National Institutes of Health). 2002. Public Health Service policy on humane care and use of laboratory animals. Office of Laboratory Animal Welfare, US Department of Health and Human Services, NIH, Bethesda, MD.

NIH (National Institutes of Health). 2010. NOT-OD-10-120: Revised policy on applicant institution responsibilities for ensuring just-in-time submissions are accurate and current up to the time of award. Office of Laboratory Animal Welfare, NIH, Bethesda, MD.

NIH (National Institutes of Health). 2014a. Frequently asked questions: PHS policy on humane care and use of laboratory animals: Is the IACUC required to review the grant application? Office of Laboratory Animal Welfare, NIH, Bethesda, MD. http://grants.nih.gov/grants/olaw/faqs.htm#proto_10.

NIH (National Institutes of Health). 2014b. Frequently asked questions: PHS policy on humane care and use of laboratory animals: Does the IACUC have to review proposed animal research activities at the time of grant award if the animal research activities will not be conducted until year 4 or 5 of a grant? Office of Laboratory Animal Welfare, NIH, Bethesda, MD. http://grants.nih.gov/grants/olaw/faqs.htm#proto_20.

NRC (National Research Council). 2011. *Guide for the Care and Use of Laboratory Animals.* 8th edn. Washington, DC: National Academies Press.

PRIM&R (Public Responsibility in Medicine and Research). 2014. PRIM&R home page. http://www.primr.org/.

SCAW (Scientists Center for Animal Welfare). 2014. SCAW home page. http://www.scaw.com/.

USDA (U.S. Department of Agriculture). 2013. *Animal Welfare Act and Animal Welfare Regulations* (Animal Care Blue Book). Code of Federal Regulations (CFR), Title 9, Chapter 1, Subchapter A, Parts 1–4.

USDA (U.S. Department of Agriculture). 2014. USDA Animal and Plant Health Inspection Service enforcement actions: 2010–2014. USDA, APHIS http://www.aphis.usda.gov/wps/portal/enforcementactions.

USDL (U.S. Department of Labor). 2014. The whistleblower protection programs. USDL, Washington, DC. http://www.whistleblowers.gov/.

CHAPTER **10**

Interactions with Other Institutional Panels

William G. Greer

CONTENTS

10.1 INTRODUCTION

The research, teaching, and testing programs of institutions frequently include regulated activities. For example, scientists conducting research that involves animal or human participants, recombinant or synthetic nucleic acids, hazardous materials, or human embryonic stem cells (hESCs) must adhere to federal standards. Regulations vary according to the type of research conducted, but the common theme is the federal requirement for self-monitoring. The philosophy of self-regulation is to afford a diverse group of institutions the necessary flexibility to develop oversight programs that support the scientific expertise and research initiatives of the organization while satisfying the governing responsibilities (Bartle and Vass 2005).

The responsibilities of oversight committees frequently overlap since a single research design may include more than one regulated component. The intent of this chapter is to discuss the interactions of the Institutional Animal Care and Use Committee (IACUC) with other oversight panels and regulatory agencies. It will also identify situations when compliance committees have shared oversight responsibilities, and the methodologies that are employed to maximize the overall efficiency of institutions' compliance programs.

10.2 REGULATORY OVERSIGHT OF RESEARCH

10.2.1 The Institution's Responsibilities

When the management of an institution decides to establish a research program, they must first commit the necessary financial and human resources to develop the programmatic framework and facilitate the related activities.

If animal use activities are to be funded by any Public Health Service (PHS) Agency or involve U.S. Department of Agriculture (USDA)-covered species, the institution must develop a program that complies with applicable regulatory standards such as the *Guide for the Care and Use of Laboratory Animals* (the Guide) (NRC 2011), the PHS Policy on Humane Care and Use of Laboratory Animals (NIH 2002), and the Animal Welfare Act Regulations (AWRs) (USDA 2013). For example, the Guide (p. 14) and the PHS Policy (IV,A,1,f) require institutions to establish, as part of their overall Animal Care and Use Program (ACUP), an Occupational Health and Safety Program (OHSP) that mitigates personnel risks associated with animal-based research.

In addition to establishing program oversight committees, institutions are frequently required to make formal (i.e., in writing) commitments to governing agencies of their adherence to federal mandates and policies. For example, institutions that are interested in conducting PHS-supported activities involving vertebrate animals must formally assure the Office for Laboratory Animal Welfare (OLAW) that animal use activities will comply with applicable federal policies. The Animal Welfare Assurance specifically includes the statement that: "This Institution will comply with all applicable provisions of the Animal Welfare Act and other Federal statutes." The Assurance is also reviewed and approved by OLAW, and describes specifically how the institution will comply with applicable federal policies. In addition, and as part of the USDA annual reporting requirements, each institution assures the USDA that "The facility is adhering to the standards and regulations under the Act" when USDA-covered vertebrate animals (9 U.S.C., Chapter 1, Subchapter A, Part 1, §1.1) are used. In other circumstances, research facilities make ongoing compliance assurances with regulating bodies (e.g., the Office of Biotechnology Activities [OBA] and the Office for Human Research Protection [OHRP]) through annual reporting and frequent communication.

10.2.2 Health and Safety of Research Staff and Animals (i.e., Occupational Health and Safety)

According to the standards governing animal-based research (NRC 1983), each institution must establish an OHSP as part of its overall ACUP. The OHSP includes components for identifying, assessing, and mitigating animal-related risks. All personnel who are engaged in activities that support the institution's ACUP must participate in the OHSP.

The OHSP should include provisions to protect individuals from zoonotic diseases, animal allergens, physical injuries (e.g., bites, kicks, and scratches), and any other related hazards. As part of the OHSP, an institution may purchase personal protective equipment (PPE) such as respirators and laboratory coats and require personnel to use it. Workers may also be immunized against common diseases such as tetanus. Although the responsibility for establishing the OHSP lies with the institution, the IACUC is specifically charged with the oversight and evaluation of the ACUP. Since the OHSP is part of the overall ACUP, the IACUC also has to assume at least partial responsibility for the OHSP.

10.2.2.1 Risk Assessment, Awareness, and Mitigation

The institution must establish processes to assess and mitigate the level of risk associated with its ACUP. It must also develop personnel training programs to educate staff members on the risks that are inherent in animal research and methods to minimize them.

To ensure that quality risk assessments are conducted, the institution must engage appropriately trained individuals. The assessment team may include personnel from health-care management, environmental health and safety, veterinary services, risk management, and the IACUC. Health-care personnel may medically evaluate each individual to determine his or her unique susceptibilities; an industrial hygienist may identify and quantify environmental hazards; veterinary staff members may focus on the specific zoonotic diseases of each animal species; and risk management employees may define the amount of risk that the institution is willing to accept.

The assessment process involves identifying both physical and biological hazards presented by animals and animal-based research (NIH ARENA 2002). It should consider the medical predisposition of each employee and his or her exposure levels to the animals. In addition, the assessment process must include an evaluation of the risks associated with the equipment (e.g., cage washers, autoclaves, and feed storage silos) that is required to maintain and operate the program. The assessment process must be ongoing and include periodic evaluations. Each research activity that may introduce a new hazard to the program must be assessed. The OSHP should include an ongoing monitoring program, which may involve reevaluating existing hazards. In addition, occupational health incidents and the history of those employees who have been actively engaged in animal-based research over the years at the institution may be considered during the ongoing evaluation.

10.2.3 Protecting the Environment

In addition to ensuring the health and well-being of animal program personnel, the institution must also protect the environment from hazards that are generated from animal-based research. Animal-based research may involve the use of hazards such as recombinant nucleic acids, carcinogens, toxins, infectious agents, or radioactive materials. During the assessment of research activities, the IACUC frequently works in conjunction with the Institutional Biosafety Committee (IBC) and other institutional safety committees to ensure that hazards are effectively managed and disposed of appropriately. The committees collectively develop processes for containing, categorizing, and eliminating hazards.

10.3 OVERSIGHT PANELS' RESPONSIBILITIES

The standards specifically mandate that institutions establish committees to assess and oversee research program activities and components. The OHRP, within the U.S. Department of Health and Human Services (HHS), enforces the requirement for establishing an institutional review board (IRB) to oversee human participant research supported by or otherwise subject to regulation by the HHS (Penslar 1993). OLAW, within the National Institutes of Health (NIH), implements a similar requirement to establish an IACUC to oversee all PHS-conducted or supported activities involving vertebrate animals. Similarly, the OBA, within the NIH, ensures that institutions establish an IBC to oversee research involving recombinant or synthetic nucleic acid molecules. In addition to establishing federally mandated committees, institutions frequently establish other groups to oversee and administer internal policies and guidelines. For example, an Embryonic Stem Cell Research Oversight (ESCRO or SCRO) committee is established to oversee human embryonic stem cell research, and various safety committees are formed to oversee research involving radioactive materials, hazardous chemicals, nanoparticles, or toxins.

The NIH Guidelines for Research Involving Recombinant or Synthetic Nucleic Acid Molecules (NIH 2013) require IBCs to include individuals with skills that enable them to assess the safety of recombinant or synthetic nucleic acid molecule research, and to identify any potential risk to public health or the environment. Consequently, and depending on the institution's research profile, the IBC must include individuals with expertise in plant and animal containment principles, the institution's biological safety officer (BSO), and two members not affiliated with the institution. The National Academy of Science (NAS) Guidelines for Human Embryonic Stem Cell Research (NRC 2005) require ESCRO members to be, at a minimum, scientists with collective expertise in the areas of stem cell research, developmental biology, molecular biology, assisted reproduction, and ethics and law; and a member who is unaffiliated with the institution. In addition, other oversight committees (i.e., the IRB and the radiation and safety committees) and internal departments (i.e., Environmental Health and Safety [EHS] and Occupational Medicine) at an institution typically include individuals with varying backgrounds to facilitate a complete and adequate review and oversight of research activities that are commonly conducted by the institution. The overall objective of committee diversification is to ensure that institutions, through their committee membership, have the necessary expertise to maintain compliant research programs, and have the ability to adapt to emerging trends associated with research activities.

The authorities of the research committee oversight panels are granted by federal law and policy. The PHS Policy and the AWRs specifically identify and define the responsibilities of the IACUC. Its service to the institution is essential since it ensures that the ACUP remains compliant with the governing standards and institutional policies. On behalf of the institutions, the chief executive officer (CEO) or the institutional official (IO) and senior management team are charged with identifying and interpreting the regulations, and developing animal care and use-relevant policies that reflect the responsible research initiatives of the organization.

10.4 PRINCIPAL INVESTIGATORS' RESPONSIBILITIES

The Guide indicates that: "Both researchers and institutions have affirmative duties of humane care and use that are supported by practical, ethical and scientific principles" (NRC 2011). Since the federal mandates were established to facilitate scientific principles, while ensuring the humane care and treatment of animals, researchers, as well as institutional leaders, share the responsibility of complying with federal standards governing research. Studies must be conducted according to regulatory standards, thus the researchers should work together with the compliance oversight committees to remain compliant.

10.5 HARMONIZING INSTITUTIONAL PANELS

As stewards of the institution, and on occasion by institutional policy, IACUC members have a shared responsibility of ensuring that animal-based research activities comply with not only the governing standards on animal use, but also all other relevant regulations. At times, animal-based research may involve nucleic acid recombination techniques that must be registered with or reviewed and approved by the institution's IBC. The research may include interactions between animals and human subjects that must be reviewed and approved by the IACUC and the IRB. A key component of harmonizing oversight panel interactions is to develop clear and concise methods of communication. Institutions must identify and implement ways to efficiently coordinate the committees' shared oversight responsibilities. At some institutions, the IACUC and IBC members conduct concurrent reviews, with each committee satisfying its specific responsibilities. In this scenario, the IACUC only approves the project after the IBC completes its assessment, and if necessary, approves of the recombinant procedures identified in the project. In addition to oversight committees conducting parallel reviews, some institutions may establish a team (i.e., a subcommittee) of the same individuals with specific qualifications to serve on both the IACUC and the IBC. The team members may contribute to satisfying the membership requirements of both committees, and may include expertise, for example, in animal health and containment procedures, viral vectors, human health and safety, and governing regulations. The subcommittee members often conduct both the IACUC and IBC reviews. Members may serve as an IACUC designated member reviewer, or summarize and answer committee questions about a submission during the full committee review (FCR) process.

10.5.1 Biosafety Committee

Like the IACUC, the IBC is an oversight committee that by federal mandate oversees government-regulated research involving recombinant or synthetic nucleic acid molecules. Thus, the IBC reviews, approves, and monitors all such research. It ensures that recombinant nucleic acid research is safe for the environment, animals, and humans. Animal-based research often involves recombinant nucleic acid research, for example, research involving transgenic animals. Institutions frequently assign additional responsibilities to the IBC. For example, an IBC may be designated to oversee research involving infectious agents, hazardous chemicals, or nanoparticles. In such situations, the IACUC and the IBC must establish systematic processes to ensure that the NIH Guidelines, the PHS Policy, the Guide, and the AWRs are satisfied. In all circumstances, the committee should be properly constituted with the expertise that is needed to conduct a sound assessment of the research.

10.5.1.1 Recombinant Nucleic Acid (e.g., DNA and RNA) Research

Through federal statutes, various government agencies oversee activities involving recombinant nucleic acid research. Nucleic acid molecules include both DNA and RNA. DNA provides the genetic code to produce the organism, and RNA interprets and converts the genetic code to proteins that comprise the organism's biological systems.

If an institution conducts NIH-supported recombinant or synthetic nucleic acid molecule research, all regulated nucleic acid technology, whether NIH funded or not, will be governed by the OBA. The OBA uses the NIH Guidelines for Research Involving Recombinant or Synthetic Nucleic Acid Molecules (NIH 2013) as the oversight standards. Section 1A states: "The purpose of the NIH Guidelines is to specify the practices for constructing and handling: (i) recombinant nucleic acid molecules, (ii) synthetic nucleic acid molecules, including those that are chemically or otherwise modified but can base pair with naturally occurring nucleic acid molecules, and (iii) cells, organisms, and viruses containing such molecules." Simply stated, the primary objectives of the NIH Guidelines are to ensure that recombinant technology is conducted safely, and that all nucleic acid molecules are adequately contained.

The Food and Drug Administration (FDA) controls animals that are exposed to recombinant or synthetic nucleic acid molecules under the provisions of the Federal Food, Drug, and Cosmetic Act (FFDCA) and FDA regulations. In the FFDCA, the FDA defines the term *drug* as "articles (other than food) intended to affect the structure or any function of the body of man or other animals" (Sec. 201. [21 USC §321]). A segment of nucleic acid placed inside an organism is intended to affect the structure or function of that organism and consequently meets the definition of a drug. If the nucleic acid construct is placed inside an animal, the FDA considers the construct to be a new animal drug and regulates it accordingly. As a result, any recombinant or synthetic nucleic acid molecule that is to be used commercially must first be approved by the FDA in accordance with the FFDCA and the FDA regulations.

Additional government agencies overseeing activities involving recombinant DNA technology include the Animal and Plant Health Inspection Service (APHIS), the Food Safety Inspection Service (FSIS), and the Environmental Protection Agency (EPA) (Mendelsohn et al. 2003). The FSIS is responsible for ensuring that concentrations of new animal drug residues do not exceed the FDA's acceptable levels, while the EPA ensures that the environment is not adversely affected by, for example, genetically engineered (GE) plants and animals.

Scientists frequently use nucleic acid research to alter the genetic profile of an organism (i.e., genetically engineer). The process is initiated when laboratory practices are used to isolate or synthesize a segment of nucleic acids, which may code for a specific characteristic or the production of a protein of interest. The molecule is produced either by isolating a segment of nucleic acids from the genes of naturally occurring organisms or by synthesizing it from scratch in the laboratory. Once developed, scientists often integrate it into the genetic profile of an organism so that new or altered traits can be expressed. Recombinant technology is routinely used in biomedical research. For example, the DNA of a bacterium such as *Escherichia coli* can be altered to include a segment of nucleic acid that codes for insulin production. Consequently, the human pharmaceuticals industry can produce large quantities of *E. coli* that produce insulin as a by-product. In addition, scientists studying human breast cancer can incorporate a segment of nucleic acid into the DNA of a mouse, resulting in the animal acquiring breast cancer. The researcher can then use the mouse model to identify treatments and cures. Recombinant technology may also be used to develop wheat and corn that has an increased resistance to drought conditions or pests.

In the course of reviewing animal-based research, IACUC members often encounter research activities that must be overseen by both the IACUC and the IBC. For example, a researcher may use a viral vector to incorporate a specific segment of DNA into the genome of a mouse. Since viral particles execute at the molecular level by efficiently incorporating their genome into cells, they are frequently used as vectors to introduce nucleic acid segments into living organisms. To produce viral vectors, scientists alter the genome of a virus to regulate the expression of genes that then might result in disease or illness in the animal. In cases such as this, the IACUC and the IBC must collaborate to ensure that the AWRs, the PHS Policy, the Guide, and the NIH Guidelines are satisfied.

10.5.1.2 Transgenic Laboratory Animals

The NIH Guidelines define a transgenic laboratory animal as one in which its "genome has been altered by the stable introduction of recombinant or synthetic nucleic acid molecules, or nucleic acids derived therefrom, into the germ-line" (NIH 2009b). The OBA and the FDA regulate traditional transgenic laboratory animals.

10.5.1.3 OBA

The OBA regulates the production and containment of traditional transgenic laboratory animals using the NIH Guidelines as the standards. The NIH Guidelines (Section III-D-4-a) include a mandate that requires assigning a risk level to transgenic animals that are produced. They define a process for classifying transgenic animals that is comparable with the Biosafety in Microbiological and Medical Laboratories (BMBL) classification system (BL1–BL4) for propagating or physically containing etiological agents. The NIH Guidelines ask scientists to classify transgenic animals into risk groups (RG) according to their potential to cause disease in healthy adult humans (NIH 2013). Those animals posing minimal risk (RG1) would not be associated with disease in healthy adult humans; with the extreme being those animals posing maximum risk (RG4) and would likely cause serious or lethal human disease. The NIH Guidelines define risk classification as a subjective process, and require the scientists and the IBC to identify the level of risk. Once the risk assignments are made, the institution, under the oversight of the IBC and the IACUC, must house the animals according to both animal care and use standards (USDA 2013, NRC 2011) and the NIH Guidelines (Appendix Q, Physical and Biological Containment for Recombinant or Synthetic Nucleic Acid Molecule Research Involving Animals) (NIH 2013).

10.5.1.4 FDA

All animals containing nucleic acid constructs are subject to FDA regulation under the new animal drug provisions of the FFDCA. In general, FDA oversight for very-low-risk laboratory animals is minimal, but the level of agency oversight increases with risk.

10.5.1.5 Transgenic "Food" Animals

The OBA applies the NIH Guidelines consistently to all species of animals, but the FDA increases the level of its oversight when agricultural species are used, especially animals that are traditionally consumed by humans as food. It is important to note that the FDA does not consider the transgenic animal the new animal drug, but rather the nucleic acid construct that the animal contains. Likewise, although the FDA defines a nucleic acid construct as an investigational drug, it is only regulated when it enters an animal's system. The FDA has identified all animals receiving nucleic acid constructs as GE animals. There are multiple ways that the construct can enter the animal: (1) consumed as part of the animal's feed, (2) injected into the animal, or (3) experimentally incorporated into the animal's genome.

The FDA ensures that products entering the human food supply are safe. This process includes ensuring food animals only receive drugs that have been determined "safe for use" by the FDA. Drug safety is determined during an FDA-prescribed investigational phase. During the investigational phase, GE animals are evaluated to determine whether they can enter the food supply. The investigational phase involves: (1) evaluating the construct's purpose and molecular structure; (2) determining how the construct entered the animal's system and the impact that it will have on the animal's health; (3) conducting an environmental impact assessment; and (4) determining whether the GE animal is safe for human and animal consumption. The FDA has imposed strong statutory requirements during the investigational phase, and has currently not approved any GE animals to enter the food supply.

Institutions with scientists who are engaging in GE animal research must maintain comprehensive records and register each study with the FDA. For example, scientists must maintain a list of all GE animals produced and document the disposition of each. The records should document, for example, that an animal is still part of an ongoing investigational study, was euthanized and incinerated, or was shipped to a different location. Each GE animal must be clearly labeled "not for human use." The records must be maintained for two years after the investigation is concluded, or the new drug is approved for use.

APHIS has a federal mandate to oversee and protect the health of animals that are used for commercial purposes (i.e., species of livestock) in the United States. Since the potential effects that GE animals might have on the overall health of U.S. livestock remain unknown, APHIS prohibits animals exposed to recombinant or synthetic nucleic acid molecules from being introduced into commercial herds of livestock, and from being sold for commercial purposes.

10.5.1.6 Infectious Disease Research

Animal-based research often involves the use of agents (i.e., viruses and bacteria) that can cause disease in healthy adult humans or animals or both. Many scientific studies focus on organisms that have the potential to cause disease in animals, but not humans. This research should prompt the IACUC to work together with the facility manager and veterinarian to establish a biosecurity plan that will protect naïve animals from infection. The containment plan may list, for example, the required attire for entering the animal suite, the appropriate measures for disposing of contaminated bedding and dead animals, and the methods for disinfecting contaminated rooms and caging.

When research involves animals and human pathogens, the institution's IACUC and IBC must review and approve the protocol (HHS 2009). During the review process, both committees should assess the risk and ensure the well-being of workers. In each situation, the institution may develop a process for quantifying the risk that each agent poses to the health of personnel and the animals. The Centers for Disease Control and Prevention (CDC) have developed a Biological Risk Assessment Worksheet, available on the CDC's website (http://www.cdc.gov/biosafety/publications/BiologicalRiskAssessmentWorksheet.pdf), which helps institutions facilitate the risk assessment process. Questions from the CDC assessment tool are frequently incorporated into more complex assessment methodologies that are used by an institution. Animals alone present unique circumstances that are not typically associated with standard microbiological research laboratories. They can infect handlers with zoonotic or research-derived agents through generated aerosols, bites, or scratches. The CDC and the USDA (HHS 2009) (Appendix D, 343) employ containment levels that include additional precaution criteria not typical of a standard microbiology laboratory.

During assessment and containment planning for infectious disease research involving animal models, the IACUC and other units within the organization must collaborate. The IACUC, personnel from the Office of Occupational Medicine, the EHS, and Animal Resources must collectively develop plans to protect the health and safety of research staff. The plans frequently include, for example, a standard operating procedure for entering the vivarium, and the appropriate use of biohazard signage, which may be posted on the room entry door. In addition, the team may develop intensive training that educates technicians on topics such as the proper handling of infected animals, the use of laminar flow equipment, and the appropriate disposal of contaminated materials. In addition, the IACUC and the institutional health professional may develop medical information cards to be carried by principal investigators (PIs) and their staff working with infectious agents. A card may identify the infectious agent and symptoms of an infection, as well as provide specific information that would be useful to medical care professionals.

10.5.1.7 Potential Sources (e.g., Human-Derived Tissues) of Blood-Borne Pathogens

The Occupational Safety and Health Administration (OSHA) standard, 29 CFR, defines blood-borne pathogens as "pathogenic microorganisms that are present in human blood and can cause disease in humans. These pathogens include, but are not limited to, hepatitis B virus (HBV) and human immunodeficiency virus (HIV)" (OSHA 2014a).

The OSHA standard, 29 CFR 1910.1030(c), and the OSHA publication 3127 (USDL 1996) also include provisions for establishing a blood-borne pathogens exposure control program. In addition, the NIH Guidelines require individuals working with human immunodeficiency virus (HIV), hepatitis B virus (HBV), or other blood-borne pathogens to comply with 29 CFR. These federal standards require employees who are exposed to human-derived materials to be included in a blood-borne pathogens exposure control program, which includes participation in required training, and a hepatitis B vaccination program.

Animal-based research often involves exposing animals to tissues of human origin—in other words, potential sources of blood-borne pathogens. For example, neoplasia studies may include injecting animals with human breast or prostate cancer cells to induce tumor development (Hutchinson and Muller 2000). In situations such as these, the human tissues are handled and contained as potential sources of infectious disease—blood-borne pathogens. The IACUC frequently partners with the institution's Health and Safety Office or occupational medicine department by facilitating the enrollment of staff members working with sources of blood-borne pathogens into the institution's blood-borne pathogens exposure control program. Although methodologies vary from institution to institution, a common practice is for the IACUC to withhold protocol approval until the blood-borne pathogen requirements are satisfied.

10.5.1.8 Animal Research and Invertebrate Vectors: Culicidae and Arachnids (i.e., Mosquitoes and Ticks)

Humans are at risk from viral and bacterial infections transmitted by mosquitoes, ticks, fleas, and other invertebrate vectors. Vector-borne diseases common to the United States include Lyme disease, West Nile virus, and Rocky Mountain spotted fever (CDC 2014). In addition, other vector-borne diseases such as malaria and dengue fever are global problems (Benedict et al. 2003). Scientists and the CDC are actively focused on identifying prevention and control strategies for these diseases. For scientists to achieve their research goals, they frequently must use invertebrate vectors such as mosquitoes or ticks as part of their animal-based research design. Consequently, scientists may need to contain colonies of, for example, mosquitoes, some of which may be carrying disease agents such as West Nile virus or the causative agent of malaria. Institutions engaged in this type of research should consider appointing scientists with expertise in vector-borne diseases to the IACUC. Scientists experienced in this type of research are frequently knowledgeable in arthropod containment guidelines and can assist the institution in establishing and maintaining an insectary that can be used to contain the arthropod vectors used in animal-based research.

10.5.1.9 Nanomaterials

At the 1857 Bakerian Lecture, Experimental Relations of Gold (and Other Metals) to Light, Michael Faraday first described nanoparticles scientifically

(Faraday 1857). Since that time, advancements in nanotechnology have set the stage for cutting-edge research with unforeseen potential. A primary concept of nanotechnology is to advance human knowledge by experimenting at the molecular level. In biological systems, a shared theme for scientists is to develop atomic size particles (i.e., nanoparticles) with specific molecular recognition properties. Modern science has led to the development of nanoparticles with specificity (i.e., molecular recognition) to cancer cells, for example. As a result, nanoparticles can be used to deliver chemotherapeutic drugs, fluorescent dyes, or radioactive therapeutics specifically to cancer cells (Hanley et al. 2009). Researchers are also developing nanoparticles that can be used to treat infectious diseases, diabetes, and neurological disorders. For nanotechnology techniques to evolve toward treatments for human disease, animal-based research will be necessary.

In 1983, the National Research Council (NRC) published *Risk Assessment in the Federal Government: Managing the Process* (NRC 1983). Congress mandated that federal agencies use this document as the standard approach for conducting risk assessments. A paradigm for assessing chemical-, drug-, or agent-related risks was standardized, but whether it can be applied to nanoparticles is currently under consideration. The risk assessment is based on (1) evidence that a substance is toxic; (2) the dose required for a substance to be toxic; (3) the level of exposure that a population may experience; and (4) whether the population exposure level is toxic. The innovative use of nanotechnology has resulted in extensive application research data with only limited information produced on nanoparticle safety. Campaigns are underway to gather data on human health and safety risks associated with nanoparticles. For example, the International Council on Nanotechnology maintains a virtual library of scientific papers associated with nanoparticle health and safety topics. However, whether adequate information exists for government agencies to conduct risk assessments remains questionable.

Congress has identified federal agencies to assess product risk levels and regulate their use accordingly. For example, the FDA regulates human consumables such as food and drugs, and the OSHA ensures the safe use of chemicals in the workplace. In 2007, an FDA task force concluded that nanoparticles pose no significant public safety risk; consequently, no specific government agency has been identified to regulate the use of nanoparticles in research.

IACUC members who are considering animal-based research that involves nanotechnology will be forced to consider the uncertainties, which cannot be discounted when a risk assessment is conducted. Considering that nanoparticles are able to pass through cellular membranes, how they enter a biological system is unclear. The potential may exist for individuals to be exposed through respiration, by contact, or ingestion (MacPhail et al. 2013). Consequently, the institution and the IACUC should share the responsibility of ensuring the health and welfare of those individuals who are engaged in nanoparticle animal-based research with other experts at the institution. In order to best consider the uncertainties, committees may seek advice from the EHS, Occupational Medicine, and the research community members (i.e., a scientist experienced in nanotechnology). In each case, the team should consider the specific physical characteristics of each nanoparticle. Collectively, the combined expertise of this group may be better equipped to consider, for example, that some nanoparticles entering a biological system may quickly degrade and pose little risk while others may be very stable and accumulate within the system having long-term unknown consequences. In addition, they may define specific safety equipment and PPE that must be employed during nanoparticle use. The group may also define how nanoparticle-exposed animals and animal bedding will be discarded.

10.5.1.10 Select Agents

In the event that animal-based research includes the use of select agents, the institution must comply with the federal select agent regulations (42 CFR Part 73 [HHS 2005], 7 CFR Part 331 [USDA 2005a], and 9 CFR Part 121 [USDA 2005b]), which are enforced through the HHS and the USDA. The HHS defines select agents as "biological agents and toxins that have the potential to pose a severe threat to public health and safety, to animal health, or to animal products" (HHS/USDA 2014). The list of select agents is updated as necessary and maintained directly in 42 CFR Part §73.3, HHS select agents and toxins; and Part §73.4, overlap select agents and toxins.

Institutions that are interested in pursuing research activities involving select agents must successfully complete an intensive registration and approval process through the appropriate regulatory agencies. The institution must establish a multifaceted select agent program that includes, for example, a high-level security program, a thorough training program, and a comprehensive record-keeping system. In addition, each institution must establish a written biosafety program that describes the select agent containment procedures, and an occupational health component for individuals having access to select agents. The written plan must be reviewed and revised at least annually by the institution.

When animal-based research involves select agents, both the IACUC and the institution share the responsibility of ensuring that both the animal welfare and the select agent regulations are satisfied. For example, during the IACUC's semiannual assessment of the OHSP, committee members should ensure that the OHSP includes a component for assessing potential individual exposures to a select agent. The committee may confirm that the animal care and use training program includes a select agent training module and methodologies to ensure that all relevant animal users are trained. In addition, during protocol assessment, the IACUC and the IBC may need to establish processes to ensure that animals exposed to select agents are no longer considered infectious and have been appropriately decontaminated before they leave the containment areas.

10.5.2 Institutional Review Board (Human Subject Panel)

Research may involve both animals and human participants. Consider an investigation that determines whether dogs have a positive impact on the health and well-being of nursing home patients. As an example, human research participants who physically interact with therapy dogs receive scheduled health assessments, and complete an emotional wellness self-assessment survey at the end of the study. Since this study involves both animals and human participants, a collaborative effort between the IACUC, the IRB, and the institution may be required to ensure compliance with both the animal welfare and the human participant (45 CFR Subpart A Section 46) regulations.

By law, the IRB will determine whether human subjects will experience more than minimal risk as a result of participating in research. The human participant regulations indicate that, "Minimal risk means that the probability and magnitude of harm or discomfort anticipated in the research are not greater in and of themselves than those ordinarily encountered in daily life or during the performance of routine physical or psychological examinations or tests." Based on the health status of the nursing home patients, the IRB may determine that participants in the study will experience greater than minimal risk and mandate oversight. In this case, the IRB would require the scientist to inform each potential participant of the risks associated with the research. For example, participants would be informed that by interacting with dogs there is a risk that they may experience allergic reactions, acquire zoonotic illnesses, or physical injuries, such as bites and scratches; only then will consenting participants be enrolled in the study.

Since the activity involves dogs in research, IACUC oversight may also be required. IACUC members aware of the IRB's goals and objectives can assure compliance with the AWRs, the PHS Policy, and the Guide, and help to protect the interest of the institution by reinforcing the IRB's objective of minimizing risks to human participants. The IACUC, for example, could mandate that only dogs with current vaccinations qualify to be used in the research. It may require the researcher to use only trained therapy dogs that must be leashed during dog and participant interactions. Institutional policy may require a collaborative review between the IACUC and the IRB, or written communication between both committees can be used to formalize the process.

10.5.3 Human Embryonic Stem Cell Research Oversight Committee

Human pluripotent stem cells (hPSCs) is a broad term that describes continuous human cells that are capable of developing into a variety of tissue types (e.g., nerve, muscle, and organ tissues). A subtype of hPSCs is hESCs, which are derived from the inner cell mass of a human embryo. Since the production of human embryonic stem cell lines requires destroying human embryos, their use in research has a contentious history in the United States, reflecting various religious and political viewpoints, as well as ethical issues.

A 2009 Executive Order (EO) (Obama 2009) from President Barack Obama required the NIH to review its policies and guidelines on human stem cell use. On July 7, 2009, the NIH Guidelines for Human Stem Cell Research (NIH 2009a) were issued and are based on two guiding principles: "(1) Responsible research with hESCs has the potential to improve our understanding of human health and illness and discover new ways to prevent and/or treat illness. (2) Individuals donating embryos for research purposes should do so freely, with voluntary and informed consent" (NIH 2009a). Consequently, the use of hESCs in research requires oversight and is restricted when used in federally funded research. As a result of the Obama EO, federal funding can support research involving hESCs, provided the cell lines are part of the NIH federal Human Embryonic Stem Cell Registry. In addition, an institution must establish an ESCRO. The ESCRO shall review and approve all proposed uses of hESCs using the National Academies' Guidelines for Human Embryonic Stem Cell Research (NRC 2005).

In the course of reviewing animal-based research, IACUC members may encounter projects that include the use of hESCs. In addition to IACUC review and approval, the committee frequently requires an ancillary review and approval by both the ESCRO and the IBC since the hESCs are of human origin (i.e., a potential source of blood-borne pathogens) before the IACUC can grant approval to initiate the research.

10.5.4 Radiation Safety Committee

Title 10 of the Code of Federal Regulations defines, "Radiation (ionizing radiation) as alpha particles, beta particles, gamma rays, x-rays, neutrons, high-speed electrons, high-speed protons, and other particles capable of producing ions" (USNRC 2014). The same directive requires institutions to establish a radiation safety committee to oversee research involving radiation. A federal mandate for each institution is to develop a radiation program that includes provisions for training and qualifying scientists and staff members to use radioactive materials. Animal-based research may involve the use of radioactive materials. For example, a scientist may use a gamma-ray detection system to follow a food that has been labeled with a radioactive isotope through the digestive system of a living model (e.g., a rat or mouse). In this particular instance, the IACUC review and approval would be contingent on an ancillary review and approval conducted by the radiation committee. The radiation committee would ensure that all 10 CFR mandates are satisfied.

10.5.5 Biological Toxins and Chemical Safety

According to OSHA Laboratory Standard 29 CFR 1910.1450, a hazardous chemical

means a chemical for which there is statistically significant evidence based on at least one study conducted in accordance with established scientific principles that acute or chronic health effects may occur in exposed employees. The term "health hazard" includes chemicals which are carcinogens, toxic or highly toxic agents, reproductive toxins, irritants, corrosives, sensitizers, hepatotoxins, nephrotoxins, neurotoxins, agents which act on the hematopoietic systems, and agents which damage the lungs, skin, eyes, or mucous membranes. (OSHA 2014b)

Chemical hazards create health risks for employees. The OSHA requires institutions to develop methods to mitigate the risks. Consequently, institutions frequently facilitate chemical safety through either an office of the EHS or a chemical safety committee. By federal law, a chemical safety program must include an effective hazard communication plan (29 CFR, 1910.1200) (OSHA 2014b), which is used to educate and provide employees with resources explaining the hazards. The plan also discusses the effective use of warning signs, and how PPE (29 CFR, 1910, Subpart 1) (OSHA 2014b) can be used to minimize related risks.

In the course of conducting animal research, scientists frequently use chemicals that meet the OSHA's hazardous chemical definition. When hazardous chemicals are used in conjunction with animals, the IACUC frequently relies on the expertise of a chemical safety program manager to ensure that the chemicals are used according to federal regulations. The IACUC may ask the chemical safety committee to conduct an ancillary review of the protocol concurrent with its review. The chemical safety committee may review chemical handling and disposal and the appropriate use of hazard communication signage (e.g., on animal cages) and PPE. The IACUC may ask that the chemical safety committee approve its portion of the protocol before final IACUC approval is granted. In addition, the approval process may include an expert from chemical safety visiting the vivarium to ensure that all appropriate safety measures are in place.

10.6 CONCLUSION

Although the IACUC is not specifically charged with performing human health risk assessments regarding the use of hazardous agents (i.e., biological, chemical, ionizing radiation) in animals, it is charged with making sure that there are processes and expertise (i.e., other compliance panels) in place for those assessments to occur. The same goes for research involving animals and human subjects or hESCs. Most institutions allow these reviews to take place in parallel, but it is often the IACUC that serves as the "gatekeeper"—withholding final approval and preventing the research from commencing until all regulatory requirements have been met, and compliance panel approvals have been obtained. Open communication between compliance panels with shared oversight responsibilities is essential in maximizing the overall efficiency of the process.

REFERENCES

Bartle, I. and P. Vass. 2005. *Self-Regulation and the Regulatory State: A Survey of Policy and Practice*. Bath: University of Bath.
Benedict, M. Q., W. J. Tabachnick, S. Higgs, A. F. Azad, C. B. Beard, J. C. Beier, A. M. Handler, A. A. James, C. C. Lord, and R. S. Nasci. 2003. Arthropod containment guidelines (Version 3.1): A project of the American Committee of Medical Entomology of the American Society of Tropical Medicine and Hygiene. *Vector-Borne and Zoonotic Diseases 3* (2):63.
CDC (Centers for Disease Control and Prevention) 2014. Division of vector-borne diseases (DVBD). http://www.cdc.gov/ncezid/dvbd/.
Faraday, M. 1857. The Bakerian lecture: Experimental relations of gold (and other metals) to light. *Philosophical Transactions of the Royal Society of London* 147:145–181.

Hanley, C., A. Thurber, C. Hanna, A. Punnoose, J. Zhang, and D. G. Wingett. 2009. The influences of cell type and ZnO nanoparticle size on immune cell cytotoxicity and cytokine induction. *Nanoscale Research Letters* 4 (12):1409–1420.

HHS (Department of Health and Human Services). 2005. Possession, use and transfer of select agents and toxins. 42 CFR Part 73. Vol. 70, No. 52.

HHS (U.S. Department of Health and Human Services). 2009. Code of Federal Regulations Title 45, Part 46. Basic HHS Policy for Protection of Human Research Subjects.

HHS/USDA (Department of Health and Human Services, U.S. Department of Agriculture). 2014. Select agents and toxins list. Centers for Disease Control and Prevention, Animal and Plant Health Inspection Service. http://www.selectagents.gov/SelectAgentsandToxinsList.html.

Hutchinson, J. N. and W. J. Muller. 2000. Transgenic mouse models of human breast cancer. *Oncogene* 19 (53):6130–6137.

MacPhail, R. C., E. A. Grulke, and R. A. Yokel. 2013. Assessing nanoparticle risk poses prodigious challenges. *Wiley Interdisciplinary Reviews: Nanomedicine and Nanobiotechnology* 5 (4):374–387.

Mendelsohn, M., J. Kough, Z. Vaituzis, and K. Matthews. 2003. Are Bt crops safe? *Nature Biotechnology* 21 (9):1003–1009.

NIH (National Institutes of Health). 2002. Public Health Service policy on humane care and use of laboratory animals. Office of Laboratory Animal Welfare, U.S. Department of Health and Human Services, NIH, Bethesda, MD.

NIH (National Institutes of Health). 2009a. NIH guidelines on stem cell research. http://www.ncbi.nlm.nih.gov/pubmed/.

NIH (National Institutes of Health). 2009b. NIH guidelines for research involving recombinant DNA molecules. *Federal Register* 74 FR 48275.

NIH (National Institutes of Health). 2013. NIH guidelines research involving recombinant or synthetic nucleic acid molecules. Office of Biotechnology Activities (OBA). http://osp.od.nih.gov/office-biotechnology-activities/biosafety/nih-guidelines.

NIH, ARENA (National Institutes of Health, and Applied Research Ethics National Association). 2002. *Institutional Animal Care and Use Committee Guidebook.* 2nd edn. Bethesda, MD: Office of Laboratory Animal Welfare.

NRC (National Research Council). 1983. *Risk Assessment in the Federal Government: Managing the Process.* Washington, DC: National Academy Press, Committee on the Institutional Means for Assessment of Risks to Public Health.

NRC (National Research Council). 2005. Guidelines for human embryonic stem cell research. National Academies of Science, Committee on the Guidelines for Human Embryonic Stem Cell Research.

NRC (National Research Council). 2011. *Guide for the Care and Use of Laboratory Animals.* 8th edn. National Academies Press: Washington, DC.

Obama, B. 2009. Executive order 13505—Removing barriers to responsible scientific research involving human stem cells. *Federal Register* 74 (46):10667.

OSHA (Occupational Safety and Health Administration). 2014a. 29 CFR Bloodborne pathogens 1910.1030. https://www.osha.gov/pls/oshaweb/owadisp.show_document?p_table=STANDARDS&p_id=10051.

OSHA (Occupational Safety and Health Administration). 2014b. 29 CFR Occupational safety and health standards 1910.1450. https://www.osha.gov/pls/oshaweb/owadisp.show_document?p_id=10106&p_table=STANDARDS.

Penslar, R. L. 1993. *IRB Guidebook*. Washington, DC: U.S. Department of Health & Human Services.

USDA (U.S. Department of Agriculture). 2005a. Possession, use and transfer of select agents and toxins. 7 CFR Part 331. Vol. 70, No. 52. http://www.ecfr.gov/cgi-bin/retrieveECF R?gp=1&SID=6a987ee202807616763c96ca969fb6a9&ty=HTML&h=L&r=PART&n =pt7.5.331.

USDA (U.S. Department of Agriculture). 2005b. Possession, use and transfer of select agents and toxins. 9 CFR Part 121. Vol. 70, No. 52. http://www.ecfr.gov/cgi-bin/retrieveECF R?gp=1&SID=b41d47931e349cdb66b8b92cf47cf7b5&ty=HTML&h=L&r=PART&n =pt9.1.121.

USDA (U.S. Department of Agriculture). 2013. *Animal Welfare Act and Animal Welfare Regulations* (Animal Care Blue Book). Code of Federal Regulations (CFR), Title 9, Chapter 1, Subchapter A, Parts 1–4.

USNRC (U.S. Nuclear Regulatory Commission). 2014. NRC Regulations, Title 10, Code of Federal Regulations. http://www.nrc.gov/reading-rm/doc-collections/cfr/.

USDL (U.S. Department of Labor). 1996. Occupational exposure to bloodborne pathogens. OSHA Form 3127.

CHAPTER **11**

The IACUC and Laboratory Animal Resources

Stephen A. Felt and Sherril L. Green

CONTENTS

11.1 INTRODUCTION

Many different names exist to attempt to encompass and define the workforce, facilities, equipment, and resources that an institution commits to animal husbandry and care (e.g., resources, centers, cores, services, departments, divisions, units, groups, etc.). Regardless of the name, Institutional Animal Care and Use Committees (IACUCs) are mandated by regulations such as the Animal Welfare Act (AWA) to have oversight of these organizations from both programmatic and facilities perspectives. This chapter explores some of the more common resource facility–related and programmatic issues encountered by IACUCs and delves further into some of the unique challenges presented by areas managed by the principal investigator (PI). In addition, it provides suggestions on ways that IACUCs can deal with the many sources of information and topics of animal research and welfare needed to assure knowledgeable oversight of animal facilities.

A number of internal and external references are available to guide IACUCs in identifying and addressing animal facility–related issues. The regulations of the AWA, the Public Health Service (PHS) Policy on Humane Care and Use of Laboratory Animals (the PHS Policy), and the *Guide for the Care and Use of Laboratory Animals* (the Guide) require IACUCs to thoroughly evaluate physical plant and programmatic issues associated with animal resources at regular intervals (USDA 2013b). Two types of standards are described in applicable regulations and guidelines: engineering and performance. Engineering standards describe a detailed approach for achieving a desired outcome; they provide little to no room for interpretation or modification of the technique should an alternative be equally acceptable. Conversely, performance standards provide a description of a detailed outcome and provide measurable criteria for assessing whether the outcome is achieved. This gives IACUCs a lot of flexibility. As noted in the Guide, the performance approach "requires professional input, sound judgment, and a team approach to achieve specific goals" (NRC 2011). Research in laboratory animal management and science provides new information, which should be used to update the performance standards on an ongoing basis at an institution.

This does not mean that all IACUC members must be completely familiar with all of the details listed by every applicable regulatory or accrediting agency. It would be ideal, but hardly practical, to expect everyone on the committee to have a thorough level of knowledge. Relying solely on the professional laboratory animal staff to provide guidance and to have expertise on animal-related issues, however, is not the answer. Memorizing every rule and regulation would be impractical, if not impossible, and because rules and regulations continue to change over time, either in content or in interpretation, specific citations still need to be referenced. It is essential, therefore, for IACUC members to be familiar with the rules and regulations, where they can be found, and who can provide expertise or assistance in understanding and implementing both the letter and the spirit of the laws and guidelines.

11.1.1 Who Governs What?

Animal Care and Use Programs (ACUPs) and their associated vivaria may be regulated by the following international, federal, state, and local agencies and accrediting organizations:

- The U.S. Department of Agriculture (USDA) administers the AWA.
- The National Institutes of Health (NIH) Office of Laboratory Animal Welfare (OLAW) oversees compliance with the PHS Policy and the Guide (NRC 2011).
- The Association for Assessment and Accreditation of Laboratory Animal Care (AAALAC) International (AAALAC International) utilizes the Guide and the Guide for the Care and Use of Agricultural Animals in Research and Teaching (the Ag Guide) (FASS 2010).
- The European Convention for the Protection of Vertebrate Animals Used for Experimental and Other Scientific Purposes (ETS 123) and the Council of Europe oversee European programs.
- The Drug Enforcement Administration controls the use of potentially abusive substances, including some of the anesthetics and analgesics used for animals.
- The Food and Drug Administration (FDA) oversees good laboratory practices (GLPs) and good manufacturing practices that may impact research conducted on animals in some facilities.
- For programs that import and export animals and animal tissues internationally or nationally, national and state regulations, respectively, may apply,
- The importation of nonindigenous or detrimental species into certain states may require special permits through the U.S. Fish and Wildlife Service (FWS).
- Laws at the county or city level may also require special permits for housing certain research animal species. Additionally, these permits may regulate the types of species housed, the types of manipulations (invasive versus noninvasive) that can be performed on animals, and the disposal of animal waste and carcasses and may also dictate the types and quantity of hazardous agents and their storage, use, and disposal.

It is incumbent upon IACUCs to determine which of the many regulations and guidelines apply to their institutions, familiarize themselves with the content of the applicable statutes and policies, and oversee compliance by ACUP participants. They may have to enlist the help of someone, often a laboratory animal veterinarian, who is familiar with the regulatory mandates of a particular location. Many institutions have dedicated research compliance offices with staff whose function is to advise the institution on applicable rules and regulations and to assist in compliance oversight.

11.1.2 Who Can Help?

Large institutions may have many internal resources, including dedicated staff, to assist IACUCs with animal facility issues. Veterinarians and other IACUC members who have expertise in a particular species of animal or area of research can provide insight on the proper husbandry, care, and use of many laboratory animals. Additionally, biosafety, occupational health, statistical, and legal experts can serve as valuable resources for an IACUC. Librarians can provide assistance in alternative searches for the replacement of live animals, the reduction of animal numbers, or the refinement of techniques (the three Rs of animal research: replace, reduce, and refine). Computer support groups can create customized programs or assist in the acquisition of commercially available software that can organize much of the information needed by the IACUC. Computer resources can be used to electronically send notices, record, and store information about animal protocols; animal procurement; animal populations; animals' physical location (through radio-frequency identification); types and numbers of animals (pain/distress categorization) used on particular projects; animal census information; animal morbidities (alert notices and medical records); laboratory diagnostics; personnel access (security) to specified rooms, corridors, and buildings; occupational health information (including clearances); and delivery (online) and documentation of personnel training. The technologies available today facilitate the integration of much of this information. For example, it is common practice for protocols not to be approved until researchers' occupational health requirements and institutional specified training have been completed and for researchers not to gain access to animal holding rooms (security) until their protocols are approved. Depending on the size of the program and the type of research conducted within the institution, it might also be appropriate for the IACUC to communicate and integrate with other oversight committees (biosafety, stem cell, radiation safety, and so on).

Smaller institutions may not have sufficient internal resources to resolve animal facility–related questions or other issues that need to be addressed by the IACUC. In these instances, outside consultants can be solicited to provide the committee with expertise. Many institutions are willing to share their templates for everything from animal research proposal (protocol) forms to semiannual inspection forms. Much information can also be obtained from the web pages of institutions that have placed information concerning aspects of their ACUP on the World Wide Web. Should an investigator request a new species of animal not previously housed in the animal facility, or an alternative type of housing or care, information on the proposed change can be solicited from other institutions or outside experts. Dialogue with accrediting and regulatory agencies can provide additional resources. AAALAC International has developed a number of position statements and frequently asked questions (FAQs), both available on the AAALAC website, that can help IACUCs navigate through a number of animal facility and program topics. Similarly, OLAW has made a number of tutorials, FAQs, online seminars, and sample documents (including a customizable facility inspection checklist template) available to users on the OLAW website. The USDA has made the Animal Welfare Inspection Guide (USDA 2013a), the Animal Care Policy Manual (USDA 2014), and a number of fact sheets and checklists available on its website. In addition to these references, numerous valuable textbooks have information that can help guide IACUCs with regard to facility and program oversight. Two of the more popular guides are the Institutional Animal Care and Use Committee Guidebook (ARENA/OLAW 2002), prepared by OLAW and the Applied Research Ethics National Association, and *The IACUC Handbook* (Silverman et al. 2014).

11.2 ANIMAL FACILITY–RELATED ISSUES

The majority of animal facility–related physical plant issues are brought to the attention of the IACUC during routine inspections. New building construction and preexisting building renovations present another opportunity for the IACUC to become exposed to these issues.

The PHS Policy and AWA regulations require that IACUCs evaluate their ACUPs (including conducting physical plant inspections) at least once every six months. The Guide allows increased flexibility with regard to the scheduling of inspections, specifying an annual minimum. Of greater importance to AAALAC International is evidence that the IACUC is highly engaged, conducts thorough evaluations of the facilities, and ensures corrective measures are taken in a timely manner and that "the program and facilities are adequately supporting the research, testing and teaching objectives of the institution" (AAALAC International). Agencies or organizations, such as the USDA, the Department of Defense (DOD), and OLAW, may also conduct inspections of animal facilities and programs. AAALAC International performs triennial visits and program assessments.

As renovation or new vivarium opportunities arise, it is prudent to keep IACUCs engaged throughout all phases of the project—planning, design, construction, commissioning, and reoccupation. IACUC involvement in these processes can assist in addressing concerns regarding animal welfare, including adherence to mandated requirements for animal facilities and required components of survival surgical facilities for nonrodent species.

Physical plant facility issues usually have more defined, quantifiable parameters than programmatic issues. IACUC members can obtain information on animal facility concerns and other relevant issues from a variety of resources. They can obtain guidance by reading applicable federal publications that specify rules and regulations, viewing available documents and tutorials, and attending relevant meetings or workshops (such as those sponsored by Public Responsibility in Medicine and Research, the American Association for Laboratory Animal Science, the National Association for Biomedical Research, OLAW, the USDA, and AAALAC International).

Every IACUC member has the responsibility to oversee the ACUP and inspect the animal facilities at his or her institution, but there is tremendous flexibility on how this can be achieved. For instance, smaller institutions often include semiannual inspections as an agenda item during a regularly scheduled IACUC meeting. Ideally, all IACUC members would tour all facilities involved in the ACUP, but this is not always practical (see Table 6.2 for a discussion of regulatory requirements for conducting a semiannual facility inspection). Large institutions with multiple, decentralized animal research facilities may, through preference or necessity, use small teams of IACUC members (subcommittees) to visit different animal facility sites. This "divide and conquer" approach is one practical way to handle the time-consuming IACUC task of visiting all animal facilities at least once every six months. However, caution needs to be exercised to assure that all subcommittees conduct inspections at different sites according to standardized criteria and formats. In this scenario, designated personnel (often IACUC administrative staff) need to collect all necessary paperwork from different subcommittees and formulate coherent communications to be forwarded to the institutional official (IO), as well as to individuals who need to know of or act on the inspection committee's findings. *Ad hoc* consultants may also be employed to assist in conducting semiannual inspections, but, as stated in the USDA regulations, at least two IACUC members must be present at inspections of facilities where USDA-covered species are housed. On occasion, the USDA will approve a request for one of the two semiannual inspections conducted at a distant site (e.g., a satellite facility that would require overnight travel) to be carried out via a live video feed to the IACUC members conducting the review. The USDA looks at these requests on a case-by-case basis.

Regardless of the approach to semiannual inspections (full committee or subcommittee), it is necessary that the IACUC members conducting the inspection understand what they should look for and how they should document their findings. A checklist approach to most facility inspections is highly recommended, since the ultimate determination for evaluations should be based on actual regulatory requirements, and these inspections should be done in a comprehensive and consistent manner. OLAW has published a very useful checklist, available on its website, which many institutions either use "as is" or use as a template to develop a customized form. The following is a brief commonsense overview of items that should be evaluated during animal facility inspections:

11.2.1 Animal Facilities: General Considerations

Animal facilities should meet the following general conditions:

- The facilities should have regularly scheduled, documented pest control programs for vermin (e.g., rodents, birds, insects, etc.).
- Overall, the facilities should be in good repair.
- The facilities should provide for separation of species and isolation of sick or quarantined animals.
- The interior surfaces of animal facilities should be impervious to moisture and easily sanitizable; there should be no exposed, unsealed wood.

- The lighting should be sufficient for thorough cleaning and inspection.
- Emergency provisions, including a supply of backup power for vital operations, should be readily available. Information on personnel to be contacted and steps to be taken in case of emergencies should be posted in the animal facility.
- Appropriate procedures should exist for the collection, storage, and disposal of animal waste, animal carcasses, and hazardous waste.
- A program for veterinary care, including provision for emergency/weekend/holiday care, disease surveillance and control, diagnosis, and treatment should be established and implemented under veterinary supervision.

11.2.2 Animal Housing Rooms

For the purpose of this chapter, the term *animal housing room* will be used. This term is considered synonymous with *animal holding room*. The following topics should be considered by IACUCs as they assess animal housing rooms:

- Overall, environmental variables such as temperature, humidity, ventilation, light cycles, vibration, and noise level should be monitored, controlled, and documented. These variables, including reproductive biological needs, should be appropriate for the species and the research project design.
- The dry-bulb temperatures in animal rooms should be set below the animals' lower critical temperature to avoid heat stress (NRC 2011). Similarly, animals need to be provided adequate resources for thermoregulation (nesting material, shelter) to avoid cold stress. The dry-bulb temperatures for common adult laboratory animals can be found in the Guide (NRC 2011).
- A 30%–70% humidity range is considered acceptable for most mammalian species. In climates where it is difficult to provide a sufficient level of environmental relative humidity, animals should be closely monitored for negative effects.
- A 10–15 air-changes-per-hour range is an acceptable guideline to maintain animal housing room (macroenvironmental) air quality by constant volume systems. This range can be appropriately adjusted based on "heat loads; the species, size, and number of animals involved; the type of primary enclosure and bedding; the frequency of cage changing; the room dimensions; or the efficiency of air distribution both in the macroenvironment and between the macro- and microenvironments" (NRC 2011).
- The lighting should be diffused throughout an animal holding area and provide sufficient illumination for the animals' well-being while permitting good housekeeping practices; adequate animal inspection, including the bottom-most cages in racks; and safe working conditions for personnel (NRC 2011). Light levels of about 325 lux (30 ft candles) approximately 1 m (3.3 ft.) above the floor appear to be sufficient for animal care and have not been reported to cause clinical effects in known photosensitive terrestrial species (e.g., albino rats).
- In general, activities that generate noise should be conducted in areas separate from animal housing areas. Exposure to sound louder than 85 dB can have detrimental health effects to animals (and people). Noisy animal species should be segregated away from quieter ones.
- Excessive vibration has been associated with detrimental health effects in laboratory animals and can become an uncontrolled variable for research experiments.

The two main sources of vibration in vivaria are ground-borne and equipment-generated. Attempts should be made to prevent the generation of excessive vibrations when possible and to avoid (or limit) animals' exposure when prevention is infeasible. Furthermore, it is recommended that major sources of vibration be considered during the planning, design, and construction phases of a building project.

- Daily observations of animals, including weekends and holidays, should be practiced and appropriately documented.
- It is recommended that animals be physically separated by species to prevent interspecies disease transmission and anxiety due to the potential for interspecies conflict. Mixing of species within a room may be acceptable if specialized equipment (e.g., ventilated caging systems) is used.

11.2.3 Cage Space and Density Considerations

- Important considerations for determining space needs include age, sex, number of animals to be co-housed, housing duration, use (e.g., production vs. experimentation), and species-specific biological or physiological needs (e.g., vertical space for arboreal species or thermal gradient for poikilotherms).
- IACUCs need to look to, and comply with, all national or regional regulations, policies, and guidelines, as well as funding agency specifications, regarding cage space requirements. Requirements regarding space needs for various laboratory animal species can be found in the Animal Welfare Act Regulations (AWRs), Guide, Ag Guide, and ETS 123.
- Caging should contain animals securely and safely, protect them from other animals or extreme environmental conditions, and maintain animals in a clean and dry state (terrestrial animals), as well as minimize scientific variables. Caging should allow easy access to nutritious, palatable, and noncontaminated food and potable water.
- Cages and food/water receptacles should be sanitized at regular intervals—often weekly for solid-bottom caging. For rodents maintained on ventilated racks, this interval may be lengthened. The IACUC should review cage-changing practices for individually ventilated cages based on current literature and other factors (rodent strain, bedding type, housing density, etc.).
- Animals (and in many cases their cages/pens) should be properly identified. In addition, records as to the source, dates of acquisition and disposition, and assigned project should be maintained.

11.2.4 Enrichment Program

- Enrichment programs should consist of species-specific written plans that are reviewed by the IACUC regularly to ensure that they are beneficial to animal well-being and are consistent with the goals of animal use. They should be updated as needed to ensure that they reflect current knowledge.
- The USDA mandates that written programs and documentation of implementation should exist for the exercise of dogs and the psychological enrichment of nonhuman primates.
- The personnel responsible for animal care and husbandry should receive training in the behavioral biology of the species they work with to appropriately monitor the

effects of enrichment, as well as to identify the development of adverse or abnormal behaviors.

- The primary aim of environmental enrichment is to promote psychological and physical well-being in the animals by providing them with sensory and motor stimulation through structures and resources that facilitate the expression of species-typical behaviors.
- The implementation of environmental enrichment should also take into account the scientific goals of the study for which the animals are used; enrichment should be considered an independent variable and, thus, suitably controlled (AAALAC 2014).
- Ideal enrichment should provide animals with choices and control over their environment, thereby improving their ability to cope with stress. For instance, ample bedding together with nesting materials allow mice to better control their internal body temperature and thereby avoid cold stress (Gaskill et al. 2009, 2012, 2013).

Social species considerations:

- The Guide states that single housing of social species should be the exception and allowed only when appropriately justified by social incompatibility, veterinary health concerns, or scientific necessity approved by the IACUC.
- Full-time social housing is the optimal way to provide an ideal social experience. However, when full-time housing with conspecifics is not possible, other opportunities for social experiences should be explored (e.g., overnight, when the animals are between studies, defined periods of time during the day, etc.) to allow full contact with conspecifics or restricted contact that allows interaction (e.g., mesh panel, grooming bars, etc.) on either a part- or full-time basis.

11.2.5 Feed and Bedding Storage

The following practices for feed and bedding storage should be maintained:

- Means of feed and bedding storage should protect against spoilage, contamination, deterioration, and vermin infestation and should allow proper sanitation of the area. Storing feed and bedding away from perimeter walls and on nonporous pallets, carts, or racks can help achieve this. Nonporous materials tend to allow for proper sanitation and last longer. If wooden pallets are chosen, they should be assured to not be a source of contamination or vermin into the facility.
- Purchasers are encouraged to consider manufacturers' and suppliers' recommended storage procedures and practices. In particular, perishable food items (e.g., meat, fruit, and vegetables) require extra precautions (e.g., refrigeration).
- Upon receipt, bags of feed and bedding should be examined to ensure that they are intact and unstained to help ensure that their contents have not been potentially exposed to vermin, penetrated by liquids, or contaminated prior to arrival.
- Stocks should be carefully monitored and rotated to ensure that the oldest food is used first.
- Opened bags of food should be stored in vermin-proof containers to minimize contamination and to avoid the potential spread of pathogens.
- It is recommended that natural-ingredient diets be stored at less than 21°C (70°F) and below 50% relative humidity.

- Most natural-ingredient, dry laboratory animal diets, when stored properly, can be used up to six months after manufacture. Nonstabilized vitamin C in manufactured feeds generally has a shelf life of only three months, but commonly used stabilized forms can extend the shelf life of feed (NRC 2011).
- Purified and chemically defined diets are often less stable than natural-ingredient diets, and their shelf life is usually less than six months. They should be stored at 4°C (39°F) or lower (NRC 2011).
- Food and bedding storage containers should be cleaned and sanitized regularly and should not be transferred between areas of differing contamination risks without appropriate decontamination.

11.2.6 Cage Wash

The following sanitary/safety conditions should be practiced:

- Physical plant construction or management practices should exist to minimize contamination of clean equipment by dirty equipment.
- Quality control procedures should be in place and documented to assure adequate sanitation of caging and equipment.
- Emergency eyewash/shower stations and appropriate personal protective equipment, including hearing, vision, and respiratory protection, should be available based on risk assessment, and training on these practices should be provided to personnel.
- The safety of walk-in cage/rack washers and bulk sterilizing equipment must be assessed. How easily can a person get out in the event that he or she becomes trapped inside? Is there an emergency off switch (or "de-energizing mechanism")? Are personnel operating the machine properly trained? It is very important that safety features are clearly identified at their location and signage is posted with instructions for use.

11.2.7 Surgery

The following criteria should be evaluated at institutions performing animal surgeries:

- When determining whether a surgery should be performed within a dedicated operating room/suite or laboratory area (that provides separation from other activities), the choice will depend on the species, the nature of the procedure (major, minor, or emergency), and the potential for physical impairment or postoperative complications (e.g., infection).
- Surgical areas should be maintained and operated in a manner that ensures cleanliness and minimizes unnecessary traffic and noise. If it is necessary to use an operating room for other purposes, it is imperative that the room be returned to an appropriate level of hygiene before its use for major survival surgery. Under the AWA, dedicated surgery suites for nonrodent, USDA-regulated species should only be used for conducting surgeries, not for "other purposes," and should be maintained and operated under aseptic conditions (9 CFR 2.31(d) (1)(ix).

- The IACUC and veterinary staff are responsible for determining that the surgeons are appropriately qualified and trained. Researcher-maintained surgical training logs, aseptic technique workshop completion, and direct observation by qualified veterinary or compliance staff as a component of the postapproval monitoring program are all useful tools that can be used to help promote a high-quality surgical-based research program.
- Adequate pre-, intra-, and postoperative monitoring records should be maintained for all species, including rodents and aquatic species. The selected physiological criteria, frequency of monitoring, and required record keeping should be reflective of the species; the invasiveness, complexity, and duration of the surgery; and the anesthetics and other drugs used. These records provide a valuable resource for IACUC members when they are assessing compliance and for veterinary clinical staff when they are troubleshooting unexpected complications.
- Controlled substances should be appropriately stored, with records of inventory and use and monitored expiration dates.
- Gas cylinders should be adequately stored/secured and anesthetic waste gases scavenged.
- Aseptic procedures should be practiced for all survival surgeries. It may be appropriate to require aseptic techniques for nonsurvival surgeries as well, particularly those of longer duration, to mitigate the potential of intraoperative sepsis and the subsequent impact on data collected.
- Functional areas for surgical support (instrument preparation), surgeon preparation, animal preparation, surgical procedures, and postoperative recovery should be physically separate, or carefully separated by stringent management practices.
- Established programs for the effective sanitation of facilities and sterilization of surgical instruments should be in place and monitored.
- A mechanism should be in place to document the qualifications of the personnel performing surgery or anesthesia.
- Anesthetic machines and vaporizers should be evaluated for proper operation on an established schedule that is consistent with the manufacturers' recommendations. Manufacturers publish recommended on-site calibration schedules, as well as off-site maintenance schedules that require the vaporizer/machine be sent to the manufacturer.

11.2.7.1 Rodent Surgery Considerations

The following principles apply to rodent surgery:

- Sites for rodent surgery need to be clean and not used for other purposes during surgeries. Separate, dedicated surgery rooms are not required, but it is important to choose the alternate locations very carefully, as it is of paramount importance to avoid exposing nonessential personnel to surgeries—and other *in vivo* manipulations, for that matter—from both occupational health and psychological risk perspectives.
- Aseptic technique and practices (e.g., sterilization of the instruments, proper preparation of the surgical site, and proper attire and preparation of the surgeon, including surgical gloves) should be utilized.
- The monitoring of rodents during surgery is critical to ensure that animals are at an appropriate plane of anesthesia. Perioperative assessment of physiological

parameters (such as body temperature, respiratory rate, heart rate, blood pressure, blood gases, ECG, etc.), along with the anesthetic depth, can be valuable metrics for this purpose. The level of detail contained in the records should accurately reflect the monitoring being performed as well as the length and complexity of the procedure.

- Cage-side monitoring cards can be effective tools for researchers to document the monitoring and care provided to surgical subjects and communicate the information to caretaking, veterinary, and IACUC personnel.

11.2.8 Husbandry Standard Operating Procedures and Sanitation Schedules

- Appropriate species-specific husbandry standard operating procedures (SOPs) should be developed and implemented by the animal care management in consultation with veterinarians and researchers. These should be reviewed by the IACUC during inspections. Housing should provide for the animals' health and well-being, while meeting the intended objectives of protocol. When necessary, outside expertise should be sought when new species are added or unfamiliar housing practices arise (e.g., hazardous agents). Objective assessments should be made to substantiate the adequacy of the animals' environment, housing, and management. Routine procedures for maintaining animals should be documented to ensure daily consistency of management and care.
- All components of the animal facility, including the animal rooms and support spaces (e.g., storage areas, cage-washing facilities, corridors, and procedure rooms), should be regularly cleaned and disinfected as appropriate to the circumstances, at a frequency based on the use of the area and the nature of likely contamination. Vaporized hydrogen peroxide or chlorine dioxide can be used effectively as a room decontaminant following the completion of studies using susceptible infectious agents or as an outbreak control measure.
- Cleaning implements should be made of materials that resist corrosion and withstand regular sanitation. They should be assigned to specific areas and should not be transported between areas with different risks of contamination without prior disinfection. Worn items should be replaced regularly. The implements should be stored in a neat and organized fashion.

11.2.9 Environmental Sanitation and Sterilization Effectiveness Monitoring

Due to the risks of potential contamination of housed animals from a variety of sources (e.g., other animals, caretakers, equipment, feed, water, pests, air, etc.) (Thigpen et al. 2004), the IACUC should ensure that the laboratory animal resources unit has an established and comprehensive quality assurance (QA) program that assesses the effectiveness of common vivarium decontamination processes. Internal or external experts may need to be consulted initially when first establishing a QA sanitation program to help answer the following questions: Who is responsible? What to monitor? When to monitor? How often to monitor?

- If autoclaved feed and bedding are being used, is sterilization being verified?
- Are there methods to assess the sanitation practices applied to the animal room (e.g., cubicles, floors, walls), supply (e.g., cages, water bottles, sipper tubes, enrichment devices), and equipment (e.g., cage racks)?
- Are there established methods to ensure water quality?

Whether the sanitation process is automated or manual, regular evaluation of sanitation effectiveness is recommended. This can often be accomplished by evaluating processed materials using microbiologic culture or organic material detection systems (e.g., adenosine triphosphate).

11.2.10 Pest Control

Programs designed to detect, prevent, control, or eliminate the presence of pests are essential in an animal environment. A regularly scheduled and documented program of control and monitoring should be implemented. The ideal program should prevent the entry of vermin altogether but also eliminate potential harborage sites within the facility. When animals are housed in outdoor facilities, exposure to predatory species should be taken into consideration.

Approved pesticides should be used in animal areas only when necessary, and investigators whose animals may be exposed to them should be consulted beforehand. Types and applications of pesticides should be coordinated with the animal care management staff and properly documented. Those chosen should be in compliance with applicable regulations. Whenever possible, nontoxic means of pest control should be used. If kill traps are used, they should be maintained in proper working order; if live traps are used, they need to be checked frequently, followed by delivery of a humane method of euthanasia.

11.2.11 Animal Population Management

With the ever-changing research funding landscape, researchers often manage their animal colony or colonies to maintain adequate numbers of animals in as small a footprint as possible, since that footprint often determines their animal per diem costs. What constitutes "adequate numbers" will depend on a number of intrinsic and extrinsic factors, including approved numbers in protocol, experimental needs, breeding characteristics of given strains/species of animals, and detrimental phenotypes. However, the creation and characterization of novel mouse strains remain expensive and time consuming. Along with the financial drain of maintaining live breeding colonies, there are potential devastating risks associated with keeping animals solely in this way—loss due to earthquake, fire, flood, outbreaks, genetic contamination, and genetic drift. With these in mind, it is prudent to consider cryopreserving all valuable mouse strains as a matter of standard mouse management. Cryopreservation is a powerful colony management tool, assuring strains are available when needed and enabling the resumption of projects placed on hiatus, the verification of previous data, collaborations and so on. For researchers who do not have the willingness, time, facilities, labor force, or other resources to maintain and manage their own mouse colonies, there are other options. Lab members tasked with the responsibility of breeding management can greatly improve organization and efficiency using off-the-shelf commercial and customizable breeding management software programs that are available. Many institutions may employ in-house colony managers who can temporarily or permanently assume this function from laboratory personnel. This is often done on a fee-for-service basis. A more drastic, but certainly viable, approach is to outsource the entire maintenance of the breeding colony to one of several reputable commercial sources, letting them ship research animals as needed for experiments.

11.2.11.1 Breeding and Cage Overcrowding

Finding effective ways to prevent and manage overcrowding of mouse cages is often a huge challenge. Many institutions will refer to the IACUC for guidance. A viable recourse might be to develop IACUC-approved housing, density, overcrowding, breeding, and/or weaning policies that are designed to prevent mouse overcrowding. Oftentimes, these policies can be ineffectual unless programs also seek to proactively communicate this information in a consistent, clear, and frequent fashion; encourage and support access to applicable training (e.g., in-house or outside breeding/colony management workshop training); closely monitor for noncompliance; and ensure that a robust process exists through which identified overcrowded cages are corrected expeditiously. Some programs have found that charging fees/fines directly to the investigator for cage separations of weaned offspring can help serve as an effective deterrent for recidivism, but IACUCs need to be prepared in case more drastic measures might be necessary (e.g., suspension of breeding procedures within a protocol or of the entire protocol). A number of different strategies used by other programs are available through professional colleagues and online.

11.2.12 Cryogen Gas Storage and Magnetic Resonance Scanners

Both cryogen storage areas and magnetic resonance (MR) scanner rooms contain a potential oxygen depletion hazard that should be thoroughly risk-assessed to determine if additional safeguards (e.g., O_2 sensors) should be installed. The hazards associated with metallic projectiles and pacemaker malfunction in the presence of MR scanners also need to be carefully assessed and safeguarded.

11.3 ANIMAL RESOURCES PROGRAMMATIC ISSUES

Along with the requirement that facility inspections be conducted by the IACUC, the committee is also charged with overseeing other aspects of the ACUP. This involves reviewing policies, guidelines, and SOPs related to animal care and use and animal health records; reviewing the biosafety, chemical safety, radiation safety, and occupational health program; and reviewing the findings/outcomes from outside agency inspection/visits (USDA, AAALAC International, DOD, OLAW, FDA, and Department of Veterans Affairs). If they are noted, deficiencies are identified, and the IACUC needs to review responses to those deficiencies in order to ensure compliance with the AWA, the Guide, and the PHS Policy, and, perhaps to a lesser extent, GLP standards and DOD directives, as applicable. Some of the most common general programmatic topics related to laboratory animal resources fall under the categories of occupational health and safety programs and veterinary care.

11.3.1 Occupational Health Considerations for Animal Care Personnel

An occupational health and safety program must be part of the overall ACUP, as working with animals poses inherent health dangers—zoonoses, allergens, radiation, physical and chemical hazards, and specific protocol- related hazards. The foundation of a program includes hazard identification and risk assessment, personnel training and protection, written procedures and policies regarding hazard use and monitoring, and medical evaluation and preventive medicine. To be successful often requires coordination between the IACUC, the IO, the Environmental Health and Safety Program, the Occupational Health and Safety (OHS) services, the administration staff (e.g., human resources, finance, and facility maintenance personnel), and research personnel. The extent and level of participation of personnel in the program should be based on the hazards posed by the animals and materials used; on the exposure intensity, duration, and frequency; on the susceptibility of the personnel; and on the history of occupational illness and injury in the particular workplace. Because laboratory animal resources personnel are often working on the "front lines" in terms of exposure risk, it is appropriate to collectively designate them the highest risk category, thereby affording them the appropriate protections and safeguards. A health history evaluation is advisable before work assignment to assess the potential risks for individual employees. Periodic medical evaluations and appropriate immunization schedules are advisable for some risk categories. Day-to-day responsibility for safety in the laboratory animal research workplace often resides with the facility supervisor(s) and is largely dependent on employees following safe work practices.

11.3.1.1 Medical Clearances

It is incumbent upon programs to have a mechanism in place that prevents an employee from working unsupervised prior to the release of the medical clearance. Oftentimes, in addition to notifying the employee, institutions elect to involve a supervisor or other key dedicated staff (training, compliance, OHS, human resources), or both, in the notification process as an additional safeguard.

11.3.1.2 Medical Questionnaires

A laboratory animal occupational health questionnaire is often used by occupational health professionals as an important tool in the medical evaluation process. The formats vary widely from program to program; a sample Animal Exposure

Health Surveillance Questionnaire is given in Appendix A6. Automating many aspects of the occupational health process (Animal Exposure Health Surveillance questionnaire submission and review, appointment scheduling, automatic reminders, clearance notifications, data mining, etc.) from a historical paper-based system has greatly improved capability, efficiency, compliance, and turnaround times for many programs. Furthermore, currently available integrative automation systems allow for medical clearances to be linked with the protocol approval, facility access, and training requirements.

11.3.1.3 Safety Training

Formal safety programs should be established to "ensure that staff has the necessary training and skills and facilities are adequate for the safe conduct of the research" (NRC 2011). There are a number of safety training topics that may be of particular relevance to laboratory animal resources staff. Laboratory animal allergies, preventive control measures, early recognition and reporting of allergy symptoms, and proper techniques for working with animals should be a requirement of any animal-focused safety training. In conjunction, institutions may need to offer formal respirator training (and fit testing) to symptomatic employees. Hearing protection, back care, and repetitive motion injury can be important topics for institutions that maintain animals, equipment, and supplies that can be associated with injuries from noise (e.g., cage washing, pigs, dogs, etc.), lifting (e.g., rodent racks, nonhuman primate [NHP] caging, feed bags, etc.), and repetition (e.g., cage change). Institutions housing macaques should require any personnel working with or around these animals to be educated about the risks associated with Macacine herpesvirus 1 and the proper use of a bite/scratch/splash emergency care kit, as well as required annual TB testing. Institutions housing pregnant ruminants may require *Coxiella burnetii*–focused training. When new hazardous agents are added to research protocols, it is always appropriate to work closely with the researchers and respective safety officials (biohazard, chemical, and radiation) and consider whether agent-specific training should be provided to the involved laboratory animal resources personnel (in addition to the lab members).

11.3.1.4 Facility and Equipment Safety Considerations

The workplace facilities and equipment necessary to properly support the OHS program will vary greatly from one program to the next. In order to minimize exposure to potential hazards, the use of engineering controls/equipment should be emphasized over individual control measures. Of particular relevance are engineering controls and equipment that target exposure to ergonomic injuries (heavy lifting of animals and equipment/supplies, repetitive motion from rodent cage handling) and animal allergens (dump stations, change hoods). To avoid or limit exposure to animal allergens, a high level of personal hygiene is essential, which requires access to appropriate change rooms, showers, laundry, and supplies.

11.3.2 Veterinary Care

The attending veterinarian is responsible for the health and welfare of the animals used in research. This responsibility extends to monitoring and promoting animal well-being at all times during animal use, and during all phases of the animal's life. An adequate veterinary care program consists of the assessment of animal well-being and the effective management of (NRC 2011)

* Animal procurement and transportation
* Preventive medicine (including quarantine, animal biosecurity, and surveillance)
* Clinical disease, disability, and related health issues
* Protocol-associated disease, disability, and other sequelae
* Surgery and perioperative care
* Pain and distress
* Anesthesia and analgesia
* Euthanasia

11.3.2.1 Animal Procurement and Transportation

Procurement and transportation of animals must be in accordance with local, state, federal, and international regulations. The AWRs set standards for the movement of regulated species within the United States. The International Air Transport Association regulations define the safe and humane transport of animals by air. The Centers for Disease Control and Prevention and the USDA regulate the movement of animals and animal products to safeguard against harbored zoonotic and other communicable diseases. The FWS regulates the movement of wild animals and their tissues. The Convention on International Trade in Endangered Species of Wild Fauna and Flora lists species that are captive bred (e.g., NHPs). In addition to accompanying animal shipments, procurement and transportation documents may need to be maintained for animals acquired by an institution for its investigators. Associated records may include health certificates, point of contact information from the sending and receiving institutions, contingency plans, emergency procedures, veterinary contact information, and agency permits.

Procurement also needs to be tightly bound to the approved protocol in terms of animal number usage. Sources of animals need to be critically considered. Establishment of a breeding colony should be based on need. Vendor-derived animals need to be evaluated carefully for quality. It is important for the veterinarian to be involved in determining whether an animal source is appropriate and its animals meet the health status requirements of the institution. Regardless of transportation mode, planning should be of paramount importance to ensure animal safety and well-being. The transportation should provide for the "animals' physical, physiological or behavioral needs and comfort" (NRC 2011), maintain the animals' health status (e.g., biosecurity level), and minimize potential hazard exposure risk to personnel (e.g., zoonoses, allergens, and physical trauma).

11.3.2.2 Preventive Medicine

A robust, comprehensive preventive medicine program will enhance the value of research animals by promoting animal health and limiting outside (confounding) health status variability. Preventive medicine programs consist of various combinations of policies, procedures, and equipment related to quarantine and stabilization and the separation of animals by species, source, and health status (NRC 2011). A quality preventive medicine program starts well before animal orders are placed (via the critical evaluation and selection of animal suppliers) and continues throughout the animals' entire stay in the facility.

11.3.2.3 Clinical Care and Management

To be effective in providing clinical care, the veterinary staff needs to be familiar with the housed species and how they are used in research and teaching. Health and welfare concerns need to be reported to veterinary staff in a timely and accurate manner. The veterinary staff is responsible for performing an objective assessment of the animal(s) to determine the best course of action. Some things to consider are

- Protocols with clearly delineated humane end points will help ensure that animals' health and welfare needs are being met.
- Establishing *standing orders* or SOPs for recurrent common health problems can be effective in delivering consistent and expedited care.
- Persistent or significant problems involving experimental animal health and welfare need to be communicated to the IACUC.
- Diagnostics, treatments, and outcomes should be documented.
- Emergency veterinary care needs to be accessible, both during and outside regularly scheduled hours.
- Veterinarians must have the authority, delegated by the IO and the IACUC, to treat an animal, including removing it from study, relieving pain or distress, or performing euthanasia if necessary (e.g., unavailable researcher, disagreement regarding course of action) (NRC 2011).
- Controlled drug records and storage procedures should be reviewed during facility inspections.

11.3.2.4 Anesthesia and Analgesia

Appropriate anesthesia and analgesia procedures must be established to ensure that clinical, welfare (humane end points), and research requirements are met. Some specific drug selection criteria are species, age, type of surgery/procedure and associated type and level of pain, drug safety/side effects/pharmacological interactions and so on. In general, the benefits of multimodal analgesia (using different classes of analgesics to achieve a synergistic effect) and preemptive analgesia (delivery of analgesics before or during surgery) are well established at this point, and these methods are becoming the recommended approach for protocols likely to result in moderate to severe postprocedural pain. The alleviation of chronic pain can be especially challenging to control.

Opiate slow-release dermal patches, extended release formulations, and implantable osmotic pumps may be viable options. It is important to emphasize that there can be wide variation among individual animals within the same species and among tissue handling practices between surgeons, so, regardless, breakthrough pain must always be assessed for and appropriately controlled to ensure appropriate analgesic management. Nonpharmacological pain control techniques (e.g., applying padding to resting boards/flooring, wound/bandage management, increasing ambient temperature) and supportive care can be effective adjunctive or alternative therapies.

11.3.2.5 Euthanasia

The IACUC, together with veterinary staff, should ensure that researchers and other personnel involved in performing euthanasia are qualified to perform requested euthanasia techniques humanely; if they are not, it is the institution's responsibility to ensure that they are properly trained prior to commencing live animal work. Unless a deviation is justified for scientific reasons on an approved protocol, methods should be consistent with the American Veterinary Medical Association Guidelines for the Euthanasia of Animals (AVMA 2013). IACUCs may wish to consider the following specific rodent euthanasia-related areas that that may involve laboratory animal resources:

- Carbon dioxide is currently considered an acceptable method for rodent euthanasia, but there is some controversy regarding its use and the potential that it invokes pain and distress in exposed animals (AVMA 2013). IACUCs need to reassess its acceptability on an ongoing basis as new scientific data becomes available.
- Carbon dioxide must come from a controlled source (i.e., compressed gas cylinder).
- Carbon dioxide should be precisely regulated using a flow meter device so that CO_2 displaces 10–30% of the chamber volume/min. Prefilled chambers are unacceptable (AVMA 2013).
- Ideally, carbon dioxide euthanasia should be conducted in the animal's home cage to minimize distress.
- Carbon dioxide is not recommended for neonates. Alternative methods, such as decapitation, should be considered for euthanasia of neonatal rodents. If CO_2 must be used, prolonged (e.g., up to 50 min) exposure to the gas is required.
- Cervical dislocation and decapitation are acceptable for rodent euthanasia if the following conditions are met: (1) personnel are trained, proficient, and competent; and (2) for decapitation, scissors/guillotines are well maintained.

11.4 CHALLENGES WITH PI-MANAGED HOUSING

According to the Guide, "animals should be housed in facilities… not in laboratories merely for convenience" (NRC 2011). In addition to regulatory oversight, there are a plethora of other reasons for discouraging this practice wherever possible— staffing; consistency of husbandry care; logistical, financial, or occupational health–related issues and so on. Despite these disincentives, under certain circumstances (e.g., experimental necessity, experiments that require specialized equipment, species that require unique housing conditions), it may be appropriate for laboratory housing to occur. From a regulatory perspective, most IACUCs will treat such an area as a *satellite area*, which specifies institutional oversight responsibilities when animals are held longer than a certain period (12 h for the AWRs; 24 h for the PHS Policy). Prior to housing animals in a satellite facility, the IACUC must review the justification of the need for satellite housing and inspect and approve that specific site. All satellite facilities must meet the requirements of the Guide, the PHS Policy, and the AWRs if the institution is AAALAC International–accredited, PHS-assured, and USDA-licensed. This can prove challenging for some laboratories when dealing with older facilities and equipment, or when personnel tasked with providing the daily care have other responsibilities within the laboratory. It is important to make sure the expectations and requirements are clear. It is also important to emphasize that this housing approval is subject to change, including revocation, in the event that additional facilities become available, regulations and guidelines evolve, experiments finish, and so forth.

Some of the more common topics to emphasize in these PI-managed areas are

- The scientific justification for the satellite housing request must be compelling. Specific literature to support the scientific justification may be required. Distance from the vivarium is not a compelling justification unless there is a scientific need (e.g., hazardous material containment, short half-life reagent, specialized equipment access).
- The expectation should be that the husbandry/care management procedures follow institutionally established SOPs or that custom procedures are developed that are approved by qualified veterinarians and the IACUC.
- The PI or his or her designee must serve as the main contacts for the lab and agree to be accountable for the care of the housed animals. Given the size and complexity of the operation, it may be prudent to identify a backup individual. The job description of this "responsible person" should adequately reflect these important duties.
- The facilities need to be validated in terms of ventilation, availability of emergency power supply, light control, temperature/humidity control, and so on. This validation should be done prior to approval and should include members of the IACUC and veterinary and husbandry staff.
- The animals should have access to appropriate environmental enrichment consistent with central vivarium practices.
- Housing must be segregated from all other laboratory activities, including areas containing personnel who do not need to have animal contact.
- Euthanasia or surgeries should not be performed in close proximity to the housed animals.
- Chemical hazards should not be stored near the animal cages or biosafety cabinets or fume hoods, when animals are present.
- For rodents, specifically, the PI-managed housing application or protocol should be explicit in terms of maximum number of cages, particularly if using microisolator caging. If caging densities need to be increased, transferring these animals into individually ventilated caging might alleviate problems related to animal allergen exposure, cage-changing frequency, and animal health.
- PI-managed housing areas are subject to IACUC semiannual inspections.

11.5 CONCLUSION

IACUCs are faced with a number of broad and sometimes complex physical plant and programmatic issues related to animal facilities. Notwithstanding the complexity and occasional confusion surrounding these issues, it is the responsibility of IACUCs to provide thoughtful institutional oversight of animal facilities and related ACUPs. It is unrealistic to believe that all IACUCs can include voting members with expertise in all of the areas that need discernment. However, the judicious use of internal resources (members of other units within the institution who can serve as advisors) and external resources (consultants, members of regulatory agencies, etc.) can broaden the capabilities of the committee and assist in addressing many of the issues facing IACUCs today and in the future. The task may seem overwhelming at times, but it is possible, with dedicated effort, to achieve comprehensive, effective, and rational oversight of animal facilities and programs.

REFERENCES

AAALAC (Association for Assessment and Accreditation of Laboratory Animal Care International). 2014. AAALAC home page. http://www.aaalac.org/index.cfm.

ARENA/OLAW (Applied Research Ethics National Association and Office of Laboratory Animal Welfare). 2002. *Institutional Animal Care and Use Committee Guidebook*, 2nd edn. Bethesda, MD: National Institutes of Health.

AVMA (American Veterinary Medical Association). 2013. *Guidelines for the Euthanasia of Animals*. Schaumburg, IL: AVMA.

FASS (Federation of Animal Science Societies). 2010. Guide for the care and use of agricultural animals in agricultural research and teaching. Consortium for Developing a Guide for the Care and Use of Agricultural Animals in Agricultural Research and Teaching. Champaign, IL: FASS.

Gaskill, B. N., C. J. Gordon, E. A. Pajor, J. R. Lucas, J. K. Davis, and J. P. Garner. 2012. Heat or insulation: Behavioral titration of mouse preference for warmth or access to a nest. *PLoS One* 7 (3):e32799.

Gaskill, B. N., K. R. Pritchett-Corning, C. J. Gordon, E. A. Pajor, J. R. Lucas, J. K. Davis, and J. P. Garner. 2013. Energy reallocation to breeding performance through improved nest building in laboratory mice. *PLoS One* 8 (9):e74153.

Gaskill, B. N., S. A. Rohr, E. A. Pajor, J. R. Lucas, and J. P. Garner. 2009. Some like it hot: Mouse temperature preferences in laboratory housing. *Applied Animal Behaviour Science* 116 (2):279–285.

NIH (National Institutes of Health). 2002. Public Health Service policy on humane care and use of laboratory animals. Bethesda, MD: Office of Laboratory Animal Welfare, U.S. Department of Health and Human Services, NIH.

NRC (National Research Council). 2011. *Guide for the Care and Use of Laboratory Animals*, 8th edn. Washington, DC: National Academies Press.

Silverman, J., M. A. Suckow, and S. Murthy. 2014. *The IACUC Handbook*. Boca Raton, FL: CRC Press.

Thigpen, J. E., K. D. R. Setchell, H. E. Saunders, J. K. Haseman, M. G. Grant, and D. B. Forsythe. 2004. Selecting the appropriate rodent diet for endocrine disruptor research and testing studies. *ILAR Journal* 45 (4):401–416.

USDA (U.S. Department of Agriculture). 2013a. *Animal Welfare Inspection Guide*, 1st edn. Washington, DC: USDA. http://www.aphis.usda.gov/animal_welfare/downloads/Inspection%20Guide%20-%20November%202013.pdf.

USDA (U.S. Department of Agriculture). 2013b. *Animal Welfare Act and Animal Welfare Regulations* (Animal Care Blue Book). Code of Federal Regulations (CFR), Title 9, Chapter 1, Subchapter A, Parts 1–4.

USDA (U.S. Department of Agriculture). 2014. USDA/APHIS Animal care policy manual. Washington, DC: USDA. http://www.aphis.usda.gov/animal_welfare/policy.php.

CHAPTER 12

International IACUCs and Outside Collaborations

Patrick Sharp

CONTENTS

12.1 LAWS, REGULATIONS, AND REGULATORY COMPLIANCE IN OTHER COUNTRIES

The responsible and ethical use of laboratory animals is unique to each nation's regulatory matrix and complements its individual, yet complex, national/regional culture, religion, ethics, customs, economic status, politics, and values toward animals and, specifically, laboratory animals used in research, teaching, and testing.

Published regulatory perceptions state that the "European approach emphasizes detailed regulations that tend to be inflexible … U.S. and Canadian approaches … encourage new approaches and flexibility. The Japanese approach is more cultural and is based on respect of animals and Buddhist philosophy" (NRC 2004). It seems that more countries are adopting the North American approach of self-monitoring and performance standards at some level. Regarding science-based performance standards, Klein and Bayne (2007) point out that "implementation of an organizational culture of care is not unique to the animal research enterprise," and "leadership at the institutional level must be accountable and responsible for the integrity of new information generated from its research programs." Failing to set the proper "culture of care," accountability, and responsibility can result in "science's ultimate post-publication punishment: retraction, the official declaration that a paper is so flawed that it must be withdrawn from the literature" (Van Noorden 2011), or in the case of a pharmaceutical compound or medical device, human/animal morbidity or mortality. or in the case of a pharmaceutical compound or medical device, human/animal morbidity or mortality.

There are general concerns in areas outside North America and Western Europe about animal welfare. Numerous articles have been published about developing national laws and regulations in Asia, applying the three Rs (reduce, replace, refine), and hosting numerous conferences on "hot button issues" pertaining to animal welfare and the use of animals in research, teaching, and testing. Some contend that the animal welfare issue in China, in particular, has no or limited opportunities for acceptance or success because of a long list of issues, including human rights, animal-based traditional Chinese/Asian medicines and foods (e.g., bear bile collection, shark fin and bird's nest soup, tiger bones) (Curren 2012, Lu et al. 2013), and corruption (Bloomberg 2014). Many contract research organizations (CROs) use the Association for Assessment and Accreditation of Laboratory Animal Care (AAALAC) International accreditation to highlight the quality of their Animal Care and Use Programs (ACUPs); AAALAC-accredited facilities undergo an announced site visit once every three years. The resulting site-visit report is entirely confidential and without transparency. Likewise, there is very little transparency with regard to non-U.S.-based government regulators and their findings; the U.S. Department of Agriculture (USDA) does publish final inspection reports for U.S. institutions and has investigated (and fined) foreign organizations when covered species have died in transit to the United States. Readers may find the article by Goodman et. al (2015) of interest concerning the ability of AAALAC accreditation to facilitate or enhance regulation of USDA-licensed facilities. The AAALAC has published a response on their website and has communications pending in various scientific publications (Newcomer, 2014).

What value is assessment and accreditation without transparency? Many sponsoring organizations hire external laboratory animal specialists as consultants to perform CRO and vendor visits to enhance the transparency and oversight of cross-border biomedical research programs. Due to visa requirements, these visits may be announced to the CRO and vendor without the sponsoring research organization's knowledge.

Religion is a motivator for the ethical conduct of research, with a Judeo-Christian approach in North America and Europe. The religious influence in Asia, east of the Ural Mountains, is diverse and includes Islam, Buddhism, Taoism, Confucianism, and Hinduism. The religious influence on Asian animal care and use has been discussed by Chapple (2000), Gharebaghi et al. (2007), Izmirli et al. (2010), Aldavood et al. (2013), Kagiyama and Nomura (NRC 2004), and Naderi et al. (2012). Islam and Christianity predominate on the African continent.

12.2 THE THREE RS

Internationally, Russell and Burch's *The Principles of Humane Experimental Technique* (1959), in which they described the three Rs (replacement, reduction, and refinement), is an important and frequently cited document. Briefly, replacement is using *in vitro* or *in silico* models instead of live animals; reduction is using the minimum number of animals; and refinement is, among other things, using analgesia, anesthesia, and minimally injurious methods and procedures. Rollin (2007a) gives special significance to minimizing pain (refinement) when stating, "animal pain might be even worse than human pain; after all, humans have hope." While pain is not the point of the study, it is well known that there are many consequences associated with pain that can interfere with research.

A given nation's regulations frequently discuss or refer to the three Rs, animal welfare, and a host of other essential items, including cage size requirements, husbandry practices, veterinary care, research proposal review (e.g., Institutional Animal Care and Use Committee [IACUC], Animal Ethics Committee [AEC]), and facility/physical plant requirements. Some animal regulatory requirements include strong considerations for animal, human, and environmental health matters. Rollin (2007b) states, "for thinking people, ethics is far more valuable than regulation." Rollin puts forward the idea that the three Rs are a marriage of science and ethics, rather than "science is value-free in general, and ethics-free in particular" (Rollin 2007a).

Historically, the three Rs have been incorporated into voluntary standards and legislation in North America and Western Europe. More recently, China (Kong and Qin 2010), India (Sankar and Kandasamy 2013), Korea (Han and Lee 2013), Brazil (Trez 2010), Turkey, and Iran (Izmirli et al. 2010) have implemented the three Rs into voluntary standards and/or legislation. Hudson-Shore (2011) indicates that little progress has been made with the three Rs in Great Britain and later (Hudson-Shore 2012) points out, "scientists are positive about the Three Rs, they may not be spending enough time searching for information on them, and that this search is not yet a structural part of the research process." In van Luijk et al.'s 2011 survey of researchers in the Netherlands regarding three Rs searches and implementation, they summarize, "specialized Three Rs databases and websites are hardly known, and, when used, are difficult to search due to differences in content, quality and search profiles."

Several biomedical research publications provide ethical use requirements and expectations when research animals are used; this may result in the rejection of manuscripts that have not undergone some form of an ethical review process (Rollin 2007b). Franco and Olsson (2013) also identify a role for journal editors and reviewers in ensuring that the three Rs are implemented. Simple compliance statements highlighting the guidelines applied, or providing proof of IACUC approval, may not be sufficient in ensuring the three Rs were implemented or were implemented properly. Rollin (2011) reveals a discussion with Dr. Albert Koltveit regarding the power of editors when research is conducted using lax regulations, "biomedical editors were 'guardians of the gate,' who are a very powerful force for ensuring adherence to that ethic. People will not do the research if we do not publish it," he affirmed. "Therefore, it is up to us to assure that any research we publish, regardless of where it is done, meets North American Standards."

Kong and Qin (2010) identify "governmental forces" as "the most important reason" for implementation of the three Rs in China, mandated through the Ministry of Science and Technology and the Ninth Five-Year Project of Laboratory Animal Science. According to Lu et al. (2013), domestic Chinese animal rights groups (e.g., the Chinese Animal Protection Network) seem to play a minor role.

12.3 NATIONAL LEGISLATION

Because of the ever-evolving regulatory continuum, a comprehensive regulatory review in this chapter is not feasible; recent changes to the Australian Code of Practice for the Care and Use of Animals for Scientific Purposes (NHMRC 2013), the U.S. Guide for the Care and Use of Laboratory Animals (NRC 2011), and the Council of Europe's European Treaty Series (ETS) 123 (EPCEU Union 2010) are presented as examples of recently updated guides and regulations. Likewise, *de novo* animal regulations have recently emerged in Singapore (NACLAR 2004), Turkey (2004), Tanzania (2008), Brazil (2008), and Korea (2008, 2009, 2011). A general overview is provided in this chapter (Table 12.1). In addition to national laws, there may be state or provincial laws directly impacting the care and use of laboratory animals (e.g., Western Australia's Animal Welfare Act) (WA 2002), some of which may have more authority than the corresponding national guidelines (e.g., Australian Code). Furthermore, local, state, and national legislation and regulations indirectly impacting animal care and use (e.g., biohazard, occupational health) may apply to and affect biomedical research.

Table 12.1 Select National Experimental Animal Welfare Guidance Documents and Legislation

Country	Document (Year) [English]
Australia	Australian Code of Practice for the Care and Use of Animals for Scientific Purposes (2013)
Austria	Bundesgesetz über den Schutz der Tiere (Tierschutzgesetz, TSchG) (2004) [Federal Act on the Protection of Animals (Animal Protection Act, TSchG)]
Brazil	Law 11794/08, Arouca Law (2008)
Chile	Sobre Protección de Animales (2009) [Animal Protection Law]
Croatia	The Animal Protection Act (2006)
Cyprus	The Bioethics Law of 2001
Czech Republic	Animal Protection Act 283/1992
Estonia	Animal Protection Act (2000, 2002) Government Regulation No. 187 (2003)
Finland	Animal Welfare Act (2006)
Germany	Tierschutzgesetz (2010) [Animal Welfare Law]
India	Prevention of Cruelty to Animals Act (1960) Animal Welfare Act (draft, 2011)
Kenya	Prevention of Cruelty to Animals Act (1983)
Liechtenstein	Total ban on animal use in experimental procedures
Malaysia	Animals Act (1953), Amendments (2006), The Revision of Laws Order (2006)
New Zealand	Animal Welfare Act (1999)
Norway	Norwegian Animal Welfare Act (2010)
Peru	[Protection of Domestic Animals (2009)]
Philippines	Act to Promote Animal Welfare in the Philippines (1998)
Poland	Polish Animal Protection Act (1998)
Romania	Law No. 205/2004 on the protection of animals (2004)
Russia	"… no special laws protecting animals from cruelty, nor has it a legislative base for regulating animal-based research." (Loukianov 2011)
South Africa	Veterinary and Para-veterinary Professions Act (1982) South African National Standard (SANS) for the Care and Use of Animals for Scientific Purposes (SANS 10386:2008)
South Korea	Animal Welfare Act (2011) Laboratory Animal Act (2009)
Sweden	Svensk författningssamling djurskyddslagen (2009:303) Svensk författningssamling djurskyddsförordningen(2009) [Swedish Animal Welfare Act] (2009:303) [Swedish Animal Welfare Ordinance] (2009)
Switzerland	Swiss Federal Act on Animal Protection (1978)
Taiwan, ROC	Taiwan Animal Protection Law (1998)
Tanzania	Animal Welfare Act (2008)

(Continued)

Table 12.1   (Continued) Select National Experimental Animal Welfare Guidance Documents and Legislation

Country	Document (Year) [English]
Turkey	The Regulation of the Protection of Animals Used for Experimental and Other Scientific Purposes, the Breeding Place of Experimental Animals, the Establishment, Operation, Inspection, Procedures and Principles of the Laboratories Which Make Experiments (2004) The Animal Protection Act. Act (2004)
Zimbabwe	Prevention of Cruelty to Animals Act (1986) Scientific Experiments on Animals Act (1963)

Legislative and regulatory compliance requires strong support for the institution's ACUP from the institutional official (IO). Although complex and expensive, an inappropriately supported ACUP is frequently ineffective and is a source of frustration to the animal users, the IACUC members, the attending veterinarian, and the IO. In addition to regulatory compliance, voluntary accreditation (e.g. AAALAC International) will be equally frustrating. The cost of placing programs back into compliance is always greater than maintaining a compliant, voluntarily accredited program.

12.3.1 National/Provincial Laws and Regulations

The IACUC, IO, veterinarian, and researcher functions occur consistently throughout various countries' national and provincial research animal laws and regulations, although the specific terms referring to each group differ slightly (e.g., AEC versus IACUC, chief executive officer [CEO] versus IO, researcher versus principal investigator, nonscientist versus community member). With the globalization of today's biomedical research, researchers frequently conduct research at more than one institution simultaneously.

12.3.2 Voting versus Consensus

In some laws and regulations, the development of consensus is stressed, while others discuss the importance of voting members. Consensus may not be easily or quickly achieved, which will cause frustration among the research team when there are protracted delays to starting research projects. Voting permits a true assessment of consensus and allows those in the minority to render a *minority view* regarding the research proposal. The minority views should be included in the IACUC/AEC programmatic review, which, in turn, is forwarded to the institutional CEO/IO and subsequently to any regulatory bodies, if required.

12.3.3 Legal "Binding": Institution versus Investigator

Most national/provincial laws and regulations bind with the institution and hold the IACUC responsible for the institutional ACUP. In these legislative settings, the

IO is the individual with the ultimate and legal responsibility for the institution's program for the care and use of laboratory animals.

Some nations' legislation pursues a parallel and complementary legal binding with the individual researchers in an attempt to augment regulatory compliance. This is seen in the United Kingdom, where the Animals (Scientific Procedures) Act (Hollands 1986) requires three separate instruments to maintain compliance with the Home Office. The certificate or licenses apply to a place ("scientific procedure establishment"), a person ("personal license"), and a project ("project license"). China has employed a similar system; however, licenses only apply to a place and a person.

12.4 INTERNATIONAL GUIDELINES

In addition, the Council for International Organizations of Medical Sciences (CIOMS) and the Office International des Epizooties (OIE) provide guidance on the ethical use of animals in biomedical research. Guidance from these organizations is perhaps most important when research is conducted in countries without national laboratory animal care and use legislation but is supported by a country with national animal care and use legislation requesting programmatic oversight. An example of this would be a U.S. National Institutes of Health (NIH)-funded project occurring outside the United States in a country or an area of a country without laboratory animal care and use legislation.

12.4.1 Council for International Organizations of Medical Sciences (CIOMS)

The United Nations Educational, Scientific, and Cultural Organization and the World Health Organization established the CIOMS to develop wide-ranging programs on bioethics and other topics. The current International Guiding Principles for Biomedical Research Involving Animals (CIOMS/ICLAS 2012) is a collaboration between CIOMS and the International Council for Laboratory Animal Science (ICLAS) and provides 10 principles for use "by the international scientific community to guide the responsible use of vertebrate animals in scientific and/or educational activities."

According to CIOMS and ICLAS, the Guiding Principles "reflect current best practices and standards of care in laboratory animal medicine and science and provide a touchstone or framework of responsibility and oversight to ensure the appropriate use of animals. They also may serve as a benchmark for advancing international collaboration in biomedical sciences." The current Guiding Principles are available from the organization's website, www.cioms.ch.

12.4.2 Office International des Epizooties

The OIE maintains the organization's original moniker, although it became the World Organization for Animal Health (WOAH) in 2004. Annually, the OIE publishes the Terrestrial Animal Health Code (WOAH 2014b) to set the "standards for the improvement of animal health and welfare and veterinary public health worldwide." The Terrestrial Code currently includes a chapter entitled Use of Animals in Research and Education to

> provide advice and assistance for Member Countries to follow when formulating regulatory requirements, or other form of oversight, for the use of live animals in research and education… A system of animal use oversight should be implemented in each country. The system will, in practice, vary from country to country and according to cultural, economic, religious and social factors. However, the OIE recommends that Member Countries address all the essential elements identified in this chapter in formulating a regulatory framework that is appropriate to their local conditions. (WOAH 2014b)

The OIE also publishes an Aquatic Animal Health Code (WOAH 2014a) annually; however, this document differs from the Terrestrial Code in that it currently lacks a chapter on using animals in research and education. Furthermore, the document's goal is to set "standards for the improvement of aquatic animal health and welfare of farmed fish worldwide, including through standards for safe international trade in aquatic animals (amphibians, crustaceans, fish and mollusks) and their products" (WOAH 2014a). The document does include a chapter entitled Welfare of Farmed Fish. As fish continue to play a greater role in biomedical research, this oversight will require rectification; the recent development of fish health sentinel programs and significant expansion of aquatic species in the U.S. Guide are a clear indication of their research significance.

12.4.3 Institutional Animal Welfare Audits

Many global institutions conduct animal welfare audits of CROs and other facilities where part or all of their preclinical research occurs, as "Sponsors see them as a mechanism to ensure that their standards are being adhered to and CROs see them as an opportunity to continually improve their processes and gain knowledge about industry standards and trends" (Pritt 2008a). These audits may be performed by the organization sponsoring the research or through third-party consultants. While such animal welfare audits had previously been performed on non-AAALAC-accredited institutions, the audits now include AAALAC-accredited CROs and other facilities. The "other facilities" that may be audited include animal suppliers, in part, because these companies "breed" animals and may be outside the regulatory purview of research facilities in some country's legislation. The author has both "audited" and "been audited." Although each organization being audited is different, each auditing organization typically has a "script," but the auditor has the ability to deviate if warranted. Unlike an AAALAC site visit, there may be additional questions and requests after the auditor has visited the facility.

Regarding the animal welfare and animal facility audits, some countries require individuals performing such business (audits) to obtain a visa. As mentioned previously, in the process of obtaining the visa, the country may confirm that the visiting auditor will be traveling to a given company (e.g., a CRO). In the process, the company being audited is alerted of the auditor's travel and, in essence, the audit may not necessarily be "unannounced."

12.4.4 Voluntary Compliance Relevance

Critics of voluntary compliance point to its relevance and consistency with regulatory standards. In the United States, USDA inspection reports are available either online or through the Freedom of Information Act. The USDA Animal and Plant Health Inspection Service (APHIS) conducts unannounced facility inspections and generates a report highlighting noncompliant items, linking them to a specific section of the Animal Welfare Act Regulations, which "excludes birds, rats of the genus *Rattus*, and mice of the genus *Mus*, bred for use in research."

Outside the United States, when a voluntary accrediting agency (e.g., AAALAC International) evaluates an animal research facility, a given country's research animal facility inspection reports are most likely unavailable for public view. The absence of government-issued research facility inspection reports should be taken into account when evaluating a facility that is accredited by a voluntary accreditation agency. This is an area of particular concern for organizations sponsoring biomedical research overseas where government inspections may be announced, and, unlike they are in the United States, the associated inspection reports are unavailable directly from the given country's inspecting government agency. While on the surface these voluntary compliance site visits appear equivalent, all too frequently organizations sponsoring research evaluate or require auditors to appropriately and effectively evaluate the organization conducting the research (e.g., the CRO) in Asia versus North America or Europe, where these additional, and costly, organizational evaluations are far less likely to occur.

12.5 IACUC OR ETHICAL REVIEW REQUIREMENTS

Most countries have legislative provisions for some form of an AEC, generally referred to as an IACUC in this chapter. The committee is typically constituted by an institutional CEO, generally referred to as an IO in this chapter. The IO is not allowed to serve on the IACUC in some countries but is permitted in other countries. Many countries request that the IO meet regularly with the IACUC chair and take animal care and use direction or suggestions from the IACUC. Various reports, including regulatory reports generated by the IACUC, are forwarded to the IO for the IO's information and action on IACUC matters. Some institutions have moved to create a deputy IO role to specifically address the numerous and unique issues concerning an institution's ACUP.

The committee's constitution may be capped at a specific number of individuals from a given unit within an organization (e.g., three in the case of Singapore's Guidelines on the Care and Use of Animals for Scientific Purposes). It may require a minimum membership, as in the Australian Code where "Categories C (Animal Welfare representative) and D (Community Member) together must represent at least one-third of those members present" (NHMRC 2013). Contingencies are made for alternate or deputy members, even though this is not specifically stated in national legislation; generally, the same appointment practices apply. Likewise, alternates must have a direct relationship to the "regular" member's role (e.g., scientist, veterinarian, nonscientist/community member, etc.). Alternate members must "vote their conscience" and not be "voting for" the "regular" IACUC member. Most countries require a quorum of members to be present for an IACUC meeting, and some legislation specifically requires the presence of the nonscientist(s)/community member(s) and a quorum. This underscores the importance for IACUCs of utilizing alternate members, where it is feasible and not restricted by law or regulation, and of having appropriate and adequate community representation.

Few countries specifically grant the institution the ability to perform a designated member review as outlined in the Animal Welfare Act (AWA). This is unfortunate, in that the "simpler" protocols tend to take time away from "complex" protocols. In many countries, this may be due to the fact that the IACUC process is relatively new, and those developing the legislation and regulations want a proper inventory and assessment of existing protocols previously not subjected to an ethical review.

Many countries lack the mechanism, used in the United States, whereby feedback occurs between the IACUC and the sponsoring research funding agency to ensure compliance. Noncompliance reporting in the United States, from the IACUC, through the IO, to the funding agency, facilitates regulatory compliance. Noncompliance carries the risk that research funding can be suspended or removed entirely. Likewise, AAALAC International also has noncompliance reporting requirements. Rollin's article (2007a) highlights the additional benefits of the IACUC system regarding public trust and researcher support.

Some national legislation explicitly encourages the use of multiple IACUCs. At the outset, this seems like a great idea to share the workload; however, it can quickly lead to institutional complexity, when similar procedures are handled differently within an institution, or when one IACUC appears "easier" to obtain research protocol approval from. Multiple IACUCs reviewing fewer research proposals lose the economy of scale seen with fewer, larger IACUCs or a single IACUC. Furthermore, if there is a noncompliant matter, is it the single IACUC's issue, or can it affect the other IACUCs or the institution as a whole? Can an equivalent IACUC policy or guideline be approved by multiple IACUCs? For the IO, there are now multiple "masters" and potential sources of institutional oversight. Therefore, the need for multiple IACUCs should be carefully weighed and evaluated.

12.6 OCCUPATIONAL HEALTH AND SAFETY

Many national regulations, including the AWA, are silent on personnel occupational health and safety (OHS). However, other government organizations within a given country may cover ACUPs directly, indirectly, or both. Employee hazards take many forms in research-based ACUPs and require proper management using engineering controls, administrative/workplace controls, and personal protective equipment.

Readers may find the following texts useful in developing an OHS program:

- Occupational Health and Safety in the Care and Use of Research Animals (NRC 1997)
- Occupational Health and Safety in the Care and Use of Nonhuman Primates (NRC 2003)

Providing OHS in some countries may be challenging due to the lack of physician assistants, nurse practitioners, and trained occupational health physicians. Furthermore, some countries lack appropriately trained and credentialed laboratory animal veterinarians to appropriately assist medical professionals.

12.7 ANIMAL WELFARE REGULATIONS

12.7.1 Foreign Regulation Resources

There are few single sources serving as a resource for foreign regulations, and such sources could quickly become dated in today's ever-changing regulatory landscape. Besides using published resources, interested individuals may glean sufficient information by conducting an Internet search on a particular country and other relevant search keywords. Readers are directed to the following resources: CompMed LISTSERV, AAALAC.org, Legislation and Oversight of the Conduct of Research Using Animals: A Global Overview (Bayne et al. 2010), *Laboratory Animals: Regulations and Recommendations for Global Collaborative Research* (Guillen 2013), and *The Laboratory Rat* (Sharp and Villano 2012). See Table 12.1 for select national experimental animal welfare guidance documents and legislation information.

12.8 ANIMAL USAGE RESTRICTIONS

Animal usage restrictions fall into three general categories: regulatory, religious, and animal health. Regulatory restrictions are those affecting the use of specific animals in biomedical research. For example, the use of primates and chimpanzees is severely restricted or forbidden in some countries, while other countries limit the use of primates and chimpanzees to domestic sources. Similar restrictions apply to threatened and endangered animals. Religious restrictions may be a consideration when hiring an individual; the employee must not be discriminated against, but must be made aware of the duties and obligations of the job and aware of the species that he or she will be working with.

Religious restrictions, particularly those relating to pigs, have been discussed in Islam and Judaism. Izmirli et al. (2010) point out that, "the use of pigs in medical research may be difficult for some members of the Muslim populations." Furthermore, Gharebaghi et al. (2007) indicate that "the Quran, the holy book of Islam, as well as Hadiths contain the obligatory ways to keep and treat animals since more than 1400 years ago." The Holy Bible, in the books of Leviticus and Deuteronomy, outlines "impure" and "acceptable" animals. Other religions may have restrictions against other animals that are understood to be "unclean" or "impure"; there also may be religious restrictions preventing some individuals from euthanizing healthy animals.

The available health status of an animal may present a problem or source of frustration for some researchers. In the United States, specific pathogen–free pigs are readily available, but this is not the case in other parts of the world. Given pigs' susceptibility to pneumonia, among other research-altering conditions, they would not necessarily be the best anesthetic risk when undergoing a surgical or other procedure requiring anesthesia. In addition, pigs (and other animals) may pose a risk for some zoonotic diseases. For instance, in the 2009–10 H1N1 influenza outbreak, pigs in Canada and Indonesia, independently, became infected with H1N1; the Indonesian pigs were exported to Singapore for food and biomedical research. Other diseases, such as Nipah virus, can affect both pigs and humans.

12.9 NIH CONSIDERATIONS FOR OUTSIDE COLLABORATIONS AND SUBCONTRACTS

12.9.1 Foreign Assurances

Foreign and domestic organizations receiving U.S. Public Health Service (PHS) funds must maintain an Assurance with the NIH Office of Laboratory Animal Welfare (OLAW). The funds may be received directly, as part of a contract or grant, or indirectly (e.g., performance site through a primary institution).

OLAW uses the International Guiding Principles for Biomedical Research Involving Animals (CIOMS/ICLAS 2012), in part, when foreign institutions apply for an Animal Welfare Assurance. The Foreign Assurance acts to accomplish three tasks: (1) it ensures the institution's compliance with the PHS Policy on Humane Care and Use of Laboratory Animals (NIH 2002) or other acceptable humane care and use of animals standards; (2) it ensures compliance with a country's laws, regulations, and policies for humane care and use of animals; and (3) it commits the foreign institution to following International Guiding Principles for Biomedical Research Involving Animals (NIH 2013).

12.9.2 Examples of Frequently Contracted Studies

12.9.2.1 Toxicology/Good Laboratory Practices (GLP) Studies

Briefly, preclinical studies are conducted with the goal of getting a device or drug to market, with the early stages of the process being heavily animal dependent. Animal-dependent toxicology and GLP studies—preclinical studies—are a major area of concern with respect to the care of animals and their ethical use in the studies, not to mention the fidelity of the resulting data and reports. For many reasons, institutions (e.g., pharmaceutical companies) have outsourced portions of studies or entire studies to external organizations—that is, CROs. The Food and Drug Administration (FDA) broadly defines the relationship as either a "sponsor" or a "CRO"; specifically, a sponsor is "a person who takes responsibility for and initiates a clinical investigation. The sponsor may be an individual or pharmaceutical company, governmental agency, academic institution, private organization, or other organization. The sponsor does not actually conduct the investigation unless the sponsor is a sponsor-investigator," while a CRO is "a person that assumes, as an independent contractor with the sponsor, one or more of the obligations of a sponsor, e.g., design of a protocol, selection or monitoring of investigations, evaluation of reports, and preparation of materials to be submitted to the Food and Drug Administration" (FDA 2011).

The FDA and other oversight agencies worldwide scrutinize the organizations conducting preclinical studies. As stated in *Animal Research in a Global Environment: Meeting the Challenges* (ILAR 2011), "Foreign CROs face the challenge of establishing credibility. Western companies have scrutinized the different CROs that are being established in Asia. There have definitely been some bad outcomes, some disappointing facilities and programs. Sometimes that record is used to make presumptive judgments about new CROs."

Several articles are available that discuss CROs and CRO selection/audit considerations; for instance, Stark (2006), McCallum (2008), Pritt (2008b), Underwood (2007), Anderson and Taylor (2005), and Brower (2004). The primary CRO market has moved toward Asia (principally China), and the region will continue as a focus for the foreseeable future; this outsourcing trend is noted by sponsors in North America and Europe. Although there are several CROs operating in various countries, the market is relatively new and will eventually undergo consolidation and vertical integration to further maximize profits. Suffice it to say, assessing a potential CRO is a group process for the sponsor, where "It is the responsibility of the researcher and the laboratory animal science professional … to ensure that high standards of care and use are understood and implemented" (Stark 2006).

The FDA has established permanent posts in India, China, Europe, and Latin America. According to the FDA website (2011), the organization is working to

establish a presence in the Middle East. FDA's foreign presence will help improve product safety by:

- Gathering better knowledge about the production and transport of products;
- Leveraging the knowledge and resources of trusted counterpart agencies;
- Building regulatory capacity in countries where such assistance is needed;
- Working closely with regulated industry so they understand FDA requirements; and
- Expanding our ability to perform inspections and in a more timely manner.

12.9.2.2 Animal Import

The authority to import animals and animal products is divided among federal agencies, with jurisdiction depending on the animal or animal product involved. Federal jurisdiction may involve the FDA, the PHS, the U.S. Fish and Wildlife

Service, and APHIS. The USDA maintains the Animal Product Manual, which offers guidance and flowcharts regarding the particular types of items being imported (e.g., vaccines, antivenom), Veterinary Services permits or declaration requirements and actions that might be taken by the USDA. The manual also contains information regarding human materials, vaccines, and so forth. It is always prudent to check with the various government agencies, even if readers are repeating a recent import process, as rules and regulations, and their interpretations, do change.

U.S. state and local agencies may also require involvement or notification, or both. Each state has a State Veterinarian supervising the various animal health matters, including the regulation of animal movement. It may be prudent to contact the state veterinarian's Office regarding these matters, too. A list of state veterinarians may be obtained from the American Veterinary Medical Association's website.

12.10 MEMORANDA OF UNDERSTANDING

A memorandum of understanding (MOU), in this context, is a document between two or more organizations that are conducting research, teaching, and testing. These agreements outline methods for each institution to properly meet its animal care, use, welfare, and other obligations. MOU benefits include minimizing the duplication of effort, reducing regulatory burden, and promoting harmonization and the sharing of compliance and training/education resources. "OLAW and APHIS agree that review of a research project or evaluation of a program or facility by more than one recognized IACUC is not a federal requirement. Institutions should have a formal written understanding (e.g., memorandum of understanding) that addresses responsibilities for animal care and use, ownership, and IACUC review and oversight" (NIH 2006).

The MOU generally includes the following:

- Institutions/facilities included
- Animals included
- Inclusive dates
- Veterinary care
- Protocol review and approval process
- Personnel qualification/training
- Regulatory and other reports
- Animal transport
- Animal housing
- IACUC participation
- Hazardous agent(s) use

12.11 TRANSPORTATION

The International Air Transport Association (IATA) is the world airlines' trade association. Standards published by the IATA provide member airlines with animal transportation guidance. This guidance includes container requirements, marking and labeling, and temperature ranges for shipping animals. The Animal Transportation Association is another organization associated with safe and humane animal transportation.

Animal transportation is a matter deserving attention due to the strong international impact it has on primates and rodents used in biomedical research worldwide. Live rodents are shuttled around the globe on passenger and cargo air carriers, the majority on passenger air carriers. In recent years, and moving forward, nonhuman primate air transportation remains uncertain, and this could negatively impact rodents and other animals used in biomedical research should the same transportation (un)availability that affects nonhuman primates be carried over to other species.

Although ground transportation (e.g., climate-controlled truck) offers more control than air transportation, air transportation—ideally—is faster and has fewer logistic issues when transporting animals over long distances between continents. Intercontinental transportation relies almost exclusively on air transportation. This has caused significant concern, primarily over nonhuman primate shipments by air and the dwindling number of air carriers willing to undergo the negative publicity associated with transporting nonhuman primates. There is concern that the negative impact on the pace of biomedical research will cause nonhuman primate biomedical research and, possibly, research with other species to migrate toward countries with ready access to primates and, perhaps, with less developed animal welfare concern and regulatory oversight (Balls 2012).

There are few publications discussing the transportation of animals in biomedical research—Syversen et al. (2008), Quigley (2013), Balls (2012), the National Research Council (2002), and Landi et al. (1982). The articles by Syversen et al. and Landi et al. evaluate the transportation environment and transport-related immune implications, respectively. Special attention should be drawn to a statement in the Syversen et al. article: "During air shipment, mice are exposed to multiple stressors: absence of the normal light cycle, jet lag, pressure variations, and, in all likelihood, loud noises, vibrations, and unusual odors." The effects of animal transportation warrant the need for greater understanding, scientifically, of what happens to animals as they are transported from point A to point B and of how to enhance an animal's assimilation into the new environment. Furthermore, what is the interval after which relevant and reliable scientific data can be obtained?

Quigley (2013) discusses transporting fresh/frozen embryos, ova, and sperm as an alternative to live animal transport. Although this is an alternative, it still requires animal use. Movement in this direction will depend on the source and destination institutions' technical expertise; such techniques as the nonsurgical embryo transfer device may support the further use of fresh/frozen gametes and embryos as a viable means of transferring animals (Steele et al. 2013).

The USDA-APHIS also maintains information on animal and animal product export from the United States on the USDA-APHIS website.

ACKNOWLEDGMENT

The author wishes to acknowledge Mr. Ibrahim Faseeh for his assistance in preparing a portion of this chapter.

REFERENCES

Aldavood, S. J., R. M. Fard, and F. Naderynezhad. 2013. Laboratory animal ethics course planning in Iran. *Alternative to Laboratory Animals: ATLA* 41 (4):40–41.

Anderson, L. C. and K. Taylor. 2005. Outsourcing of animal care and biomedical resources. *Contemporary Topics in Laboratory Animal Science/American Association for Laboratory Animal Science* 44 (2):66.

Balls, M. 2012. The international transport of laboratory animals: No excuse for biased extremism of any kind. *Alternative to Laboratory Animals: ATLA* 40 (3):133–136.

Bayne, K., T. H. Morris, and M. P. France. 2010. Legislation and oversight of the conduct of research using animals: A global overview. *The UFAW Handbook on the Care and Management of Laboratory and Other Research Animals.* Chichester, UK: Wiley, pp. 107–123.

Bloomberg. 2014. Glaxo probe shows China graft endemic since czar executed. July 18. Bloomberg News.

Brower, V. 2004. Going global in R&D. *EMBO Reports* 5 (4):333.

Chapple, C. K. 2000. Asian religious views on animals: Implications for bioethics and the use of laboratory animals, In A. L. Kraus and D. Renquist (eds) *Bioethics and the Use of Laboratory Animals.* Chester, NH: American College of Laboratory Animal Medicine, pp. 45–56.

CIOMS/ICLAS (Council for the International Organization of Medical Sciences and International Council for Laboratory Animal Science). 2012. International guiding principles for biomedical research involving animals. CIOMS/ICLAS.

Curren, R., Jones, B. 2012. China is taking steps toward alternatives to animal testing. *Alternative to Laboratory Animals: ATLA* 40 (1):1–2.

EPCEU (European Parliament and the Council of the European Union). 2010. Directive 2010/63/EU of the European Parliament and of the Council of 22 September 2010 on the protection of animals used for scientific purposes. *The Official Journal of the European Union* 276.

FDA (U.S. Food and Drug Administration). 2011. Office of Global Regulatory Operations and Policy. Silver Spring, MD: FDA. http://www.fda.gov/AboutFDA/CentersOffices/OfficeofGlobalRegulatoryOperationsandPolicy/.

Franco, N. H. and I. A. Olsson. 2013. Is the ethical appraisal of protocols enough to ensure best practice in animal research? *Alternative to Laboratory Animals: ATLA* 41 (1):5–7.

Gharebaghi, R., M. R. Vaez Mahdavi, H. Ghasemi, A. Dibaei, and F. Heidary. 2007. Animal rights in Islam. *AATEX* 14:61–63.

Goodman J. R., A. Chandna, and C. Borch. 2015. Does accreditation by the Association for the Assessment and Accreditation of Laboratory Animal Care International (AAALAC) ensure greater compliance with animal welfare laws? *Journal of Applied Animal Welfare Science* 18(1):82–91.

Guillen, J. 2013. *Laboratory Animals: Regulations and Recommendations for Global Collaborative Research.* Waltham, MA: Academic Press.

Han, J. S. and G. H. Lee. 2013. Laboratory animal welfare and the three Rs in Korea. *Alternative to Laboratory Animals: ATLA* 41 (4):45–47.

Hollands, C. 1986. The Animals (Scientific Procedures) Act 1986. *The Lancet* 328 (8497):32–33.

Hudson-Shore, M. 2011. The latest statistics of scientific procedures on living animals reveal little three Rs progress in Great Britain in 2010. *Alternative to Laboratory Animals: ATLA* 39 (4):403–411.

Hudson-Shore, M. 2012. Searching effectively for three Rs information. *Alternative to Laboratory Animals: ATLA* 40:22–23.

ILAR (National Research Council Institute for Laboratory Animal Research). 2011. *Animal Research in a Global Environment: Meeting the Challenges: Proceedings of the November 2008 International Workshop*. Washington, DC: National Academies Press.

Izmirli, S., S. J. Aldavood, A. Yasar, and C. J. Phillips. 2010. Introducing ethical evaluation of the use of animals in experiments in the Near East. *Alternative to Laboratory Animals: ATLA* 38 (4):331.

Klein, H. J. and K. A. Bayne. 2007. Establishing a culture of care, conscience, and responsibility: Addressing the improvement of scientific discovery and animal welfare through science-based performance standards. *ILAR J* 48 (1):3–11.

Kong, Q. and C. Qin. 2010. Laboratory animal science in China: Current status and potential for adoption of three R alternatives. *Alternative to Laboratory Animals: ATLA* 38 (1):53–69.

Landi, M. S., J. W. Kreider, C. M. Lang, and L. P. Bullock. 1982. Effects of shipping on the immune function in mice. *American Journal of Veterinary Research* 43 (9):1654–1657.

Lu, J., K. Bayne, and J. Wang. 2013. Current status of animal welfare and animal rights in China. *Alternative to Laboratory Animals: ATLA* 41 (5):351–357.

McCallum, A. 2008. How to conduct an audit of an outsourcing provider. *BioPharm International*. April 2. http://www.biopharminternational.com/biopharm/article/articleDetail.jsp?id=507456.

NACLAR (National Advisory Committee for Laboratory Animal Research). 2004. Guidelines on the care and use of animals for scientific purposes. NACLAR.

Naderi, M. M., A. Sarvari, A. Milanifar, B. S. Borjian, and M. M. Akhondi. 2012. Regulations and ethical considerations in animal experiments: International laws and Islamic perspectives. *Avicenna Journal of Medical Biotechnology* 4 (3):114–120.

Newcomer, C.E. 2014. A note from AAALAC International regarding the recent article in Science Daily News.... News from AAALAC. AAALAC International. 28 August. http://www.aaalac.org/news/index.cfm.

NHMRC (National Health and Medical Research Council). 2013. *Australian Code for the Responsible Conduct of Research*, 8th edn. NHMRC.

NIH (National Institutes of Health). 2002. Public Health Service policy on humane care and use of laboratory animals. Bethesda, MD: Office of Laboratory Animal Welfare, U.S. Department of Health and Human Services, NIH.

NIH (National Institutes of Health). 2006. Frequently asked questions: PHS policy on humane care and use of laboratory animals: When institutions collaborate, or when the performance site is not the awardee institution, which IACUC is responsible for review of the research activity? Bethesda, MD: Office of Laboratory Animal Welfare, NIH. http://grants.nih.gov/grants/olaw/faqs.htm#proto_8.

NIH (National Institutes of Health). 2013. NIH grants policy statement (2013) Part II. Bethesda, MD: NIH. http://grants.nih.gov/grants/policy/nihgps_2013/nihgps_ch3.htm.

NRC (National Research Council). 1997. *Occupational Health and Safety in the Care and Use of Research Animals*. Washington, DC: National Academies Press.

NRC (National Research Council). 2002. Guidelines for the humane transportation of research animals. *Kekkaku* 77 (10):693–697.

NRC (National Research Council). 2003. *Occupational Health and Safety in the Care and Use of Nonhuman Primates*. Washington, DC: National Academies Press.

NRC (National Research Council). 2004. The development of science-based guidelines for laboratory animal care. In *Proceedings of the November 2003 International Workshop*. Washington, DC: National Academies Press.

NRC (National Research Council). 2011. *Guide for the Care and Use of Laboratory Animals*, 8th edn. Washington, DC: National Academies Press.

Pritt, S. 2008a. The animal welfare audit concept. *ALN Magazine* 7:49–50.

Pritt, S. 2008b. Working with contract research organizations. *ALN Magazine* 7:11–13.

Quigley, C. 2013. Lost in transit: A forgotten rodent welfare issue? *Alternative to Laboratory Animals: ATLA* 41 (1):8–9.

Rollin, B. E. 2007a. Animal research: A moral science. *EMBO Reports* 8 (6):521–525.

Rollin, B. E. 2007b. Overcoming ideology: Why it is necessary to create a culture in which the ethical review of protocols can flourish. *ILAR J* 48 (1):47–53.

Rollin, B. E. 2011. An ethicist's commentary on the credibility of animal care and use committees. *Canadian Veterinary Journal* 52:584–586.

Russell, W. M. S. and R. L. Burch. 1959. *The Principles of Humane Experimental Technique*. London, UK: Methuen.

Sankar, P. and K. Kandasamy. 2013. The three Rs in India. *Alternatives to Laboratory Animals* 41:42–44.

Sharp, P. and J. S. Villano. 2012. *The Laboratory Rat*, 2nd edn. Boca Raton, FL: CRC Press.

Stark, D. 2006. Laboratory animal-based collaborations and contracts beyond the border. *Laboratory Animals* 35 (6):37–40.

Steele, K. H., J. M. Hester, B. J. Stone, K. M. Carrico, B. T. Spear, and A. Fath-Goodin. 2013. Nonsurgical embryo transfer device compared with surgery for embryo transfer in mice. *Journal of the American Association for Laboratory Animal Science* 52 (1):17.

Syversen, E., F. J. Pineda, and J. Watson. 2008. Temperature variations recorded during inter-institutional air shipments of laboratory mice. *Journal of the American Association for Laboratory Animal Science* 47 (1):31.

Trez, T. de A. e. 2010. Refining animal experiments: the first Brazilian regulation on animal experimentation. *Alternative to Laboratory Animals: ATLA* 38:239–244.

Underwood, W. J. 2007. Contracting *in vivo* research: What are the issues? *Journal of the American Association for Laboratory Animal Science* 46 (4):16–19.

van Luijk, J., Cuijpers, Y., van der Vaart, L., Leenaars, M., and Ritskes-Hoitinga, M. 2011. Assessing the search for information on three Rs methods, and their subsequent implementation. Abstract: Europe PubMed Central. *Alternative to Laboratory Animals: ATLA* 39:429–447.

Van Noorden, R. 2011. The trouble with retractions. *Nature* 478 (7367):26–28.

WA (Government of Western Australia). 2002. Animal Welfare Act. Perth: Department of Premier and Cabinet State Law Publisher.

WOAH (World Organization for Animal Health). 2014a. Aquatic animal health code. WOAH. http://www.oie.int/international-standard-setting/aquatic-code/.

WOAH (World Organization for Animal Health). 2014b. Terrestrial animal health code. WOAH. http://www.oie.int/international-standard-setting/terrestrial-code/access-online/.

CHAPTER 13

IACUCs from an Academic Perspective

Linda N. Brovarney

CONTENTS

13.1 LIVING IN A FISHBOWL

Institutional Animal Care and Use Committees (IACUCs) in an academic environment have many additional challenges that must be considered, and in this age of transparency, it may feel as if the IACUC is in a fishbowl looking out. While all IACUCs have a similar purpose and scope that is driven by federal regulations, there is some flexibility in how these regulations are applied, which may vary in degree from institution to institution. IACUCs functioning in an academic setting may pose some additional complexities that will be explored in this chapter.

The institutional official (IO) is the linchpin of the operation of the Animal Care and Use Program (ACUP) and is the primary responsible individual for its success, providing leadership and direction. The IO rarely has much to do with the ACUP's day-to-day operations, however, and relies on the coordination and cooperation of other key personnel. The relationship between the IO, the IACUC, and the attending veterinarian (AV) is critical. They need to have not only a formal relationship but a good working relationship as well. The IO must be kept informed of any serious programmatic or compliance matters that arise. Also included in this mix should be the IACUC director or other senior administrative staff. The former individual is not mandated by regulatory requirement but does play a critical role in program administration and compliance.

While communication and cooperation among the IO, the AV, and the IACUC are necessary to support a culture of compliance, other units in the institution are also important to a successful ACUP, including the Environmental Health and Safety (EHS) committee, the Institutional Biosafety Committee (IBC), the Occupational Health unit, and the animal facility director. Additional stakeholders that are helpful for the IACUC to stay in close communication with include local or university police, news services, and legal affairs.

A program will most likely suffer if there is not enough support from the highest level of leadership at the institution. The IO provides programmatic guidance and is ultimately responsible for the program's compliance with the Public Health Service

(PHS) Policy on Humane Care and Use of Laboratory Animals (NIH 2002). The IO must be engaged and promote partnership and communication among the units, which is a key component to making the animal research enterprise a strong program. The program can only be truly successful if it enlists the faculty as an active partner, and the IO can facilitate communication at that level.

13.1.1 Size and Diversity of Academic Programs

Not every academic institution is a behemoth, and while some IACUCs have more than 15 members, the majority do not. Most IACUCs, however, have more than the minimum numbers required by either the Animal Welfare Act Regulations (AWRs) or the PHS Policy (USDA 2013a; NIH 2002). Academic institutions generally have more members than those in industry as the research conducted is usually more varied and expansive in scope and requires wider scientific expertise. It is highly advantageous for an IACUC to have enough members to carry the load of protocol review and other requirements of the ACUP. However, an IACUC that is too large could pose a problem with engagement of its members. If the IACUC chair does not invest in involving every member, they may lose the feeling of belonging.

IACUCs at large academic institutions have challenges that can be directly related to the species variety at that institution. With research being conducted on species so diverse, it may be difficult to have adequate faculty representation. Some institutions have more than one IACUC, especially if there is a high volume of research activity, which makes it difficult for one IACUC to complete its duties in a timely fashion. Often the duties are divided, with each IACUC in charge of a certain part of the program, such as biomedical research and agricultural research. This also keeps the IACUCs at a manageable size to function properly. Another model could be that the research program is physically separated so that two IACUCs make sense from a logistical standpoint. A challenge with having more than one IACUC could be the consistency of review. Having one IACUC chair for both committees may help alleviate that issue, but having expertise in all areas of research that is conducted at a university can also be a challenge. For a detailed discussion of this topic, see Silverman et al. (2014, 31–35).

Ensuring that researchers and students are adequately trained is the responsibility of the IACUC (NRC 2011). IACUCs must establish training programs that meet the needs of all types of students with varying levels of experience using a variety of species, and then must be able to track the training provided. Establishing policies and procedures to provide control over this process can be accomplished by withholding personnel approval on a protocol until training is completed, which should be a part of the annual protocol review process.

13.1.2 IACUCs' Role in Taming Bureaucracy

Faculty members at academic institutions are increasingly responsible for doing much of their own administration. In addition, obtaining money to fund research is becoming much more competitive, and submitting grant proposals can be a full-time job considering the decreasing percentage of grant proposals that are funded. A researcher needs to submit many grant proposals to be competitive, but where does the time for conducting science come in? The IACUC can be seen as just another burden. With that said, although it may be difficult for the IACUC and the researcher community to develop a trusting and respectful relationship, an effort should be made to do so by both parties. This can be accomplished by transparency during the protocol review process and having clear guidelines for compliance so that researchers know what is expected. In academic institutions it is a common belief that the IACUC makes the rules for its own ease; when changes are made by regulatory agencies, it is important to inform the researchers so that they understand why new regulatory guidance is formulated and how to comply.

The IACUC should be working with the researcher to facilitate good science and promote animal welfare. By opening up lines of communication, the IACUC can work toward having a positive relationship with faculty. The inclusion of the research community in the development of standard procedures and seeking their input prior to the implementation of new policies and guidelines can provide a sense of contribution to IACUC processes that goes a long way toward forming mutual respect. The IACUC staff can be an effective liaison between the faculty and the committee because they have a better understanding of what the IACUC wants. An IACUC staff that is readily available to speak to an investigator by phone or in person facilitates a good partnership.

One way to promote a positive relationship from the beginning is to encourage new researchers to start the protocol approval process prior to arriving at the institution. Senior IACUC staff and the AV could hold meetings or have conference calls with new faculty early in the process so that questions can be answered and guidance provided. This will smooth the transition for new faculty coming on board and help develop a personal relationship promoting a culture of compliance.

There are a number of things that the IACUC can do to lessen the regulatory burden on researchers. Be wary of regulatory creep, which can occur when the interpretation of a regulation becomes more rigid over time, creating additional unnecessary burden. The National Institutes of Health (NIH) just-in-time (JIT) review, designated member review (DMR), as well as administrative review with veterinary consultation (NIH 2014b), and the use of administrative preview are methods to streamline review. The use of web-based protocol submissions that include information that is visible to the investigator on where the protocol is in the review process should be taken advantage of to decrease protocol review times (NIH 2006a). The IACUC may also consider offering training on protocol writing, including examples of good protocols on the IACUC's website.

Even after the IACUC does everything it can toward facilitating an open and cooperative relationship, not every faculty member is going to be receptive. Working with faculty that constantly pushes back and complains seems wearisome considering how busy the IACUC is. Faculty must be handled with diplomacy and tact yet with a firm and unwavering position by the IACUC. Some researchers require a bit more attention than others, and if an in-person meeting will help, then that should be done. The bottom line is that they must be required to comply with the regulations.

Meetings of this sort can be very time-consuming for IACUCs, so it is likely more effective and less contentious to hold a smaller meeting with the IACUC chair, the AV, or senior IACUC staff.

13.2 PHS ASSURANCE

The PHS Policy, Section IV.A, requires that, "No activity involving animals may be conducted or supported by the PHS until the institution conducting the activity has provided a written Assurance acceptable to the PHS, setting forth compliance with the Policy" (NIH 2002).

The PHS funding components include the NIH, the Centers for Disease Control and Prevention (CDC), and the Food and Drug Administration (FDA). The Office of Laboratory Animal Welfare (OLAW) does not oversee animal activities funded by the National Science Foundation (NSF), the Department of Defense (DOD), the U.S. Department of Agriculture (USDA), and nonprofit or for-profit organizations.

Any institution that receives PHS funding must have an approved Animal Welfare Assurance document on file with OLAW. This document, called the "Assurance," describes the institution's program for the care and use of animals in PHS-conducted or supported activities (NIH 2002). Upon receiving a grant or contract award, the institution is notified by the funding component. This is called a Notice of Award (NIH 2013a). If there is no Assurance on file for that institution, the funding component will notify OLAW that an award is pending, and OLAW will contact the institution to "negotiate" an Assurance. An institution cannot submit an Assurance without solicitation by OLAW. To obtain an Assurance, the institution's program must be in compliance with the PHS Policy (NIH 2002), the AWRs if conducting research using USDA-regulated species (USDA 2013a), and the Guide for the Care and Use of Laboratory Animals (the Guide) (NRC 2011). If the requirements in the Guide differ slightly from the AWRs, then compliance with USDA regulations must be followed as applicable. OLAW will review the institution's submission and verify that it meets all requirements. If not, OLAW will negotiate an approved Assurance with the institution by providing the institution in writing with what needs to be modified to obtain approval (NIH 2012). Even if a grant is funded, the NIH will not release funding until the institution has an approved Assurance on file. Three types of Assurances are used.

The most common is the Domestic Assurance (inside the United States) for institutions that receive PHS funds through a grant or contract award (NIH 2012). This type of Assurance is used if the institution has its own ACUP, IACUC, IO, and veterinarian with program authority, conducts research on-site, and controls its own animal facilities. Domestic Assurances are approved for a period for no longer than 4 years (NIH 2012).

The Assurance describes the program components and its compliance with the PHS Policy. There are specific areas of the program that are required to be included in the Assurance. The OLAW website has sample Assurances that should be reviewed by any institution seeking PHS funding, or one that is ready to renew its existing Assurance to ensure that the document incorporates all of the elements that OLAW expects to be included (NIH 2012). "Effective December 1, 2014, OLAW will not renew a Domestic Assurance unless the institution has current direct or indirect PHS funding for activities involving animals." Institutions without current funding from the NIH, CDC, or FDA "will receive a letter of inactivation on the expiration date of their Domestic Assurance. Lack of an Assurance will not adversely affect the institution's ability to apply for future PHS funding. If OLAW is notified by a PHS funding component that the institution has been selected for an award or is named as a performance site for another institution's PHS-supported research, OLAW will negotiate a new Domestic Assurance" (NIH 2014a).

Foreign institutions (outside the United States) that receive PHS funds directly through a grant or contract award, or institutions outside the United States that receive PHS funds indirectly and are named as a performance site by a primary awardee's institution, must have an approved Foreign Assurance. The renewal period is 5 years, but OLAW will not renew a Foreign Assurance past the expiration date unless that institution has current PHS funding for activities involving animals (NIH 2012).

The foreign institution must provide

- Components of the institution's program that will be covered by the Assurance
- Commitment to the Council for International Organizations of Medical Sciences (CIOMS) International Guiding Principles for Biomedical Research Involving Animals and listing, in English, of all other applicable laws, regulations, or policies governing animal care and use for the country of jurisdiction
- Institutional endorsement

The third type is an *Interinstitutional Assurance* (formerly termed the *Interinstitutional Agreement*). This Assurance is required when the awardee institution does not have its own ACUP, IACUC, or facilities to house animals and does not conduct animal research on-site, but instead conducts animal activities using a secondary Assured institution's site as the performance site. That secondary institution must hold a Domestic or Foreign Assurance. Interinstitutional Assurances are approved for the life of the grant/contract up to 5 years (NIH 2012).

The requirements of the Interinstitutional Assurance are

- Statement of applicability and institutional responsibilities
- Endorsement of both the awardee and the Assured institution

OLAW does send a reminder notice to institutions when their renewal is due for review, but it is incumbent upon the institution to submit its renewals in advance allowing enough time for a review of the document. OLAW requests submission 4 months prior to expiration to allow for processing of the application. If the Assurance expires but has been submitted and is in process, the Assurance remains in full effect (NIH 2012).

Some institutions review their Assurance during prescribed intervals to ensure that their program is in compliance and make adjustments during those times. At a minimum, it should be reviewed when a change in the ACUP is initiated and when there is a change in existing policy or new policy is instituted. Changes in the program should be included in the required annual report to OLAW (see Table 1.5). An amended Assurance should not be submitted for review anytime during the approval period. The only exception is notification to OLAW of a change to the IACUC chair or the IO as these are the means of communicating with the institution and must be kept current (NIH 2012).

It may be in the institution's interest to write its Assurance with broad strokes while complying with the PHS Policy. An institution may propose a program that exceeds the standards of the PHS Policy, but once OLAW approves an Assurance document, the institution will be required to meet the standards that it has proposed.

13.3 GRANT CONGRUENCY

As required in the PHS Policy and the NIH Grants Policy Statement, the institution must conduct a review and approval of those components of grant applications and contract proposals related to the care and use of animals prior to award of the grant (NIH 2013a). As part of an NIH award, it is the institution that is required to conduct a protocol/grant congruency review.

All grantee institutions must assure the NIH that they follow grants policy. By signing the grant application, the authorized organizational representative (AOR) commits the organization to meeting the terms and conditions, and the principal investigator (PI) commits that the organization will follow the PHS Policy and conduct its animal activities according to its IACUC-approved protocol (NIH 2013b). It is incumbent upon the institution to establish appropriate policies and procedures that demonstrate compliance with the PHS Policy in all PHS-supported activities, and it is the institution's responsibility to ensure that the research described in the grant is congruent with the activities described in the corresponding protocol. This is termed the *congruency review*, which by definition is not an exact match but an approximation, equivalency, or state of agreement. NIH policy dictates certain components that must be included in the vertebrate animal section (VAS) of the grant (NIH 2010a):

1. A concise but complete description of the procedures to be conducted and the proposed use of the animals, including the species, strains, ages, sex, and numbers to be used.
2. A justification for the use of animals, including the rationale for the use of the species and the approximate numbers to be used.
3. A brief description of the program for veterinary care.
4. The procedures and methods to minimize pain and distress. Humane end points may be included here.
5. The method of euthanasia.

While the NIH does not explicitly require the grantee institution to conduct a side-by-side comparison, the best model may be to develop a procedure for direct comparison of the grant and the IACUC application. By comparing the research strategy sections and the VAS of the grant with the IACUC application, it can be determined if the required components that are described in the grant are included in the IACUC application. OLAW acknowledges that research is fluid and allows PIs discretion as to the best way to perform studies within the approved scope of work. There will likely be less detail in the grant than in the protocol (NIH 2010a).

Each institution should have a process or policy that it follows outlining its program for conducting the congruency review. It is important to have an individual who is qualified to identify inconsistencies and understands the IACUC protocol review process. Many institutions conduct the congruency review in the IACUC office as part of the administrative prereview of animal use applications, but other units, such as the sponsored research office staff or compliance oversight personnel, are also equipped to perform this review. Some smaller institutions may also have IACUC members or the research department's administrative office conduct congruency reviews as part of the IACUC review process.

A grant is awarded for a period of usually three to five years. The congruency review is required for both competing and noncompeting grant applications, where competing applications are for new funds or the continuation of existing funds after the initial award period. For competing applications only, the IACUC approval date may be submitted to the NIH at any time prior to award (NIH 2013b). For noncompeting grants, the investigator must submit a progress report annually, and the date of IACUC approval is required. If a significant change in the activities involving animals is described in the progress report, there must be modifications to the IACUC application, and a congruency review must occur such that the approved protocol includes the changes described in the grant. The congruency reviewer may require additional modifications to the IACUC proposal if necessary to obtain congruence with the grant. It is the investigator's responsibility, and not the IACUC's, to submit a proposed significant change to the NIH. If there are no significant changes, the investigator must provide a statement to that effect to the NIH.

A change in scope is not the same as a significant change. A change in scope is defined as a "change in the direction, type of research or training from the aims, objectives, or purposes of the approved project" (NIH 2013a). If a change in scope is being considered, the PI and the AOR should contact the NIH in advance for approval of a change in scope. Examples include a change in species, PI, disease of study, or procedures.

A one-to-one protocol/grant ratio is not required by the PHS Policy or the NIH Grants Policy (NIH 2013a). Some institutions use a one grant per protocol system while others allow more than one grant per protocol. If there is more than one grant per protocol, the institution must ensure that PHS funds are spent as per the grant requirements. Each IACUC must decide which model works best for their institution. There can be complications with matching various aspects of protocols with multiple grants, but a one grant per protocol system could create a lot of extra work for an already overburdened IACUC.

Whichever system it chooses to use, the institution must document IACUC approval of those animal activities proposed in the grant and be able to associate each grant with the relevant IACUC protocol(s).

13.4 JIT PROTOCOL REVIEW

On September 1, 2002, the NIH changed its grants policy and implemented IACUC JIT review. The PHS Policy now permits an Assured institution to submit verification of IACUC approval subsequent to NIH peer review but prior to award (NIH 2010b). This process allows grant applicants and signing officials the ability to submit certain components of a grant application at a later date in the process, occurring after peer review and during the period that the application is being considered for funding. Prior to this date, it was necessary to have IACUC approval submitted to the NIH within 60 days of submission of a grant application. With the implementation of JIT, this important policy reduces the burden on investigators and IACUCs so that time is focused only on those projects that are more likely to be funded.

Each institution should have procedures in place to manage the JIT review process. The administration of this process is often completed within the contracts and grants or the IACUC office. Since the IACUC office is responsible for protocol review and knows the committee's workload and review cycle, the JIT review process may benefit from being managed there.

If preliminary data have been collected for a subsequent submission to the NIH for a grant that is based on further animal research, an IACUC approval for this prior activity must be on file at the institution.

The NIH has the following expectations in effect for institutions that are taking advantage of the JIT review process (NIH 2010b):

- The PHS Policy remains unchanged; the institution must have an approved Assurance and there must be verification of an IACUC-approved animal use protocol at the time that the grant funds are released.
- This process is not intended to defer IACUC approval, and the IACUC may use its discretion and review the animal use protocol at any time during the grant submission process.
- The IACUC may not be pressured to approve a protocol or be overruled on its decision to withhold approval. The institution that chooses to use the JIT review process must support the decisions of the IACUC and its responsibilities.
- It remains the responsibility of the investigator to convey in a timely manner to his or her IACUC any modifications related to the scope of the project and the usage of animals that may result from the NIH review and award process.
- It is the institution's responsibility to submit any modifications required by the IACUC to the NIH with the verification of approval.
- The NIH is responsible for ensuring that institutions are given enough notice to allow for timely IACUC review prior to the release of funds, and it must take appropriate internal measures to provide timely feedback.

Most funding agencies follow the NIH and use a JIT model for IACUC review, but some may require that the protocol be approved prior to grant submission. It is the responsibility of the investigator to know the requirements of the funding agency.

13.5 CONFLICT OF INTEREST DISCLOSURES

In order to address any conflict of interest (COI) that might exist, some institutions have also included a question in their IACUC application in which they inquire, "whether they or any other person responsible for the design, conduct, or reporting of this research has an economic interest in, or acts as an officer or a director of any outside entity whose financial interests would reasonably appear to be affected by, the research" (HHS 2011). This may be redundant if the institution has a formalized and centralized procedure to manage this requirement. Financial conflict of interest (FCOI) is not the only area where a potential COI might arise. If during the semiannual inspection, an IACUC member or veterinarian inspects his or her own research location or area of responsibility, it may appear that there is a COI or bias. One way to remove this perception could be to include an additional IACUC member on those inspections, but it is important to note that it is in the veterinarian's best interest to find and correct any problems that may be present that could impact findings during future inspections.

While there is no regulation that prevents the AV from being the IACUC chair, this can be seen as a COI because the IACUC has the responsibility to provide oversight of the entire ACUP, including all animal facilities that the AV typically oversees. If an IACUC member is personally involved in a protocol being reviewed, he or she should not be present during deliberation of the protocol other than to provide information or answer questions. In addition, he or she cannot be counted toward a quorum or be allowed to vote on that proposal (ARENA/OLAW 2002).

13.6 SUBCONTRACTS AND SUBAWARDS

A subcontractor or subrecipient, as compared with a consultant or fee-for-service vendor, is defined as an entity—often another university—that helps the grantee carry out the activities of the award by performing a portion of the research using its own institution's facilities (NIH 2013c).

If an institution receives PHS funds and has its own Assurance but chooses to conduct some or all of the animal activities at one or more secondary institutions, the activities subcontracted or subgranted to the secondary institution are funded through a mechanism referred to as indirect funding. In this case, the secondary institution must be named as a performance site by the prime awardee institution. After approving the performance site, the funding component will contact OLAW to negotiate an Assurance with the secondary institution if needed. The performance site may be included as a covered component under the Assurance of the prime awardee with the following restrictions:

- If the performance site has a different administration, the primary institution must take responsibility and have authority for the ACUP for all PHS-funded activities.
- All components of the primary awardee's Assurance apply to the performance site, including the training and occupational health and safety programs.

- The performance site must agree to follow the guidance of the IO and the IACUC of the Assured institution.
- As part of the program of institutional oversight, the performance site must be included in the semiannual site inspection cycle.

Under consortium (subaward) agreements in which the grantee collaborates with one or more other organizations, the grantee, as the direct and primary recipient of NIH grant funds, is accountable for the performance of the project, the appropriate expenditure of grant funds by all parties, and all other obligations of the grantee (NIH 2013c). The animal welfare requirements that apply to grantees also apply to consortium participants and subprojects. Grantees must establish a subaward, or consortium agreement, with any outside organization that performs any of their grant-supported research activities. They must document their agreements in writing and submit all required reports to the NIH. Each subaward must have a formal written agreement for meeting the scientific, administrative, financial, and reporting requirements of a grant, and in every agreement, the grantee must have a substantive role in the project (NIH 2013c).

The NIH holds grantees accountable for their subawardees' research, spending, and reporting actions, which must conform to all terms and conditions of a grant award (HHS 2011). Subaward organizations cannot form their own subaward agreements with other organizations and may receive funds only from the grantee. The animal welfare requirements that apply to grantees also apply to consortium participants and subprojects. The primary grantee is responsible for including these requirements in its agreements with collaborating organizations, and for ensuring that all sites engaged in research involving the use of live vertebrate animals have an approved Animal Welfare Assurance and that the activity has valid IACUC approval. The approval of more than one IACUC is not required if the grantee and the performance site(s) have Assurances; the institutions may exercise discretion in determining which IACUC reviews research protocols and under which institutional program the research will be conducted (NIH 2006f). If the prime grantee does not have an Assurance and the animal work will be conducted at an institution with an Assurance, the grantee must obtain an Interinstitutional Assurance from OLAW. Under the Interinstitutional Assurance, the grantee and the performance site agree that the research will be conducted under the auspices and the program of animal care and use of the performance site's Assurance (NIH 2011b).

13.6.1 Interinstitutional Assurances

The PHS Policy requires institutions that receive PHS support for activities involving animals to have an approved Assurance with OLAW. The Interinstitutional Assurance (formerly known as the Interinstitutional Agreement) is used when the awardee institution does not have its own ACUP, facilities to house animals, or an IACUC (see PHS Assurance) (NIH 2011b).

13.6.2 Memorandum of Understanding

As OLAW describes, there are many circumstances that involve partnerships between collaborating institutions or relationships between institutional ACUPs, and these collaborations have the potential to create ambiguity (NIH 2006f). The best way to define responsibilities is in a written agreement or memorandum of understanding (MOU). This important document establishes a framework when two groups are collaborating for the parties to mutually agree on responsibilities and activities in the scientific and regulatory areas. Such an agreement can be simple, but should proactively address the responsibilities for off-site animal care and use, animal ownership and the incorporation of applicable PHS Policy requirements for IACUC review and approval of proposed animal activities, significant changes to animal activities, and semiannual facilities review. Additionally, it should define the oversight of transportation between facilities and IACUC review of amendments that affect both institutions. This would meet the recommendations in the Guide (NRC 2011) and the requirements of the NIH Grants Policy Statement on written agreements. These documents should be reviewed by the institution's legal or sponsored research departments.

While there is no regulatory requirement for a dual protocol review, some institutions may require a dual review of protocols for the work that is being conducted at another institution. This may have an impact if a USDA-regulated species is having a surgical procedure conducted at one institution and is then transferred to or from the collaborating institution. The institution receiving an animal that has had a surgical procedure may need to ensure that it complies with the AWRs regarding multiple survival surgical procedures; therefore, IACUC review of that protocol may be important (USDA 2013a).

The PHS Policy states that both the awardee institution and the performance site must hold an approved Animal Welfare Assurance. If the performance site does not have an Assurance, the awardee institution has the option to amend its Assurance to cover the performance site, which effectively subjugates the performance site to the Assured institution, and makes the Assured institution responsible for the performance site. If both institutions hold Domestic Assurances, they may determine who will conduct the IACUC review, but it is recommended by OLAW that both institutions hold documentation of protocol review, and the IACUC conducting the review should notify the other institution if questions are raised during a semiannual program review (NIH 2006f).

13.6.3 Requirement for Institutional Protocol Dual Review

OLAW and USDA agree that review of a research project or evaluation of a program or facility by more than one recognized IACUC is not a federal requirement (NIH 2006f), and while the PHS Policy does not require a dual review of protocols, some institutions that are primary grantees and subcontract work to other institutions have specific components of the subawardees' IACUC protocol that they must verify. In some cases, it may be a function of oversight of the subawardee institution, such as a formal administrative review similar to a grant/protocol comparison conducted in the IACUC office to verify that the approved activities are covered by the grant, or that the IACUC-approved protocol incorporates all of the components that the primary grantee requires of its own researchers. Other institutions require the subawardee institution to provide only the IACUC approval letter or a copy of that institution's approval for its files or both. Still others may require IACUC review at their own institution. With that said, each institution should outline its individual responsibilities in an MOU that clarifies who conducts the IACUC review and oversight, but both institutions must retain some form of documentation.

If the institution has projects that are funded by the DOD, additional regulatory requirements apply. The Animal Care and Use Review Office (ACURO), a component of the U.S. Army Medical Research and Materiel Command Office of Research Protections (USAMRMC ORP), must review and approve all animal use prior to starting work with animals. PIs must submit the institutional animal use protocol, IACUC approval of that protocol, and a version of the animal use appendix titled "Research Involving Animals." An annual review of studies and a dual review of newly approved protocols and any modifications that have been reviewed and approved by that institution are required to be approved by the DOD prior to implementation (DOD 2005). Also, regarding any DOD-funded study, the IACUC must conduct an appropriate continuing review at least annually, even when the research study involves non-USDA-regulated species.

13.6.4 Oversight of the Animal Care Program

Continuing IACUC oversight of animal activities is required by federal laws, regulations, and policies. An institution can utilize a variety of options for ongoing protocol assessment and regulatory compliance. Postapproval monitoring (PAM) occurs after the initial period of protocol approval and can be accomplished in many ways, and it is largely dependent on the size and scope of the program (NRC 2011, NIH 2006e).

Very large academic institutions are best served by having one or more compliance specialists who understand research and animal welfare principles. They are able to discuss with researchers their opportunities to refine research procedures. Their ability to incorporate continuing protocol review during regular facilities inspections, or those conducted as separate inspections, is highly valuable. Additional inspections or observations that are conducted by veterinarians or IACUC members of selected procedures, and observation of animals by animal care staff, veterinary technicians, and IACUC staff and members, as well as external regulatory inspections and assessments, can also be considered as part of the PAM program.

Both the Health Research Extension Act and the Animal Welfare Act (AWA) require the IACUC to inspect animal care and use facilities, including sites used for animal surgeries, every 6 months (NIH 1985, USDA 2013b). The compliance specialist(s) as well as the IACUC, veterinary staff, and animal care staff may conduct PAM for locations where survival surgery is conducted outside of centralized care. By enlisting support from others in the program, inspections of these locations may be conducted more frequently than semiannually. During formal IACUC inspections, the compliance specialists must be able to access protocols for compliance purposes, and the use of computer tablets, if available, to access that information and record inspection data may prove useful. In this way, animal study sites may be reviewed concurrently with a review of animal protocols. Utilizing skilled veterinary technicians for surgical observations can be incorporated into a successful PAM program, and those findings can be reported to the IACUC for evaluation. The level of complexity must be driven by the needs of the institution. Utilizing an appropriate risk-based approach with metrics to support its decisions is paramount.

13.6.4.1 Transportation of Animals between Facilities

Many laws govern the transportation of animals. Animal transportation can occur within the institution, between institutions, or to and from vendors or other commercial or noncommercial sources. The program must have institutional policies, guidelines, and standard operating procedures (SOPs) describing how, when, where, and by whom animals are transported. Veterinarians should approve vendors and determine which animals are allowed to enter which vivarium, including the process for acclimation, holding, or formal quarantine. The minimization of transportation time, control of the environment and the spread of zoonotic diseases, and the preservation of specific pathogen-free (SPF) status is critical. The documentation of transportation and the disinfection of transportation vehicles are critical, as well as training staff to ensure animal and personnel safety and the prevention of disease transmission between sites.

When animals are being transported to another collaborating institution, an MOU that describes each institution's responsibility for animal care and use, ownership, and IACUC review should be in place. All USDA-regulated animals should be transported following the requirements of the AWRs (USDA 2013a).

13.6.4.2 Responsibilities of the Primary Grantee

The primary grantee bears the responsibility for compliance, and its IACUC would be expected to promptly report any incident of noncompliance with the PHS Policy to OLAW. Depending on the nature of the noncompliance and which site is best able to take corrective action, OLAW will determine whether the primary grantee or the performance site must submit the final report on the noncompliance and the remedies taken (NIH 2007).

Requirements that apply to the grantee, including the intellectual property requirements and the program income requirements of the award, also apply to the consortium participant(s).

13.7 DIFFICULTIES RECRUITING MEMBERS
TO SERVE ON THE IACUC

There are few committees whose members have greater responsibilities and requirements for time and effort than those serving on an IACUC. That, in and of itself, creates a challenge for the recruitment and retention of IACUC members.

Each institution has its own process of recruitment and retention of IACUC members. The number of members may vary widely from institution to institution, but both the AWRs and the PHS Policy establish a minimum standard for committee constituency, and the AWRs go further to state that no more than three members can be from one administrative unit. The regulations, however, do not limit a member from fulfilling more than one role, that is, the nonaffiliated member may also be the nonscientist member (NIH 2002, USDA 2013a). It is not only a regulatory requirement but also a fundamental institutional responsibility that each member receives adequate initial and continuing education and training to stay current with the regulatory environment and the institution's own policies and practices. This also helps members remain engaged and incorporated into their role as a member. Training programs may vary; they may consist of formal presentations at every meeting, or they may be more flexible, and information could be provided *ad hoc* depending on current events and regulatory changes, or, for example, refresher training for upcoming semiannual inspections. IACUC members should be apprised of their responsibilities prior to the formal appointment process so that they fully understand the scope of the work required and are willing to make the commitment (Greene et al., 2007). While the PHS Policy has required membership categories, it does not specify that members from each category be present in order to conduct official business or to have a quorum. If an institution is receiving DOD funding, there is an additional requirement to "have at least one member who represents the general interest of the community and is not affiliated with the institution sponsoring the IACUC. The IACUC must designate an alternate member(s) for the non-affiliated member to ensure community representation at convened IACUC meetings." Additionally, to have a quorum, at least one veterinarian and one nonaffiliated member (or his or her alternate) must be present in the review of DOD-supported research (DOD 2005).

Depending on the size of the institution and the types of research being conducted, the IACUC should have representation from as many components of the scientific community of that institution as is necessary to accomplish an adequate review of the research being conducted. The members need to understand the scientific aims of the protocols and how these may impact animal welfare. It is important that the IACUC has sufficient scientific expertise in relevant areas to be able to adequately conduct an appropriate review. There is also no regulation prohibiting the use of consultants, and, when necessary, the IACUC should feel comfortable utilizing their expertise for some difficult or complex projects that may need additional scrutiny.

Additional information and experience available from other units that impact the ACUP are important for the IACUC to utilize, and its interest would be best served by including their expertise. Information provided by these individuals may be a valuable resource for the IACUC, including members from EHS, the IBC, the Occupational Health and Safety Program (OHSP), animal resources management, and so on. They may be appointed as voting members or nonvoting consultants to the committee.

Use of alternates can be an important advantage for IACUCs. Alternates must have an official appointment the same as any other member. They may be appointed as a one-to-one designation, fulfilling a specific individual's role in their absence; or they may be appointed to serve as a category of member (i.e., scientist or nonaffiliated member acting as an alternate for multiple regular members). Alternates may also fill more than one of the specified positions on the IACUC such as a nonscientist and a nonaffiliated member; however, if that member leaves the committee, the committee may not be properly constituted to conduct official business until another individual is appointed to fulfill those roles. These appointments must always meet the requirements of the category (or categories) of membership that they are serving, and an alternate may not represent more than one member at any one time. If a regular member fills two categories, the alternate must fill those same two categories. The appointment letter should clearly state if the alternate is for an individual, which must either be named or indicated as a category of membership (i.e., scientist or veterinarian). Alternates may never contribute to a quorum at the same time as the member they are serving as an alternate for, or contribute to official IACUC business simultaneously. Alternates should be treated as any other full member receiving similar orientation, continuing education and training as required, and are expected to vote their conscience. They must not in any way be expected to represent the position of the regular member whom they replace (NIH 2011a).

13.7.1 Member Length of Service

There are no regulations providing guidance for a minimum or maximum term that an IACUC member serves, and IACUCs vary widely on their requirements for membership length. When taking into consideration that not all members attend every meeting, and that institutions vary in meeting frequency, IACUCs should determine what the minimum commitment should be. A good model may be that members serve at least 3 years to be of greatest benefit to the IACUC. It takes at least 1 year for members to become experienced in IACUC matters and protocol review, and by 2 years they are typically very knowledgeable in these matters. By year 3, they have some institutional history and should be acting in a supportive and mentoring role for new members who often have many questions about how the IACUC works and their role as a member, including protocol review and other IACUC functions, as well as what to consider while on inspections. At that point, they may also be in the process of mentorship toward service as the IACUC chair or vice-chair.

The member appointment process should be formalized so that each member's term of service has a defined beginning and end. This does not mean that a term cannot be renewed when it is completed, but there is a risk that membership that is too lengthy or open-ended could potentially create burnout in an otherwise very engaged and active member. This model also has a built-in mechanism to release problematic members who the committee may be better off replacing. Another model may be to have membership formally renewed on an annual basis or some other predetermined interval.

13.7.2 Member Compensation

Faculty service is seen as a responsibility of all faculty members and is essential to an institution's success. Many faculty members are on a tenured track, and their participation in this institutional responsibility should be recognized by their supervisor or department chair as a highly valued and important contribution to the university's mission. It should be a critical component for their review of upward mobility toward tenure and should be included in their merit review.

For the IACUC chair and vice- or co-chair, service on a regulatory committee that requires such an extensive time commitment can be especially challenging, and the institution needs to recognize this intensified level of service. As compensation the institution may wish to consider partial salary support with the department allowing for the loss of time that would otherwise be spent conducting research or other activities for that unit.

Attendance at meetings should be encouraged and supported by the IO, including costs for these activities, which should be funded by the institution. Covering travel costs and parking and providing food or refreshments at meetings should be the standard.

Regarding the nonaffiliated or public members, they should be reimbursed similarly for travel expenses, parking, and meals, and many institutions provide additional nominal stipends for attendance at meetings and inspections due to the extensive workload involved. The amount of the stipend should not be so large as to appear to influence voting or be an important source of income.

13.7.3 Pros and Cons of Using Tenured Faculty versus Assistant/Associate Professors

Senior faculty members may have more time to devote to service on the IACUC. They also provide valuable expertise that spans years of institutional and animal research experience and, as a result, may command more authority and credibility. On the other hand, younger faculty are ambitious and often more energetic and current with animal research. They are also eager to advance professionally and to do so they may need to provide university service so that they receive credit toward a tenured tract. If they are not tenured, however, they may be required by their supervisor to bring in grant dollars and conduct research, which could create a conflicted situation for the institution regarding IACUC membership.

An additional consideration is the importance of preserving the anonymity of the IACUC members regarding their protocol review so that less senior faculty members are not put in a position of prejudice for their review and commentary on IACUC applications.

13.8 INVESTIGATING ALLEGATIONS

The use of animals in research is challenged with ethical and political concerns, and when that is compounded by accusations of animal mistreatment or protocol noncompliance leading to animal welfare concerns, the IACUC must investigate these allegations in a serious and deliberate fashion. While not all allegations may be real, the IACUC's role and responsibility is a difficult one, and its members have to carefully and skillfully decipher fact from conjecture to obtain an accurate resolution. Sometimes, the findings may be somewhere in between, but every IACUC should have policies and procedures in place to follow up on issues brought to its attention.

Animal mistreatment requires a conscious decision to inflict physical pain, suffering, or death and is not necessarily the same as protocol noncompliance. Researchers may make errors by not following their protocol, which could lead to animal pain and distress, but this is rarely willful and can be corrected by modifications to the protocol, additional training, or veterinarian or IACUC oversight. Occasionally, the IACUC may believe that to prevent further animal distress, other more severe sanctions, such as protocol suspension, need to be administered to provide the time-out that the investigator may need to bring the protocol and laboratory operations into compliance before restarting the project. It is critical to have the support of institutional leadership, and the IO should be kept apprised of any serious issues that are brought forward in a timely fashion.

13.8.1 Who Can Report Animal Welfare Concerns?

It is a fundamental responsibility of an institution to protect the welfare of animals under its care. Any individual, including members of the public, can report allegations of noncompliance, and the institution must ensure that there are adequate and appropriate mechanisms to do so. The Guide requires that, "The institution must develop methods for reporting and investigating animal welfare concerns, and employees should be aware of the importance of and mechanisms for reporting animal welfare concerns" (NRC 2011).

Most institutions have reporting policies that detail procedures on how reporting a concern is processed and to whom a report should be made, including procedures on how the institution processes anonymous reports. It is important to have more than one point of contact so that the individual reporting allegations is comfortable with the process. It could be the IO, the AV, or the IACUC chair, but, more often than not, personnel are more comfortable reporting to the compliance office staff or those with whom they work on a daily basis. It is in the best interest of the institution to include individuals at this level in the process too.

Under no circumstances should an individual be punished or feel reprisal for reporting a concern. This must be clearly stated in the institution's policy and should be part of the required training provided to the research community and staff. There also needs to be a process established for ensuring that any concerns are brought to the attention of the IACUC in a timely and efficient manner. Institutions should post their policy and process for reporting concerns in prominent places in the animal facility. If animal welfare may be at stake, the AV or his or her designee must first ensure the safety and well-being of the animals in question and be empowered by the IACUC to stop an activity if necessary. According to the Guide, p. 114, "A veterinarian or the veterinarian's designee must be available to expeditiously assess the animal's condition, treat the animal, investigate an unexpected death, or advise on euthanasia. In the case of a pressing health problem, if the responsible person (e.g., investigator) is not available or if the investigator and veterinary staff cannot reach consensus on treatment, the veterinarian must have the authority, delegated by senior administration (see Chapter 2, Institutional Official and Attending Veterinarian) and the IACUC, to treat the animal, remove it from the experiment, institute appropriate measures to relieve severe pain or distress, or perform euthanasia if necessary."

If the report is not anonymous, it may be advisable to follow up with the individual so that he or she is assured that the process of reporting concerns works and that the IACUC is performing its regulatory oversight responsibility effectively.

If an allegation or a report is made from an outside source, such as a member of the public or an animal rights or extremist group, it is important to communicate this with the institution's public relations office or news services office. A good relationship between these offices and the IACUC should be established early on so that facts can be provided quickly to address any concerns about animal care and use that may be brought forth. The institution may want to include the institution's legal office as well.

13.8.1.1 Investigating and Reporting Animal Welfare Concerns to the IACUC

Once an allegation of an animal welfare concern has been made, the first action is to ensure that any needed care to the animals has been provided. The AV or his or her delegate should get involved quickly if the animals require attention. There should be an established policy or process for researching the facts quickly, including how the concerns were brought to the attention of the IACUC. Some larger institutions have compliance personnel that are trained to perform this activity, which may include reviewing the protocol, reviewing internal policies and guidelines that may apply, interviewing staff or researchers, and consulting with the veterinary and/ or husbandry staff.

Depending on the facts, a subcommittee of the IACUC may be formed quickly to review the findings, or a special session of the IACUC can be called. The latter may be difficult in a larger institution; however, if there is no immediate impact on animal welfare, the PI can be requested to halt any further activity until the IACUC deliberates on the findings at the next convened meeting. This also allows enough time to gather pertinent information that needs to be presented. An additional step that institutions should incorporate is a response from the PI. It should include how the infraction occurred, how it was corrected, and what steps were put in place to prevent the situation from recurring. This allows the IACUC to evaluate the circumstances, taking into consideration the PI's perspective and the actions taken to remedy the situation. The compliance staff is the ideal liaison for working with the PI in this instance, and researchers appreciate the opportunity to have a skilled professional review of their response. Since it should ultimately be the responsibility of the PI to self-correct, this approach will lead to better compliance in the long run and can be a proactive way to provide some guidance and training for researchers on working with the IACUC. It will also prevent the IACUC from dictating how a PI will correct a problem, which can create tension.

While it may not always be possible, it is best practice to separate the veterinary staff from compliance activities, which helps facilitate a more positive and trusting relationship between the researchers and the veterinarians. Having a unit whose responsibility is compliance benefits the entire program because the veterinary staff is not viewed as being the enforcer. The compliance process becomes an administrative function, and roles are more clearly delineated.

It is important to preserve the IACUC's efforts for more important issues, such as protocol review and compliance or policy discussion. With that said, does every item of noncompliance need to be reviewed at a convened meeting by the IACUC? Is the compliance unit delegated with freedom to act in specific circumstances? Or, to enhance efficiency, could some findings of noncompliance be reviewed at a standing subcommittee meeting in the form of a spreadsheet with recommendations for an IACUC response? Examples may include expired substances or minor deficiencies that have been identified on semiannual inspections with no animal welfare impact.

The IACUC should have a compliance policy that describes its authority and the process for evaluating issues of noncompliance involving IACUC protocols, policies, and regulatory guidelines. This provides structure and transparency for the research community as well as the public. The IACUC may also want to establish internal policies and procedures dealing with escalation of action regarding certain repeat findings of noncompliance. This promotes fairness and consistency of action, which is an area that IACUCs may struggle with.

When the findings are presented to the IACUC, the details of the investigation may be brought forward from several sources, but they should be organized and presented in a clear, concise, and summarized format. Prior history should be taken into consideration, and any IACUC policies describing the details of escalating noncompliance should be available for review. The IACUC may request additional information if necessary; however, if it is presented well, the IACUC should have the pertinent information to deliberate on and make decisions regarding additional corrective actions that it requires.

13.8.1.2 Reporting of Noncompliance to OLAW

The underlying foundation of the PHS Policy is one of institutional self-evaluation, self-monitoring, and self-reporting. The PHS Policy, Section IV.F.3, requires that

> The IACUC, through the Institutional Official, shall promptly provide OLAW with a full explanation of the circumstances and actions taken with respect to:

a) any serious or continuing noncompliance with this Policy;
b) any serious deviation from the provisions of the [Guide for the Care and Use of Laboratory Animals]; or
c) any suspension of an activity by the IACUC. (NIH 2002)

OLAW expects prompt and timely reporting of noncompliance as part of the self-regulation of programs that are covered by the PHS Policy. Prompt by definition means carried out without delay. The easiest way to comply with the prompt requirement is to perform a preliminary investigation of the findings, gathering the relevant facts, and contact OLAW directly by phone, fax, or e-mail. It is helpful to keep a log of any communications and corresponding documents that are used for preliminary reporting, as this may also be used to make additional notes that may be needed for final follow-up reporting. This will also provide structure for clear and concise reporting. Additionally, it is important for OLAW to establish a relationship with the IACUC office, and if the IO is unsure if an item is reportable, they are helpful in assisting the IO to make that determination. All documents submitted to OLAW may be requested under the federal Freedom of Information Act (FOIA). However, if the item under discussion is not required to be reported to OLAW, no record will be kept.

The necessary items for preliminary prompt reporting are

1. The name of the institution and the contact information of the person reporting
2. The Assurance number
3. A brief description of what occurred (species involved, category of personnel, and dates and times of occurrence)
4. Any corrective actions that have occurred to date
5. A plan and schedule for additional correction and prevention

An estimate of the time frame for final follow-up reporting from the IO is also requested (NIH 2013d).

After the noncompliance has been fully investigated and corrective actions have been finalized, OLAW requires final follow-up reporting on the occurrence. The final follow-up to OLAW must be in writing and signed by the IO. Institutions are required to submit signed final reports electronically to the Division of Compliance Oversight (NIH 2013e). These reports are to include

- Name of institution
- Assurance number
- Reporting requirement category: Identify the reporting requirement of the PHS Policy IV.F.3. under which the incident qualifies (i.e., serious or continuing noncompliance with the PHS Policy, serious deviation from the provisions of the Guide, or suspension of an activity by the IACUC).
- Preliminary report: Note when, by whom, and to whom a preliminary report was made, if applicable.
- Explanation of incident: Explain in detail what happened, when and where, the species of animals(s) involved, and the category (but not the names) of the individuals involved.

- Corrective actions: Describe the corrective and preventive actions taken to address the situation. Include all the short or long-term corrective plans along with the implementation schedule. Indicate whether the IACUC reviewed and accepted the corrective actions submitted by the responsible party and any ongoing actions taken by the IACUC (e.g., enhanced oversight).
- Grant/contract number: Include the relevant grant or contract number (for situations related to PHS-supported activities).
- Impact on PHS-supported activities: Describe any potential or actual effect on PHS-supported activities. This also applies to incidents that have occurred in a functional, programmatic, or physical area not supported by the PHS that could affect PHS-supported activities. (Examples include inadequate program of veterinary care, training of technical/husbandry staff, or occupational health; inadequate sanitation due to malfunctioning cage washer; room temperature extremes due to HVAC failure).
- Compliance with terms and conditions: If the incident involved PHS-supported activities and was not compliant with the terms and conditions of the grant award, confirm that the situation was reported to the funding component and that all unauthorized costs initially paid from the grant have been removed and covered by other sources. Or, certify that no unallowable costs were charged during the noncompliant period. (NIH 2013d)

Problems that occur in a relatively short time frame may be reported together, but delaying reporting does not comply with the requirements of the PHS Policy on prompt reporting. OLAW offers examples of reportable items on its website, which provides a helpful framework but it is not all inclusive, and institutions should use rational judgment in determining what situations fall within the scope of these examples.

An authorized institutional representative can be delegated to conduct the preliminary prompt reporting and could be the IACUC chair, the AV or his or her delegate, or a higher-level administrator in the compliance office. Due to the extensive record keeping that is necessary, tracking and reporting of noncompliance should be conducted by qualified administrative staff specifically trained to understand reporting requirements and processes. This function would probably be better served if administered in the IACUC office as this is more commonly the office of record for OLAW and other IACUC-related functions.

To apply uniform and consistent standards, institutions may wish to report noncompliant activities to OLAW even if they are not PHS funded. However, as all items that are reported to OLAW can be requested under the FOIA, the institution has to determine if it will report all noncompliance to OLAW no matter the funding, or only those activities that are PHS supported, as well as those that are not directly supported by the PHS but are in a functional, programmatic, or physical area that could affect PHS-supported activities.

Since all information provided to OLAW can be requested by the public, care should be taken to draft the final follow-up reporting in a clear, concise, and factual manner, avoiding editorials and embellishments and focusing on actions taken to address the noncompliance and to prevent a recurrence. An institution should never add evidentiary supporting documents, such as letters sent to the PI from the IACUC or excerpts of IACUC minutes for proof of discussion at meetings. Those details can be summarized in the report, which can be distilled to a page or less. These reports need to be stand-alone documents, and providing additional information by way of attachments may leave the institution open to public records requests for extraneously provided information.

OLAW evaluates and reviews noncompliance reports and the actions taken. OLAW may ask for clarification or other information to assess the case, or recommend certain actions to enhance compliance and prevent recurrence. After OLAW has completed its evaluation of the situation, a report of the findings and acceptance of the corrective actions are sent to the IO and are copied to the IACUC office/contact, as well as any complainants in the case.

OLAW will assist the reporting institution in developing definitive corrective plans and schedules if necessary. Compliance actions affecting an award are rare because institutions are usually able to address incidents successfully and take appropriate actions to prevent recurrence.

13.9 IACUC OVERSIGHT OF SATELLITE FACILITIES

IACUC approval to conduct research or house animals outside centralized care can pose a greater animal welfare risk than when those activities occur in centralized care due to the lack of direct oversight of external locations by various personnel that have a day-to-day presence in the facility. Therefore, adequate oversight of these activities may require additional resources that are often provided by compliance personnel. Of primary consequence, approval to conduct research outside centralized care must be adequately and scientifically justified in the approved protocol and not for the investigator's convenience. All locations should be inspected by the IACUC, the researcher, and the veterinarian prior to approval for suitability and compliance with the requirements in the Guide, and the AWRs if USDA-regulated species are involved. The inclusion of a member of EHS is advantageous to assess whether there are adequate measures to limit the exposure of personnel to anesthetic waste gases, allergens, and other hazards that may affect personnel safety. Cleanliness and lack of clutter is paramount, and a checklist to document a thorough inspection of these locations should be employed. If possible, these locations should be equipped to have the appearance and functionality of a centralized space.

13.10 ANIMALS USED FOR TEACHING

There are many ethical and political concerns regarding the use of live animals for teaching purposes. This is one area where there have been many advances in replacing living animal with nonliving models, computer-based training, video tutorials, and the use of cadavers. The regulations make clear that the institution is responsible for ensuring that all personnel must be appropriately trained to perform their duties. The regulations do not prescribe how this is accomplished, but they state that it is the responsibility of the IACUC, during protocol review, to make a determination that the training is adequate. Each institution should have a training and education policy that describes the training program and requirements prior to animal handling, care, and use. The number and species of live animals used for teaching will certainly vary between institutions due to the diversity of the species used, the types of research conducted, and, to some extent, the turnover of research and animal care personnel. The use of live animals in training is necessary to develop the skills that are required to ensure humane handling, care, and use of animals.

Animals used for teaching and education purposes should be viewed no differently than those used for research and testing, and consideration of the three Rs, reduce, replace, and refine, is very important in this instance. In many cases, animals that are required for teaching are used for a single specific purpose, such as training residents and surgeons how to perform specific surgical techniques. Due to the invasive nature of these procedures, most if not all institutions would euthanize these animals after that aim has been accomplished. Training in this area is commonly conducted by the PI, the researcher's staff, or veterinarians. Use of live animals to teach euthanasia can be an important part of any training program to ensure that those conducting euthanasia are qualified and trained to do so, and that it is performed in the most humane manner possible. For large academic programs with a high volume of researcher and staff turnover, a training program that incorporates the use of rodents already slated for euthanasia and that are donated by other researchers can be used to teach euthanasia to rodent users who are new to the campus.

If animals are used for survival training procedures, such as instructing researchers and staff on handling and basic laboratory techniques, the IACUC must consider the type of procedure being conducted and weigh any pain and distress that the animal may undergo with the number and the invasiveness of the procedures performed. "Multiple procedures that may induce substantial post-procedural pain or impairment may be conducted on a single animal only if justified by the PI, and reviewed and approved by the IACUC" (NIH 2006d). These usually consist of basic handling and common laboratory techniques, such as blood collection, injections, restraint, and anesthesia. Training for individuals who have never worked with laboratory rodents requires special training skills, not only to prevent animal bites, but also to teach gentle handling so that the animal undergoes as little stress as possible. If at all feasible, the use of more docile strains of animals is advisable for inexperienced handlers. Additionally, for most species it is important that the animals are conditioned to being handled before inexperienced personnel work with them. There must be provisions in any IACUC-approved protocol to have specific humane end points outlined for training animals. Once the animals in the training program have come to the end point of their training use, they may also be used for hands-on euthanasia training.

The responsibility for teaching researcher and animal care staff may vary depending on the size of the institution and the breadth of species used, and, in many instances, this task typically falls to the veterinarians and veterinary technicians or husbandry supervisors. In some larger institutions, the basic training may be conducted by IACUC staff simply because of the sheer volume of species-specific training that is required, but this type of program requires a specific background and skill set. Hands-on training may also be a shared task between the units, dependent on the species used and the type of training that is needed. For example, the IACUC staff may conduct rodent species–specific training due to the higher volume and standardized curriculum, while the veterinarians or veterinary technicians may conduct larger species training that may have more specificity. There is most likely no single individual who could possibly have all of the qualifications to teach every procedure that researchers may be required to learn and the ability to perform them well enough to teach. Therefore, another technique, coined *matchmaker* training, when qualified researchers train other researchers on certain techniques, can be employed.

13.11 FIELD STUDIES

All states have regulations protecting their precious animal resources, and researchers in the field must adhere to all federal, state, and local laws, regulations, or policies. The investigator must be knowledgeable of the requirements for obtaining permits to study wildlife. If conducting research outside the United States, many international laws and regulations apply.

For PHS-supported field studies that involve vertebrate animals, IACUCs need to be aware of the locations where the field studies will take place and what procedures will be involved, and be somewhat familiar with the habitat to assess the potential impact on the animal subjects. Most IACUCs lack experience and expertise for reviewing field studies and should rely on the knowledge of wildlife biologists, veterinarians, and those experienced in field studies to provide sufficient guidance. If the activity involves vertebrate animals, the IACUC is responsible for oversight in accordance with the PHS Policy.

If the activity alters or influences the normal activities of the animal that is being studied, such as in capture and release for banding, tattooing, placing of radio collars, or biological sampling, the activity must be reviewed and approved by the IACUC (NIH 2006b).

If the activity does not alter or influence the normal activity of the animal, IACUC review and approval is not required. Noninvasive manners of study include observations, photographs, collection of feces, hair snares, and use of track plates. If these studies have the potential to impact the health or safety of personnel or impact the animal's environment in any way, however, they may need IACUC oversight.

For USDA-regulated species, the USDA defines "field study" as any study done on free-living wild animals in their natural habitat, which does not involve an invasive procedure, and which does not harm or materially alter the behavior of the animals under study, and the USDA specifically exempts these studies from IACUC review and approval (USDA 2013a). However, a study on free-living wild USDA-regulated species that involves invasive procedures, or harms or materially alters the behavior of an animal under study, is covered by USDA animal welfare regulations and requires IACUC review and approval (USDA 2013a). It may be advisable for an IACUC to apply consistent policies and procedures to all animals covered by the institution's ACUP, regardless of the type of research or teaching activity involved, to promote consistent oversight.

While neither the PHS Policy nor the AWRs require IACUCs to conduct semiannual inspections of field study sites, to make assessments of compliance it may be sound practice to have the PI submit other methods for evaluation to the IACUC, such as photographs or video of the work taking place (NIH 2006b,c). Furthermore, with today's technology, it is possible to conduct a remote inspection of some components of the study via live video feed. An IACUC's decision to conduct semiannual inspections of field study sites should be considered on an individual basis, and it may depend on whether animals are being held or housed or if the location is geographically in close proximity.

A field study may be subject to a number of laws, and therefore multiple permits may be required for a research protocol. It is the responsibility of the PI to determine which laws govern the activities and to obtain the permits that are necessary to conduct the research. The IACUC should also ensure that appropriate permits are in place.

13.11.1 Permits: Endangered Species

The purpose of the Endangered Species Act (ESA) is to regulate a wide range of activities affecting plants and animals designated as endangered or threatened and the habitats on which they depend. The U.S. Fish and Wildlife Service's endangered species program issues permits for native endangered and threatened species and provides comprehensive information on the types of permits required depending on the species selection and data to be collected.

The activities authorized by permits differ depending on whether the species is listed as endangered or threatened. An endangered species is in danger of extinction throughout all or a significant portion of its range. A threatened species is likely to become endangered in the foreseeable future.

For endangered species, permits may be issued for scientific research, enhancement of propagation or survival, and taking that is incidental to an otherwise lawful activity (NOAA 2014; Wong 2013, FWS 2014). For threatened species, permits also may be issued for zoological, horticultural, or botanical exhibition; educational use; and special purposes consistent with the ESA.

For the study of endangered species outside the United States, other international permits and local and national approvals will apply. It is the responsibility of the researcher to know what the requirements are for the location and species of study.

13.11.2 Occupational Health Concerns for Participants

The occupational health and safety of laboratory animal researchers extends to those conducting research in the field. Its implementation and effectiveness depends on knowledge of situations that may occur and should include a risk assessment from occupational health professionals, veterinarians, and researchers. Since many of the occupational health concerns are not those found in a controlled environment such as a laboratory setting, the task is more challenging and requires those closely involved to make a well-informed assessment of the hazards that may be present and how those risks could be mitigated.

The Guide requires that the institutional OHSP must identify potential hazards in the work environment and conduct a critical assessment of the associated risks, including risks associated with unusual experimental conditions, such as those encountered in field studies or wildlife research (NRC 2011). The OHSP should assess safety issues, including the potential for exposure to zoonoses, and provide the IACUC with assurances that the field study will not compromise the health and safety of either animals or persons in the field. It should ensure that potential risks for injury or illness during a wildlife study are identified and personnel exposure to these risks is minimized. To aid the OHSP in its assessment, the researcher should include input from experienced individuals who are familiar with the location and the hazards at the field site. This information will guide the researcher and the OHSP in developing a disaster and contingency plan, which should include environmental challenges and risks associated with the animal species studied, including those not studied, and how they might impact personnel in an unanticipated encounter. Zoonotic disease potential and equipment failures are also matters of consideration.

There are hazards that researchers may anticipate and others they may not. It is critical for researchers to carefully consider the study environment and the experience and expertise of the other members of the team, and be as prepared as possible for any disaster or dangerous situations that may arise.

13.11.3 Invasive Procedures: Surgery in the Field

Training is necessary if a researcher plans to conduct more invasive techniques in the field, and organizations such as the American Society of Mammalogists and the Ornithological Council provide training for those that need it. Implantable telemetry is one example of a more invasive method to collect data that requires a surgical approach, which in turn necessitates IACUC approval. Invasive surgical procedures should only be conducted by properly trained personnel who are knowledgeable of the techniques necessary to successfully carry out the procedures and appropriately respond to veterinary emergencies that might arise.

13.11.4 Emergency Euthanasia

Emergency euthanasia of animals in the field is often performed under stressful situations, and those conducting the euthanasia procedure must be well trained and efficient. All euthanasia of animals in field studies must follow the American Veterinary Medical Association (AVMA) Guidelines for the Euthanasia of Animals, and these should be part of the study design and emergency contingency plan (AVMA 2013). Researchers should be well versed in AVMA-approved methods of euthanasia and be prepared to manage such emergencies while working in the field. As this would constitute an unanticipated adverse event, the IACUC would need to be apprised of the circumstances, what occurred, and how it was managed, including a plan to prevent repeat occurrences.

13.11.5 Humane Traps

The methods of data collection depend on the information requirements of the specific study, and there are a number of noninvasive ways in which data can be collected without disturbing the animals or their habitat. While conducting field research, it is often easier for the animals to come to the researcher. Stationary study paradigms, such as photography or videotaping, provide information on animal occupancy, presence/absence, abundance/density, and distribution. Hair snares and track plates provide information on the presence/absence, density, and occupancy. These studies do not require IACUC approval due to the noninvasive data collection methods. However, if live animals are to be captured and handled for any reason, the PI will need to submit a protocol for review and approval by the IACUC. Those individuals involved in the live capture of animals should have training and experience in safe capture techniques. The team should include a member with training to prevent the undue injury or death or both of animals. There are professional companies that provide training on safe capture, handling, and restraint. There are also a number of commercially available humane traps that can be used in field research (Safe-Capture International 2014). If the study is out of the country, it may not be cost effective to bring equipment, and it may need to be fabricated in the field.

13.12 FOIA AND STATE OPEN RECORDS
LAWS FOR PUBLIC INSTITUTIONS

The FOIA is a law that allows public access to the records of federal agencies, whether they were generated by the agency or obtained by the agency, and provides that any person has a right to obtain access to federal agency records. The FOIA includes nine limited statutory exemptions, which describe exceptions to obtaining these records or parts of these records (U.S. Department of Justice n.d.).

Most information describing research activities is not protected under an exemption and may not be redacted by the federal government. In general terms, some information falling under one of the following categories: (1) personnel or financial records; (2) privacy or the Health Insurance Portability and Accountability Act (HIPAA)-protected information; (3) investigatory information; or (4) trade secrets or proprietary information, may be eligible for redaction. The federal government will give the submitter an opportunity to review the documents to see if any information applies and if it is able to be redacted before the federal government releases it. It is important to include legal affairs when contacted by the NIH regarding records requested to assist in making a determination of what, if anything, can be redacted.

The release of information also includes the release of data included in federally sponsored research grants. Since the identification of the grant recipients does not fall under any of the nine exemptions, their names will be released. This is one way that animal rights or extremist groups gather personal information about animal researchers.

Most of the requirements falling under the FOIA have also been adopted by many of the states to comply with open records laws for public institutions. Each state may have some variances, so it is important that each institution checks with its legal department to determine what qualifies for redaction in that state.

13.12.1 Public Records Requests

Academic institutions receiving public funds are required by open records laws of their state to release information requested by the public. Every state has an open records law, and many states model their own laws after the FOIA. Each institution should have a formalized process for how the institution receives a request, which must be in writing, and for identifying which office is responsible for processing and tracking the progress of the request. The office must be familiar with the responsible persons or departments holding the records, and consultation with the legal department should occur to assist in interpreting the request and reviewing the documents prior to their release. Often, the information contained within institutional records can form the basis for USDA citations and media or animal rights or extremist groups' attention, so keeping the IO and the IACUC chair informed is crucial. Federal exclusions and exemptions may apply similarly to state and local laws, and it is advisable to check with the institution's legal department. All names and locations should be redacted to protect the privacy of individuals and their families, unless the legal department advises against it. If the requestor takes the institution to court over release of this information, he or she must provide a compelling reason why the withholding of this information is not in the best interest of the public. Most would argue that this is a public safety issue for researchers.

Many public institutions expend enormous man-hours preparing and producing these documents in response to public requests, and the compensation to the institution for producing these documents is insignificant. This is an example of an unfunded regulatory mandate, and, as records requests can fluctuate with scope and frequency, it is difficult to plan for this work. Additionally, skilled and trained personnel who are experienced in identifying and redacting appropriate items should be the only people performing this task.

If using an online system for protocol submission, programmers could facilitate this process by developing a redacted version that is automatically created when the protocol is approved, which hides some fields such as researchers' personal information. There are programs for creating minutes that could have a redaction function using member codes, and electronic animal medical records modules that would assist the veterinary staff in standardizing medical record entries, which could more easily be redacted. To reduce the burden of redaction, options may include placing some commonly requested and preredacted documents on the institution's website so that they are already available for the public to see. Examples are the institution's Assurance and possibly some animal use protocols, specifically the protocols that conduct research with USDA-regulated species, as those are almost exclusively requested. This also would require ongoing document management, as it would be necessary to remove outdated information and replace it with newly approved versions.

The most frequent requests are for minutes, medical records, and protocols. These documents need to be skillfully written keeping in mind what truly needs to be included. Follow regulatory guidelines for the institution's documents retention policy and regularly destroy documents that are on a predetermined schedule of removal. Do not keep documents if there is no regulatory requirement for keeping them.

Remember that the institution has control over every document it creates, but once a document has been released, that control is lost. Be mindful when reviewing protocols and drafting correspondence and minutes; and before finalizing, review them one last time as if you are a member of the public (NABR 2013).

13.13 NEWS AND MEDIA SERVICES AND UNIVERSITY RELATIONS

The key to successful media relations is multifold. Animal activists can influence public opinion, and news reporters want to have a sensational story. Institutions must be prepared to respond. To aid in transparency and good community relations, the institution needs to be proactive in sending a message about the necessity and value of animal research, including the institution's stance on the humane treatment of animals under its care. The media relations office should not hesitate to report the advances in basic science or biomedical research that have resulted from the use of animals at the institution (UAR 2009). There is something to be said for making friends before you need them, and this is a perfect example. The ACUP needs to have a close relationship with the news office so that any communication about the ACUP in response to media attention can be conveyed quickly and factually. It is helpful for the institution to have a media-trained spokesperson to address the news media who is prepared to respond to any questions that may arise. Having information prepared in advance about researchers' work that is being conducted and its benefit to medical advancements is important. It is also helpful to regularly meet with the media relations personnel, including giving them a tour of the animal facility. Do not wait for a crisis to occur and then scramble to develop a response. The bottom line is that for the institution to be prepared, a crisis communication strategy needs to be developed in advance and should be reviewed and updated regularly.

13.14 ANIMAL RIGHTS OR EXTREMIST GROUPS' ACTIVITY AND WORKING WITH THE LOCAL POLICE

It is important to distinguish between animal rights activism and animal rights extremism. An animal rights activist is a person who, from an ethical standpoint, promotes the rights of animals to humane treatment and freedom from exploitation by humans. Most institutions have experienced animal rights demonstrations and leafleting, which is a legal way to express views. An extremist, on the other hand, is a person who promotes vandalism, defamation, and intimidation in an attempt to advance his or her position (Conn and Parker 2008). Actions taken by either of these groups can rise and fall, oftentimes depending on what is requested under the FOIA or state open records laws.

The IACUC should establish a good working relationship with the local or university police. The IACUC can be the liaison between the researchers and the police, identifying for them who may be at greater risk of being targeted by animal rights or extremist groups. Most often, this would be nonhuman primate or dog researchers. Some researchers may be reluctant to discuss their vulnerability with strangers, and the IACUC can help bridge that gap. As researchers may reside in neighborhoods other than those that are serviced by the local or university police, the police departments in their area of residence should be notified that there are animal researchers in their precinct who may be at additional risk. This is one area in which the local police or university police can be of great assistance. The police are usually thought of as responding to criminal acts, but as experts on crime, they also provide valuable guidance on security measures and crime prevention that should be supported by leadership at the university.

The university police also maintain records of all animal-related activity and can periodically provide the IACUC with records of such activity. It is important for the institution to be aware of trends, and to review the uptick in or quiescence of activity and why it is occurring. It may also be important to consider whether proactive public relations management and greater transparency might positively affect the institution.

13.15 CONCLUSION

To work in an academic setting takes a lot of patience, perseverance, and, above all, flexibility. There are unique challenges that must be appropriately managed. The IACUC must stay apprised of the changing regulatory environment and strive to effectively perform all of the duties required for protocol and programmatic review. The IACUC must work closely with the AV, the IO, other stakeholders, and especially the faculty to make necessary programmatic changes with the least burden for all involved. With adequate resources, institutional support, and faculty commitment, the program will benefit and animal welfare will be ensured.

REFERENCES

ARENA/OLAW (Applied Research Ethics National Association and Office of Laboratory Animal Welfare). 2002. *Institutional Animal Care and Use Committee Guidebook*, 2nd edn. Bethesda, MD: National Institutes of Health.

AVMA (American Veterinary Medical Association). 2013. *Guidelines for the Euthanasia of Animals*. Schaumburg, IL: AVMA.

Conn, PM and JV Parker. 2008. The animal research war. *FASEB Journal* 22 (5):1294–1295.

DOD (Department of Defense). n.d. General guidelines for awards funded by the DOD. DOD.

DOD (Department of Defense). 2005. The care and use of laboratory animals in DOD programs. Washington, DC: DOD.

FWS (U.S. Fish and Wildlife Service). 2014. Endangered Species Program: Permits. FWS.

Greene, ME, ME Pitts, and ML James. 2007. Training strategies for institutional animal care and use committee (IACUC) members and the institutional official (IO). *ILAR Journal* 48 (2):131–142.

HHS (U.S. Department of Health and Human Services). 2011. Responsibility of applicants for promoting objectivity in research for which public health service funding is sought and responsible prospective contractors. Code of Federal Regulations Title 42, Part 50. http://www.gpo.gov/fdsys/pkg/FR-2011-08-25/pdf/2011-21633.pdf.

HHS (U.S. Department of Health and Human Services). 2014. Responsible prospective contractors. Code of Federal Regulations Title 45, Subchapter A, Part 94. http://www.ecfr.gov/cgi-bin/text-idx?SID=432bdb2a9581e1cab253f3322388ca6e&node=45:1.0.1.1.51&rgn=div5.

NABR (National Association for Biomedical Research). 2013. NABR webinar: Are your IACUC records putting you at risk? October 8. http://nabr.org/IACUC_Risk.aspx.

NIH (National Institutes of Health). 1985. U.S. government principles for the utilization and care of vertebrate animals used in testing, research and training, no. 13. Bethesda, MD: NIH. http://grants.nih.gov/grants/olaw/references/phspol.htm#USGovPrinciples.

NIH (National Institutes of Health). 2002. Public Health Service policy on humane care and use of laboratory animals. Bethesda, MD: Office of Laboratory Animal Welfare, U.S. Department of Health and Human Services, NIH.

NIH (National Institutes of Health). 2006a. Frequently asked questions: PHS policy on humane care and use of laboratory animals. Bethesda, MD: Office of Laboratory Animal Welfare. http://grants.nih.gov/grants/olaw/faqs.htm.

NIH (National Institutes of Health). 2006b. Frequently asked questions: PHS policy on humane care and use of laboratory animals: Does the PHS policy apply to animal research that is conducted in the field? Bethesda, MD: Office of Laboratory Animal Welfare. http://grants.nih.gov/grants/olaw/faqs.htm#App_6.

NIH (National Institutes of Health). 2006c. Frequently asked questions: PHS policy on humane care and use of laboratory animals: Is the IACUC required to inspect field study sites? Bethesda, MD: Office of Laboratory Animal Welfare. http://grants.nih.gov/grants/olaw/faqs.htm#prorev_4.

NIH (National Institutes of Health). 2006d. Frequently asked questions: PHS policy on humane care and use of laboratory animals: Are multiple major survival surgical procedures permitted on a single animal? Bethesda, MD: Office of Laboratory Animal Welfare. http://grants.nih.gov/grants/olaw/faqs.htm#useandmgmt_9.

NIH (National Institutes of Health). 2006e. Frequently asked questions: PHS policy on humane care and use of laboratory animals: Is post approval monitoring required? Office of Bethesda, MD: Laboratory Animal Welfare. http://grants.nih.gov/grants/olaw/faqs.htm#instresp_6.

NIH (National Institutes of Health). 2006f. Frequently asked questions: PHS policy on humane care and use of laboratory animals: When institutions collaborate, or when the performance site is not the awardee institution, which IACUC is responsible for review of the research activity? Bethesda, MD: Office of Laboratory Animal Welfare. http://grants.nih.gov/grants/olaw/faqs.htm#proto_8.

NIH (National Institutes of Health). 2007. NOT-OD-07-044: NIH policy on allowable costs for grant activities involving animals when terms and conditions are not upheld. Bethesda, MD: NIH. http://grants.nih.gov/grants/guide/notice-files/NOT-OD-07-044.html.

NIH (National Institutes of Health). 2010a. NOT-OD-10-027: Instructions for completion and peer review of the Vertebrate Animal Section (VAS) in NIH grant applications and cooperative agreements. Bethesda, MD: NIH. http://grants.nih.gov/grants/guide/notice-files/NOT-OD-10-027.html.

NIH (National Institutes of Health). 2010b. NOT-OD-10-120: Revised policy on applicant institution responsibilities for ensuring just-in-time submissions are accurate and current up to the time of award. Bethesda, MD: NIH.

NIH (National Institutes of Health). 2011a. NOT-OD-11-053: Guidance to reduce regulatory burden for IACUC administration regarding alternate members and approval dates. Bethesda, MD: NIH.

NIH (National Institutes of Health). 2011b. NOT-OD-12-021: Update of sample interinstitutional assurance. No. 2014. Bethesda, MD: NIH.

NIH (National Institutes of Health). 2012. Office of Laboratory Animal Welfare: Obtaining an assurance. Bethesda, MD: NIH. http://grants.nih.gov/grants/olaw/obtain_assurance.htm.

NIH (National Institutes of Health). 2013a. NIH grants policy statement.

NIH (National Institutes of Health). 2013b. NIH grants policy statement (2013) Part I. Bethesda, MD: NIH. http://grants.nih.gov/grants/policy/nihgps_2013/nihgps_ch1.htm.

NIH (National Institutes of Health). 2013c. NIH grants policy statement (2013) Part II. Bethesda, MD: NIH. http://grants.nih.gov/grants/policy/nihgps_2013/nihgps_ch3.htm.

NIH (National Institutes of Health). 2013d. NOT-OD-05-034: Guidance on prompt reporting to OLAW under the PHS policy on humane care and use of laboratory animals. Bethesda, MD: NIH. http://grants.nih.gov/grants/guide/notice-files/NOT-OD-05-034.html.

NIH (National Institutes of Health). 2013e. NOT-OD-13-044: Notice of change to electronic submission of final noncompliance reports to the Office of Laboratory Animal Welfare. Bethesda, MD: NIH. http://grants.nih.gov/grants/guide/notice-files/NOT-OD-13-044.html.

NIH (National Institutes of Health). 2014a. NOT-OD-14-099: Notice of change in criteria for renewal of domestic animal welfare assurances. Bethesda, MD: NIH. http://grants.nih.gov/grants/guide/notice-files/NOT-OD-14-099.html.

NIH (National Institutes of Health). 2014b. NOT-OD-14-126: Guidance on significant changes to animal activities. Bethesda, MD: NIH. http://grants.nih.gov/grants/guide/notice-files/NOT-OD-14-126.html.

NOAA (National Oceanic and Atmospheric Administration). 2014. Endangered species permits FAQs. NOAA Fisheries, Office of Protected Resources. http://www.nmfs.noaa.gov/pr/permits/faq_esapermits.htm.

NRC (National Research Council). 2011. *Guide for the Care and Use of Laboratory Animals*, 8th edn. Washington, DC: National Academies Press.

Safe-Capture International. 2014. Safe-Capture International. http://www.safecapture.com/.

Silverman, J, MA Suckow, and S Murthy. 2014. *The IACUC Handbook*, Boca Raton, FL: CRC.

UAR (Understanding Animal Research). 2009. Website spotlight: A researchers' guide to communications. Understanding Animal Research. http://www.understandinganimal-research.org.uk/news/2009/05/website-spotlight-a-researchers-guide-to-communications/. Accessed 20 May 2014.

USDA (U.S. Department of Agriculture). 2013a. *Animal Welfare Act and Animal Welfare Regulations* (Animal Care Blue Book). Code of Federal Regulations (CFR) Title 9, Chapter 1, Subchapter A, Parts 1–4.

USDA (U.S. Department of Agriculture). 2013b. Animal Welfare Act of 1966 intended to regulate the transport, sale and handling of dogs, cats, guinea pigs, nonhuman primates, hamsters and rabbits intended to use for research or other purposes. *Public Law* 89 (544):2131–2156.

U.S. Department of Justice. n.d. Freedom of Information Act, 5 U.S.C., Sect. 552. As amended by public law 101–231, 110 Stat 3048. Washington, DC: US Department of Justice.

Wong, S. 2013. Chasing shadows: Conservation of small carnivores. Lecture at San Francisco Zoo, November 2. http://www.sfzoo.org/announcements/wild-places-wild- things-lecture-2.

CHAPTER 14

IACUC Issues in Industry

Marcy Brown and Jane Chambers

CONTENTS

14.1 INTRODUCTION

In the life sciences arena, several industry sectors are involved in research to improve human and animal health, including biotechnology and pharmaceutical companies, as well as contract research organizations (CRO) and preclinical drug development services. The biotechnology and pharmaceutical companies run the gamut from small, biotech start-ups to global companies often referred to as "big Pharma." CROs range from large, international full-service organizations to small, niche specialty companies that provide support to the pharmaceutical, biotechnology, and medical device industries by providing research services on a contract basis. This chapter will provide an overview of Institutional Animal Care and Use Committees (IACUCs) in industry and will review and discuss issues that may impact how these

IACUCs operate. Our observations are drawn from a combined 25 years or more of IACUC-related experience, service on global corporate IACUC and regulatory teams, and an informal survey of IACUC members at industry institutions.

14.2 BACKGROUND: THE REGULATORY FRAMEWORK

The specific regulatory framework under which IACUCs in industry operate is not significantly different from that of IACUCs in general. Depending on the species used, the source of funding, and the accreditation status, the care and use of animals in biomedical research in the United States mainly falls under the Animal Welfare Act Regulations (AWRs) or the Public Health Service (PHS) Policy on Humane Care and Use of Laboratory Animals or both. In addition, many states have their own laws or regulations and even local ordinances affecting the use of animals for research purposes. These requirements vary from state to state; the reader is encouraged to consult his or her specific state regulations for more information. The most common state laws and regulations govern the licensing of research facilities, require permits for certain species, or regulate the practice of veterinary medicine, as well as whether or not, and under what circumstances, animals from municipal pounds may be obtained for research.

In addition to federal and state regulations, organizations that wish to obtain and maintain accreditation with the Association for Assessment and Accreditation of Laboratory Animal Care (AAALAC) International must establish an IACUC and manage their programs in accordance with these regulations and policy. AAALAC International uses the *Guide for the Care and Use of Laboratory Animals* (the Guide) (NRC 2011), as well as the *Guide for the Care and Use of Agricultural Animals in Research and Teaching* (the Ag Guide) (FASS 2010) as the primary standards to evaluate Animal Care and Use Programs (ACUPs) in the United States. Although AAALAC International accreditation is voluntary, its benefit is seen as so important that many biotechs, CROs, and pharmaceutical companies consider it to be highly desirable and, in some cases, mandatory. This holds true even for privately funded organizations that do not use regulated species and are therefore exempt from the requirement to establish and maintain an IACUC. Finally, for large companies that may have multiple sites and IACUCs, there may be corporate or global guidelines that IACUCs need to incorporate and follow.

14.3 IACUC RESPONSIBILITY, COMPOSITION, AND MEMBERSHIP REQUIREMENTS

The responsibility, composition, and membership requirements for IACUCs in industry are not very different from those of IACUCs in general. Institutions that are regulated by the AWA or the PHS Policy or both are required to establish and maintain an IACUC that must review and approve (or disapprove) all activities involving animals, as well as oversee their care. All individuals involved in an ACUP, including the institutional official (IO), the attending veterinarian (AV), the animal care staff, the researchers, and the IACUC have important roles to play. However, both the Guide and the *Institutional Animal Care and Use Committee Guidebook* (ARENA/OLAW 2002) specifically outline the key role of the IACUC; no matter the size or the type of organization, the responsibility of the IACUC is to oversee and assess the institution's entire ACUP and its components (NRC 2011).

The composition and membership requirements for an IACUC vary according to the regulatory oversight agency involved (if any). If an organization receives PHS funding, it must have an IACUC with at least five members, including at least one veterinarian, one practicing scientist, one nonscientist, and one individual who is not affiliated with the organization in any way except as a member of the IACUC. If an organization is funded internally but uses an animal species that is regulated by the AWRs, its IACUC must have at least three members, including a chair, a veterinarian, and a nonaffiliated member (NAM). If an organization is not under federal regulatory oversight but wishes to obtain or maintain AAALAC International accreditation, it must follow the recommendations of the Guide (pp. 24–25), which state that IACUC membership includes a veterinarian, a scientist, a nonscientist, and at least one public member to represent the general community interest, and also that "[the] size of the institution and the nature and extent of the Program will determine the number of members of the committee and their terms of appointment." It is not uncommon to have representation from each scientific unit that conducts animal work as well as animal care staff or vivarium management. It is also useful to have alternate members to ensure a quorum if regular members are unable to attend or suddenly become unavailable for a long period of time. For additional details on the specific regulatory requirements for and responsibilities of the IACUC, the reader is referred to the AWRs (USDA 2013a) (specifically §2.31) and the PHS Policy (NIH 2002) (specifically IV.A.3.; IV.B.-C.; and IV.E.-F.). Some committee composition and membership issues create special challenges for industry, such as ensuring an adequate number of members, recruiting and training nonaffiliated IACUC members, and aligning IACUCs across multiple sites.

14.3.1 Ensuring an Adequate Number of Members

One issue, especially for smaller institutions, is ensuring that the IACUC has an adequate number of members appointed to serve. This becomes especially important for quorum purposes in cases of absence and extended leave of IACUC members, or when members must recuse themselves to avoid conflicts of interest. It is also important to ensure that all the required functions of the IACUC (NIH 2002) (review and approve proposed activities and significant changes to activities related to the care and use of animals, inspect animal facilities and study areas, conduct a semiannual review of the program for animal care and use, make reports and recommendations to the IO, review and investigate concerns involving the care and use of animals, and suspend activities as necessary) are carried out effectively without unnecessarily burdening each individual member. There can be significant problems if the number of IACUC members is too small. "IACUCs that have a small membership often have a narrower base of expertise and, depending upon the size of the program they service, may encounter an onerous workload" (Silverman et al. 2014). One way to solve this problem is through the use of alternate members who are appointed for some, if not all, of the IACUC members. The use of alternate IACUC members can provide a contingency for absences or in the event that members must recuse themselves. However, due to competing work priorities, responsibilities, and commitments, it may be difficult to persuade scientists to serve on an IACUC. When this is the case, the best solution is to engage the IO, who should have an understanding of his or her responsibility for the success of the institution's ACUP. One of the IO's primary responsibilities is to ensure that the institution has a functioning IACUC. Part of this is appreciating the critical role that the IACUC plays in ensuring compliance and the amount of time and effort it takes to fulfill the responsibilities of IACUC membership. An engaged and supportive IO will identify and recommend those individuals who have the time to participate fully and would be best suited to serve on the IACUC, and will then communicate to the prospective members the importance of service on the IACUC. The IO will also communicate to management the importance of the role of the IACUC member, to ensure support for the member's service.

In the same way, recruiting NAMs to serve on the IACUC can be one of the most difficult aspects of ensuring a fully constituted IACUC. The NAM must not be affiliated with the institution, must represent the community interests, and must be willing and able to put in the time to be an integral part of the committee. The NAM often also fulfills the role of nonscientist and should have "equal status to every other committee member and ... be afforded the opportunity to participate in all aspects of IACUC functions" (FASS 2010). The recruitment, training, and engagement of nonaffiliated IACUC members are discussed in greater detail in Section 14.3.2.

Another issue, especially in small biotech companies, is that it is not uncommon for an IACUC member to wear multiple hats in the overall ACUP. For example, the facility or operations manager may serve as IACUC chair or voting member, as well as the IACUC administrator and postapproval monitoring (PAM) coordinator. While it is permissible for one person to fill some or all of these roles, in our opinion, this practice may give the appearance of a conflict of interest, especially during an IACUC semiannual review of facilities (over which the facility manager is responsible). When one person has several overlapping roles and responsibilities, and time management becomes an issue, IACUC-related duties may be put on the back burner, or the person may experience burnout, all of which have the potential to negatively impact the program. If resources do not exist to bring in additional personnel, institutions facing this type of situation should take a hard look at their ACUP to identify areas where efficiencies may be improved or self-imposed burden lessened. There are ways to manage the balance between risk and burden, especially in cases of self-imposed regulatory burden. A good starting point is for the institution to review its IACUC practices with an eye to identifying self-imposed regulatory burden and determine first, whether it is necessary and second, whether it can be achieved in a more efficient or cost-effective manner (Haywood and Greene 2008).

In much the same way as the IACUC member wears multiple hats, the IACUC chair has additional responsibilities to keep abreast of regulatory trends and interpretations; ensure that the IACUC carries out its required mandates; educate and support the IACUC members; serve as the IACUC spokesperson and leader; and communicate regularly with the IO, AV, and researchers. Keeping up with the responsibilities of this role can become a challenge, as the position of chair is generally not this person's only responsibility. The chair will often have his own or her own research to conduct or department to manage. Staying current on IACUC regulations and industry standards can be time-consuming and take away from the chair's "day job." Besides time issues, there may be budget constraints that prohibit participation in external IACUC training or continuing education, especially in smaller institutions or start-up companies. Although it is not uncommon for IACUC chairs in academia to receive some type of compensation in the form of salary support or release time from teaching duties, the same is not generally true in industry. In industry, as well as academia, the pressures placed on individuals to complete projects can create a time management issue. For this reason, the provision of a skilled IACUC administrator or coordinator to help keep abreast of the complex regulatory environment and provide support for the committee's activities is invaluable (DeHaven 2002). Even a part-time person in such a position can have a tremendous impact on reducing the burden on the chair, as well as facilitating the work of the IACUC and reducing the burden for the researchers and animal users.

14.3.2 Recruiting, Training, and Engaging Nonaffiliated IACUC Members

The NAM is defined as an individual who represents general community interests in the proper care and use of animals, is not a laboratory animal user, is not affiliated with the institution, and is not an immediate family member of a person who is affiliated with the institution (AWA Sect. 13,b,1,B; AWRs §2.31,b,3,ii [USDA 2013b]; PHS Policy IV.A.3.b.4. [NIH 2002]; the Guide [NRC 2011, pp. 24–25]; APHIS/AC Policy #15 [USDA 2011]). One of the most frequent topics of concern for IACUCs in both academia and industry is how to find and recruit NAMs. NAMs should be active and involved, are willing to ask questions, and feel free to express their views. However, selecting NAMs should be done with the utmost care, to screen out animal extremists who might disrupt meetings, leak confidential information, or commit other offenses against the institution. "Research organizations now have to prepare for activists masquerading as potential employees, break-ins, electronic 'denial-of-service' attacks against Internet sites and e-mail systems, intimidating protests at the personal residences of researchers, threats against family members, arson, car bombs and targeting of related businesses" (NABR 2014). Although not always easy, NAMs may be found in a number of ways. A common and generally secure method is to recruit friends or contacts of the chair, members of the IACUC, the AV, the IACUC administrator, or personnel in other departments within the organization. Lawyers, ethicists, clergy, retired teachers, or public servants are often good IACUC members and may be recruited by contacting local professional societies or organizations. Many state biomedical advocacy organizations maintain lists of people who have expressed an interest in serving on a local IACUC, and in many cases these people have already been vetted by the organization. A list of statewide or regional biomedical organizations current at the time of this writing is provided in Table 14.1. Finally, contacting local veterinarians and nonprofit service organizations may be useful in the search for NAMs. Even local veterinarians themselves may serve as the NAM, as long as he or she is not a laboratory animal user, either directly or through consultation or other services (Silverman et al. 2014). No matter what source is used for recruiting NAMs for an IACUC, it is critical to conduct a complete background and security check prior to considering any individual for this important role. In addition, all IACUC members, but especially the NAM, should sign a confidentiality and proprietary information or nondisclosure agreement in which he or she agrees not to disclose or use, directly or indirectly, any confidential or proprietary information about the organization that he or she may learn in his or her service as an IACUC member.

The IACUC's role in the oversight of training, as well as the training requirements for IACUC members is described in detail in Chapter 7 of this book, the IACUC Guidebook (ARENA/OLAW 2002), and the Guide (NRC 2011). Having a strong, comprehensive training program for the IACUC is key to ensuring animal welfare, and the NAMs must receive the same training provided to all IACUC members. "With perhaps the exception of members who are laboratory animal veterinarians by training, IACUC members come to the committee without knowledge of the rules, regulations, and expectations necessary to assess whether or not the institution's program is in compliance" (Greene et al. 2007). This is especially true of the NAM. All IACUC members should undergo initial training, with an orientation to the purpose and responsibilities of the IACUC, but for the NAM this should also include an orientation to the organization and the type of research that is being performed to help him or her understand the role that animals play in this research. Introducing the NAM to the key players of the program, such as the IACUC chair,

Table 14.1 State Biomedical Research Associations

States United for Biomedical Research	www.statesforbiomed.org
Alabama Association for Biomedical Research (AABR)	
California Biomedical Research Association (CBRA)	www.ca-biomed.org
Connecticut United for Research Excellence, Inc. (CURE)	www.curenet.org
Massachusetts Society for Medical Research (MSMR)	www.msmr.org
Michigan Society for Medical Research (MISMR)	www.mismr.org
New Jersey Association for Biomedical Research (NJABR)	www.njabr.org
North Carolina Association for Biomedical Research (NCABR)	www.ncabr.org
Northwest Association for Biomedical Research (NWABR)	www.nwabr.org
Ohio Scientific Education & Research Association (OSERA)	www.osera.org
Pennsylvania Society for Biomedical Research (PSBR)	www.psbr.org
Southwest Association for Education in Biomedical Research (SWAEBR)	www.swaebr.org
Texas Society for Biomedical Research (TSBR)	www.tsbr.org
Wisconsin Association for Biomedical Research and Education (WABRE)	www.wabre.org

Note: Current as of March 2014.

the AV, the IACUC administrator, or support staff, and perhaps the animal facility manager will help him or her understand the various components of the program and how they interact. Finally, for new NAM members, providing a medical dictionary and a list of common acronyms is an essential, but often overlooked part of training.

Because of the often highly secured and protected computer and e-mail systems used in industry, providing the NAM members with access to online protocol systems, IACUC files and documents, as well as e-mail privileges, can be a challenge. In our experience, it is best practice to provide the NAM with a company e-mail account and a company-configured computer with software and systems already in place for securely accessing company programs and IACUC documents. Depending on the company firewall, hardware and software requirements, and user knowledge of computer systems, providing company intranet and e-mail access to the NAM may require extensive training, and then continual review to ensure that the NAM has appropriate access to IACUC documents.

14.3.3 Alignment of IACUCs across Multiple Sites

It is not uncommon for larger companies to have multiple sites across the nation and even the globe, each with their own IACUC. The culture and "personality" of each IACUC can differ enough that practices and procedures are not harmonized across sites, which may create unwanted inconsistencies for the business. A challenge is how to develop a mechanism to maintain consistency and quality in the individual ACUPs and to standardize, or harmonize, the major components of the programs to meet company commitments to animal welfare. This is especially important if more than one site falls under a single USDA registration or PHS Assurance. Corporate IACUC guidelines and policies, standard operating procedures, and unifying processes can and should be created to cover general IACUC-related topics, such as blood collection, dose volumes, humane end points, and multiple survival surgery guidance. The use of a standardized protocol review form and a protocol review process, as well as consistent processes regarding animal welfare investigations, postapproval monitoring, and animal user training can also ensure that multiple IACUCs are harmonized across the company. One mechanism to facilitate alignment across sites is to establish a corporate governance body, committee, or working group with individual representation from each site or location. The individual members of this group would represent "the voice of" their particular site, bringing forward site-specific issues, sharing best practices, and providing process metrics for reviewing trends across sites. Each site representative and, ideally, each site IACUC would contribute to the development of standardized documents and processes mentioned earlier.

14.4 OTHER ISSUES IN INDUSTRY

Preclinical studies often require drug dosages to be administered to animals at very high levels in order to determine the no-observed-adverse-effect level (NOAEL) that is required by regulatory agencies prior to clinical studies. This may require the animal use protocol to fall into the USDA E pain category (see Appendix G). IACUCs must evaluate the end points and the reduction of pain and distress where possible. These studies are expensive and can be of a long duration. Companies will often contract with CROs to conduct these studies as it is more cost-efficient than conducting these studies in-house. Off-site study conduct and oversight provide an additional challenge.

14.4.1 Toxicology Studies and Animal Welfare

Toxicology plays an important role in the drug discovery and development process. To determine whether a drug is safe and effective prior to clinical studies in humans, preclinical (animal toxicology/safety) studies must be conducted. Many pharmaceutical and biotechnology companies have drug safety departments or divisions that conduct such studies, which are undertaken to identify and measure a drug's adverse effect. These studies are required by the Food and Drug Administration (FDA), which will not allow unknown and uncharacterized compounds to be administered to human subjects in clinical trials before their effects have been studied in laboratory animals. Depending on the nature of a drug, its intended use, and its proposed study in clinical trials, toxicity testing may include some or all of the following types of studies: acute toxicity; subacute, subchronic, or chronic toxicity; carcinogenic toxicity; reproductive toxicity; genotoxicity; and toxicokinetic studies (Dorato and Engelhardt 2005, Mathieu 2008). Adverse effects on animals may be caused during such testing, resulting in significant pain or distress or both. The FDA supports measures that are dedicated to reducing the use of animals in toxicity testing and has research and development efforts underway to reduce the need for animal testing while working toward the replacement of animal testing. However, animal tests are often the only means by which toxicity in humans can be effectively predicted. To this end, the FDA recognizes and supports the role of the IACUC in studies involving animals. What is the responsibility of the IACUC with regard to these types of studies? The AWRs (USDA 2013a) and the PHS Policy (NIH 2002) contain almost identical language describing the responsibility of the IACUC to critically evaluate proposed animal activities to ensure pain and distress are avoided or minimized (e.g., "Procedures with animals will avoid or minimize discomfort, distress, and pain to the animals, consistent with sound research design," NIH 2002). The Guide echoes this responsibility, but also acknowledges that studies commonly requiring special consideration include those assessing toxicological effects (NRC 2011). It is the IACUC's responsibility to minimize animal pain and distress by ensuring that proposed toxicology studies have clearly defined end points describing when an animal may be removed from the study for humane reasons. The Guide lists some of the information that is critical to the IACUC's assessment of whether the end point proposed is appropriate, including:

- A precise description of the humane end point, including the criteria used for assessing the animal
- How often animals will be observed
- How personnel have been trained to assess and recognize the humane end point

It is also the IACUC's responsibility to ensure that procedures that may cause more than momentary or slight pain or distress will be performed with appropriate sedation, analgesia, or anesthesia, unless the procedure is justified for scientific reasons in writing by the investigator (NIH 2002). There are other questions that the IACUC should consider in reviewing toxicology studies, such as whether there are procedures in place to deal with unexpected or severe clinical signs, whether supportive therapy has been considered, and whether animals may be socially housed with environmental enrichment when possible without compromising the study or the data.

There have been advances in science and technology that provide opportunities to improve animal welfare and reduce animal use in testing. The Interagency Coordinating Committee on the Validation of Alternative Methods (ICCVAM) was established by law (Public Law 106-545) "To establish, wherever feasible guidelines, recommendations and regulation that promote the regulatory acceptance of new or revised scientifically valid toxicological tests that protect human and animal health and the environment while reducing, refining, or replacing animal tests and ensuring human safety and product effectiveness" (106th Congress 2000). Progress has been made in the refinement of procedures, including humane end point criteria, and a reduction in animal-based test methods (Stokes 2011, 2002); however, until the need for regulatory testing in animals is completely replaced with alternative methods, the responsibility rests with the IACUC to ensure that a sound, written scientific rationale is provided if pain or distress will not be relieved with analgesics or anesthetics, and that procedures "will avoid or minimize discomfort, distress, and pain to the animals, consistent with sound research design" (NIH 2002).

14.4.2 Outsourcing Studies to CROs

In this era of increased pharmaceutical and biotechnology industry competition, success for many companies is dependent on their ability to develop their drug or medical device products in an economical and timely manner, while also being compliant from a legal and regulatory perspective. Research institutions, whether pharmaceutical, academic, or biotechnical, are facing growing regulatory, competitive, and financial pressures to increase their productivity. These pressures include increased public scrutiny of *in vivo* research, increased federal regulations, and increased costs to develop new drugs. Therefore, with respect to *in vivo* research, institutions are evaluating all options for pursuing animal research. Industry collaborations with both academic institutions and other industry companies are on the rise. In addition, more and more often, institutions are using CROs to outsource their *in vivo* research. This trend toward outsourcing of animal research has raised some concerns about animal welfare standards, personnel qualifications, and veterinary care (Bayne et al. 2011). There are potential issues to be addressed when outsourcing animal studies, some of which are discussed here. First, the institution should develop a corporate policy or strategy for its outsourced studies (Underwood 2007) that includes a requirement that the CRO or other organization maintain the highest standards of animal care and use. Prior to initiating any studies, a risk evaluation of the CRO should be performed, including such information as

- Regulatory status (e.g., USDA, FDA, NIH-OLAW, good laboratory practice [GLP] certified, and local authority).
- Accreditations held (e.g., AAALAC International and ISO).
- The source (supplier) of the animals and whether the animals are purpose-bred for research.
- A description of the housing conditions (type of primary enclosure), whether animals are single, pair, or group housed, and whether the organization has a social housing and environmental enrichment program for all species.
- Whether the studies are reviewed by an established IACUC or an equivalent animal welfare oversight body (e.g., AWERB in the United Kingdom).
- The type of study to be performed, the species and number of animals involved, and the level of pain or distress expected as a result of the study procedures.
- The criteria for humane end points for the study.
- The method of euthanasia that will or may be used.
- Whether there is a veterinarian on-site or an established relationship with a contract veterinarian, and details regarding his or her qualifications and years of experience.
- Whether there has been any animal rights activity, demonstrations, or adverse publicity involving the organization.

Armed with this information, a risk assessment can be performed to determine whether or not an audit of the CRO and its facilities (remote or on-site) is needed. The responsibility for performing this assessment and audit may fall to the IACUC in smaller institutions or to a corporate office or regulatory team in large pharmaceutical companies. Once a determination is made to outsource a study to a particular CRO, a written contract should be executed that includes a confidentiality agreement, defines who owns the animals and who owns the data, and outlines the expectation that the CRO will comply with all applicable regulations and guidelines for animal care and use (Underwood 2007).

14.5 SUMMARY

In summary, the requirements, responsibilities, and issues for IACUCs, whether in an academic setting or industry, are similar. Multiple sites, the ancillary duties of the IACUC chair and IACUC members, the recruitment and support of NAMs, the minimization of pain and distress in toxicology studies, and strategies for outsourcing studies can be extra challenging for industry, but they are certainly not insurmountable.

REFERENCES

106th Congress. 2000. Public Law 106-545. ICCVAM Authorization Act of 2000, December 19, 2000.

ARENA/OLAW (Applied Research Ethics National Association and Office of Laboratory Animal Welfare). 2002. *Institutional Animal Care and Use Committee Guidebook*, 2nd edn. Bethesda, MD: National Institutes of Health.

Bayne, K., D. Bayvel, J. M. Clark, G. Demers, C. Joubert, T. M. Kurosawa, E. Rivera, O. Souilem, and P. V. Turner. 2011. Harmonizing veterinary training and qualifications in laboratory animal medicine: A global perspective. *ILAR Journal/National Research Council* 52 (3):393–403.

DeHaven, W. R. 2002. Best practices for animal care committees and animal use oversight. *ILAR Journal* 43 (Suppl 1):S59–S62.

Dorato, M. A. and J. A. Engelhardt. 2005. The no-observed-adverse-effect-level in drug safety evaluations: Use, issues, and definition(s). *Regulatory Toxicology and Pharmacology* 42 (3):265–274.

FASS (Federation of Animal Science Societies). 2010. *Guide for the Care and Use of Agricultural Animals in Agricultural Research and Teaching*. Champaign, IL: Consortium for Developing a Guide for the Care and Use of Agricultural Animals in Agricultural Research and Teaching.

Greene, M. E., M. E. Pitts, and M. L. James. 2007. Training strategies for institutional animal care and use committee (IACUC) members and the institutional official (IO). *ILAR Journal* 48 (2):131–142.

Haywood, J. R. and M. Greene. 2008. Avoiding an overzealous approach: A perspective on regulatory burden. *ILAR Journal* 49 (4):426–434.

Mathieu, M. P. 2008. *New Drug Development: A Regulatory Overview*, 8th edn. Waltham, MA: Parexel International Corporation.

NABR (National Association for Biomedical Research). 2014. Federal regulation of biomedical research involving animals. http://www.nabr.org.

NIH (National Institutes of Health). 2002. Public Health Service policy on humane care and use of laboratory animals. Bethesda, MD: Office of Laboratory Animal Welfare, U.S. Department of Health and Human Services, NIH.

NRC (National Research Council). 2011. *Guide for the Care and Use of Laboratory Animals*, 8th edn. Washington, DC: National Academies Press.

Silverman, J., M. A. Suckow, and S. Murthy, eds. 2014. *The IACUC Handbook*, 3rd edn. Boca Raton, FL: CRC Press.

Stokes, W. S. 2002. Humane endpoints for laboratory animals used in regulatory testing. *ILAR Journal* 43 (Suppl 1):S31–S38.

Stokes, W. S. 2011. Best practices for the use of animals in toxicological research and testing. *Annals of the New York Academy of Sciences* 1245 (1):17–20.

USDA (U.S. Department of Agriculture). 2011. Animal care manual. Policy 15: Institutional official and IACUC membership. In *Animal Care Resource Guide*. Washington, DC: USDA.

USDA (U.S. Department of Agriculture). 2013a. *Animal Welfare Act and Animal Welfare Regulations* (Animal Care Blue Book). Code of Federal Regulations (CFR), Title 9, Chapter 1, Subchapter A, Parts 1–4.

USDA (U.S. Department of Agriculture). 2013b. Animal Welfare Act of 1966 intended to regulate the transport, sale and handling of dogs, cats, guinea pigs, nonhuman primates, hamsters and rabbits intended to use for research or other purposes. *Public Law* 89 (544):2131–2156.

Underwood, W. J. 2007. Contracting *in vivo* research: What are the issues? *Journal of the American Association for Laboratory Animal Science* 46 (4):16–19.

CHAPTER 15

Perspectives of an IACUC Chair

Kathleen A. Murray

CONTENTS

15.1 INTRODUCTION

As described in the *Guide for the Care and Use of Laboratory Animals* (the Guide), the functions of an Institutional Animal Care and Use Committee (IACUC) are a component of an overall Animal Care and Use Program (ACUP) (NRC 2011). One of the primary functions of an IACUC is the assessment of a facility's animal program, facilities, and procedures. The Guide also endorses the concept of shared ACUP oversight responsibilities between the IACUC, the attending veterinarian (AV), and the institutional official (IO) as an effective mechanism to align regulatory and management authority (NRC 2011). In this shared ACUP management paradigm, the IACUC chair often represents the IACUC. While the chair performs a valuable role in facilitating and enabling the IACUC to fulfill many of the committee's responsibilities, it is also important to remember that the chair has just one vote—the same as any other member. The chair needs to be aware of the influence that his or her actions and comments may have on other members, and to always remember that it is the committee that has the ultimate authority.

15.2 SELECTION AND APPOINTMENT OF THE CHAIR

An effective IACUC chair is critical to the success of the committee. The chair represents the IACUC when interacting with the research community, the IO, and other entities such as regulatory and accrediting bodies and, depending on the institution, the general public. As the spokesperson for the IACUC, the chair must be able to explain and defend the IACUC's policies, positions, and decisions. In general, desirable characteristics and skill sets for an IACUC chair include: a general knowledge of regulations and science, prior experience conducting animal-based research, an advocate for both animal welfare and good science, sufficient seniority to be comfortable discussing issues with senior-level personnel, excellent written and verbal communication skills, an ability to maintain confidentiality, a willingness to understand and appreciate different perspectives, patience, flexibility, and someone who is respected by the research community and other stakeholders.

This list of desirable traits is not all-inclusive and is not ranked by importance. Priorities will vary depending on specific institutional needs, as well as the level and type of administrative support that is available to the IACUC and the chair. For example, if an experienced IACUC administrator supports the chair, the need for the chair to understand regulatory details may be less important as the IACUC administrator could function as an advisor on regulatory requirements to the chair and the IACUC. Finally, it is important that the chair has the time that is required to fulfill the role. At most institutions, the IACUC chair already has a full-time position within the organization, and the chair is an additional responsibility. The amount of time that is required will vary based on the type and size of the institution, as well as any administrative support provided to the IACUC and the chair. It is critical that the institution's administration understands the need for and the value of an effective IACUC chair. Management should acknowledge and recognize the chair's time, effort, and contributions to the overall success of the institution's research and ACUP when conducting overall job performance reviews.

The chair must be appointed by the chief executive officer (CEO), as specified in the Animal Welfare Act (AWA) (USDA 2013a) and the Public Health Service (PHS) Policy (see IV.A.3.a) (NIH 2002). The CEO may want to solicit input from the IO, established IACUC members, previous chairs, and other stakeholders such as the AV, when appointing a new chair. Ideally, an IACUC chair will have previously served on the institution's IACUC as an active member so that he or she is familiar with the institutional policies, IACUC practices, the ACUP, and the research community.

15.3 ROLE AND RESPONSIBILITIES OF THE CHAIR

In general, the role of the chair is to provide leadership, ensure that committee members are aware of their obligations, and that the committee complies with its responsibilities. A successful chair leads by example. The chair is responsible for making sure that the committee is properly managed and that it is functioning effectively. One of the primary responsibilities of the chair is to convene and chair IACUC meetings, as needed, to fulfill the committee's responsibilities. The chair is a voting member of the IACUC and contributes toward a quorum. This implies that the chair is present at all meetings; however, it is not a requirement, as the chair may designate an acting chair if he or she is unable to attend a meeting or participate in part of a meeting due to a conflict of interest. If the chair is also a principal investigator (PI), then it is important that the chair recuse himself or herself from voting and may not contribute toward a quorum in order to avoid a conflict of interest when his or her animal use activities are being reviewed and approved by the IACUC. Some institutions elect to formally appoint a vice or deputy chair who functions as a backup to the chair when the chair is out of the office, or otherwise unable to attend or participate in a meeting (or part of a meeting due to a conflict of interest). The chair or acting chair should always ensure that there is a quorum before calling the meeting to order.

15.3.1 IACUC Administrative Support

Other duties that are often assigned to the chair are administrative functions, which are necessary and critical to the committee's success, but can be quite time-consuming. It is strongly recommended that the chair/IACUC be provided with appropriate administrative support resources to conduct these tasks. Depending on the type of institution, the volume of animal research activities, and the size of the ACUP, these resources may vary from a part-time individual to several full-time equivalents. The chair can delegate many clerical, administrative, and professional responsibilities to an experienced IACUC administrator, including the scheduling of meetings, semiannual facility inspections, and program reviews; preparing draft meeting agendas; distributing materials to the committee; recording meeting minutes; preparing semiannual reports; assisting with new member training; coordinating and counseling PIs and the IACUC on protocol and regulatory issues; preparing required annual reports to the U.S. Department of Agriculture (USDA), the Office of Laboratory Animal Welfare (OLAW), and the Association for Assessment and Accreditation of Laboratory Animal Care (AAALAC) International; maintaining IACUC files; and assisting with the postapproval monitoring program. An effective and knowledgeable IACUC administrator can assume most of the administrative burden from the chair, which will facilitate a senior person fulfilling the role of chair. In addition, a professional IACUC administrator with regulatory expertise and familiarity with local institutional practices and policies is useful in providing program continuity when IACUC chair appointments are rotating and are of relatively short duration.

15.4 INTERACTION WITH INSTITUTIONAL OFFICIAL

The IO, as defined in the AWA and the PHS Policy, is the person at a research facility who is authorized to legally commit on behalf of the research facility that the institution will meet the requirements of 9 CFR Parts 1, 2, and 3 (USDA 2013a) and the PHS Policy (III.G.) (NIH 2002). The Guide states that the IO, as a representative of senior administration, bears ultimate responsibility for the ACUP and is responsible for resource planning and ensuring the alignment of the program goals with the institution's mission. As discussed in Section 15.1, the Guide endorses the concept of shared ACUP oversight responsibilities between the IACUC, the AV, and the IO as an effective mechanism to align regulatory and management authority (NRC 2011). In this shared ACUP management paradigm, the IACUC chair often represents the IACUC when interacting with the IO.

The CEO of the research facility appoints the IACUC to assess the facility's ACUP, facilities, and procedures. In many facilities, the CEO also functions as the IO. In large institutions, the CEO may appoint a senior-level person to assume the role of the IO. The IO relies on the IACUC's semiannual facility inspection and program review to assess the compliance of the ACUP with relevant regulations and guidelines. The IACUC chair should develop a good working relationship with the IO. The ability to have candid discussions, when needed, about IACUC recommendations regarding any aspect of the research facility's ACUP, facilities, personnel training, including deficiencies, concerns, and noncompliance, will foster a team approach, and contribute to effective oversight and continuing improvement of the ACUP.

Communication methods between the chair and the IO will vary depending on the nature of the information that is being shared. Routine updates may be provided through written material, such as copies of IACUC meeting minutes, semiannual reports, and the outcome of regulatory inspections. A regularly scheduled face-to-face meeting is recommended. The frequency of the meeting may vary based on a variety of factors, such as the size of the ACUP, the type of institution, the maturity of the ACUP, and the significance of issues with which the organization may be dealing. In addition, many institutions find it useful to invite the IO to occasionally attend an IACUC meeting or to participate in the semiannual facility inspection and program review, as well as exit meetings following regulatory inspections and accreditation visits. If the institution hosts IACUC appreciation events, such as an end-of-year banquet, pizza lunches, or other types of recognition, it should not forget to invite the IO.

Interactions between the IO and the IACUC are opportunities for the IO to observe the assessment process and to be reminded of its importance and value to the institution. The IO's presence also serves as a reminder to the IACUC members of the critical role that they fulfill in the self-regulation process and protecting the public's trust. All interactions also provide the IO with an opportunity to express the institution's thanks for the critical work that the IACUC does, and to reinforce the institution's support of and commitment to a high-quality program.

The chair should also be an advocate for the IACUC when interacting with the IO. In order to perform their functions, the IACUC needs to be provided with the appropriate resources. This may include office space, computers, IACUC management software, administrative staff, and a budget to support the continuing education of the IACUC members. The chair may also play a role in recommending new IACUC members to the IO/CEO for appointment to the committee.

15.5 ROLE IN ENHANCING INSTITUTIONAL AWARENESS OF ANIMAL WELFARE

The IACUC, through its participation in required key functions such as protocol review, semiannual facility inspections, program review, and postapproval monitoring, interacts with all PIs who are involved with animal use within the institution. These interactions are opportunities to advocate for the three Rs and share best practice information. In the past, and possibly even now at some institutions, there may have been a few curmudgeonly investigators who viewed the IACUC as a necessary evil and an administrative burden that they must comply with in order to conduct their research. The chair, by being familiar with science, can facilitate interaction with the research community and help them understand how good animal welfare compliments and supports good science.

15.6 CONDUCTING AN IACUC MEETING

The keys to conducting a successful IACUC meeting include appropriate preparation, communication of the meeting goal(s)/purpose with expected output/deliverables, assignment of action items, and follow-up. Unless the meeting is a regularly scheduled recurring event, it is useful to let participants know the reason for the meeting so that they may prepare prior to the meeting.

15.6.1 Premeeting Preparation

The IACUC administrator is generally responsible for preparing a draft agenda for the chair to review and approve. For regularly scheduled recurring meetings, if the chair reviews the draft agenda and determines that there is no reason to convene a meeting, then the chair should cancel the previously scheduled meeting.

15.6.2 Conducting the Meeting

15.6.2.1 Robert's Rules of Order

Following parliamentary procedures such as *Robert's Rules of Order* is useful in conducting effective and efficient meetings. While most IACUCs will not find it necessary to strictly implement all of the very formal procedures, the adoption of concepts and processes such as establishing a quorum, making a motion, seconding the motion, discussion followed by a vote for approval, as well as associated record keeping, will be useful and relevant. Approval requires a majority of the quorum, and minority opinions should be captured in the meeting minutes and reports. A concise description of the discussion should follow as well as a record of the vote (number in favor, number opposed, and number abstained) and a statement of whether the motion passed or failed.

15.6.2.2 Confirming That the IACUC Is Properly Constituted to Conduct Business

Only a properly constituted IACUC may conduct activities, and certain activities may only be conducted at a convened meeting of a quorum. Activities that require a convened meeting include: a full committee review (FCR) of an animal use protocol or an amendment with a significant change, a suspension of an animal use protocol, a review and approval of the IACUC semiannual facility inspection, and a program review report to the IO.

15.6.2.3 Confirming a Quorum

A quorum, defined as 50% of the voting members plus one, must be present at a convened IACUC meeting in order to approve, require modifications in order to secure approval, withhold approval, or perform other IACUC actions. After calling the meeting to order, the first order of business should be a roll call and confirmation of a quorum. If a quorum is not obtained, the committee cannot conduct its business. Since a quorum is so essential, it is useful to have the IACUC administrator check with members prior to scheduled meetings to ensure that a quorum of members will attend the meeting. In order to increase the ability to obtain a quorum of members when time-sensitive IACUC business must be addressed, many institutions formally appoint alternate IACUC members. The meeting minutes should include the meeting member attendance list, including any alternates, and a statement that a quorum was obtained.

15.6.2.4 Identifying Conflicts of Interest

When confirming that a quorum is present, it is important that the chair remembers that no member may participate in the IACUC review of an activity in which that member has a conflict of interest, except to provide information about the proposed activity. Conflict of interest considerations also include that no member can contribute to the constitution of a quorum for voting on an activity for which he or she has a conflict of interest.

15.6.2.5 Meeting "Culture"

As noted in Section 15.1, it is the entire IACUC that has the authority, and although each individual member plays an important role, no one committee member's opinion or vote carries more weight than another. This concept and a review of the appropriate conduct at meetings are useful items to address in an orientation program for new IACUC members. It is the responsibility of the chair to provide leadership to the committee and ensure that meetings are both effective and functional. The preparation and distribution of a meeting agenda and any premeeting materials prior to the meeting will set the stage for a productive meeting. This will allow each member to adequately prepare for the meeting so that he or she can participate fully in meeting discussions. The inclusion of suggested time limits for agenda items may help the committee to stay on track, particularly if there are many agenda items, or if the committee has a tendency to lose focus during discussions.

- Respect: One might think that a discussion about the need to maintain respect during an IACUC meeting would not be necessary and, hopefully, in most cases such a discussion is just restating and reminding people what should be automatic behavior. As the IACUC conducts its business, some topics such as a discussion of ethical issues or investigating alleged concerns regarding humane care can generate strong personal opinions, which may not be unanimous. It is important that committee members remember that every member is entitled to his or her opinion and everyone should be allowed and encouraged to participate in the discussion. There are no "stupid questions" or "stupid opinions." This may mean ensuring that quieter participants are given an opportunity to be heard while managing and minimizing contributions from louder participants. The committee membership has been purposely designed to encourage the representation of different perspectives and viewpoints. Discussion, interaction between the committee members, and participation by all are indications that the committee is functioning as envisioned. Attempts should be made for a constructive resolution of conflicts, but sometimes, individuals may need to "agree to disagree." Also, one should remember that the committee's decision does not need to be unanimous—a majority quorum vote determines the action taken. Minority opinions may always be formally expressed and documented.
- Preventing Sidebars: The distraction of sidebar conversations and their impact on the overall effectiveness of the meeting is one of the items that should be included in the ground rules for effective meetings that are reviewed with all new IACUC

members. The chair, as the meeting facilitator, should focus on the behavior and not on the individuals, and gently remind people to not have sidebar conversations. The chair may also invite them to share their discussion with the entire group if it is related to the current agenda item. If it is not related, then it may be useful to remind the group of the need to stick to the prioritized meeting agenda. Other topics can be placed on a "parking lot" list, which saves the issue for later discussion and allows the group to move forward with the current agenda item in a timely manner.

- Engaging Nonscientific and Community Members in Discussion: Encouraging participation by all is critical to the successful execution of the IACUC's oversight mission. During discussions, the chair should observe the body language and facial expressions of the nonscientific and community members as an indication of their understanding of the material that is being presented. It may be useful for the chair to translate key points and summarize issues using lay terms to ensure that nonscientific members understand technical/scientific discussions. Depending on their personality or comfort level or both with expressing their opinions in the meeting, nonscientific and community members may defer to committee members with animal research experience and a scientific background. The chair may need to facilitate the involvement of these members in the discussion. This can be done by reminding the committee of the importance of getting additional viewpoints, and then asking a nonscientific member what his or her thoughts are, or what questions he or she thinks are important to address. Similarly, a community member might be asked how he or she thinks the general lay community might view a specific issue. In both cases, the chair can explain that members with animal research experience or a scientific background may be too close or too familiar with an issue, and that the chair thinks that the committee would benefit from hearing the perspective of someone with a different background. Thanking all of the members for sharing their varied perspectives and viewpoints following a particularly productive discussion is useful to reinforce this type of positive interaction in the future.

15.6.2.6 Protocol Review

15.6.2.6.1 Pros of PIs Present for Protocol Discussion

Many committees use the designated member review (DMR) process to review and approve almost all of their protocols, although there may be some types of protocols where the institution prefers an FCR and has built this requirement into its IACUC policy or standard operating procedure (SOP). Examples of protocols that may automatically trigger an FCR include those with a new species, a protocol with multiple survival surgical procedures, Category E studies (more than momentary unrelieved pain/distress), and those with extended feed/water restriction or prolonged restraint.

In general, unless all protocols are reviewed by an FCR, those protocols that are tagged for an FCR (either by a committee member request or IACUC policy) are complex from an animal welfare perspective or have components that are novel for the institution. When reviewing these types of protocols it is often useful to have the PI present at the meeting. The PI can explain the need for the study design and the techniques or procedures or both. The PI can also discuss his or her experience with this type of study and answer questions about monitoring, expected outcomes, and anything else that the committee is unclear about or it would like additional information on. Having the PI present to interact with the IACUC is an efficient way to address questions and concerns, and also for the IACUC to communicate to the PI what issues the committee might have with the study design. Ideally, this type of collegial discussion will enable the PI and the IACUC to jointly develop a plan to meet the PI's research goals and provide for the highest quality of humane care during the experiment.

15.6.2.6.1 Cons of PIs Present for Protocol Discussion

In the real world, if either the IACUC or the PI does not approach the discussion at the meeting as a partnership, there may be some challenges associated with having a PI present at an IACUC meeting. As an example, the PI may be perceived by the IACUC members as egotistical and does not feel the need to explain why he or she wants to do something a certain way since he or she is the scientific expert in this area. The PI may also be perceived as not acknowledging the value of the IACUC process or not recognizing the oversight authority that resides with the committee. Similarly, the IACUC may be perceived by the PI as being a roadblock to the scientific process. Committee members may be viewed as being on a "power trip" with the authority that resides in the IACUC.

Even without any of these negative and nonproductive behaviors, some committee members may not be comfortable questioning a PI directly. As a means to address these potential challenges, it may be useful for the chair to have a brief discussion of the protocol prior to having the PI join the meeting. The chair can use this time to solicit questions or concerns from all members. If a member is not comfortable voicing his or her concerns when the PI is present, the chair can fill that role. The chair can also remind the committee that the PI is a guest at the meeting and the goal is to partner with the PI in working through any protocol issues. Similarly, when extending the invitation to the PI to participate in the IACUC meeting, the chair may find it useful to remind the PI of the goals and the desired outcome of any discussion. Finally, after the discussion it is important to thank the PI for the information and then excuse him or her from the meeting so that the committee can continue its deliberations without the PI present. The PI should not be present for the final deliberations or the motion and subsequent committee vote. The PI's presence would be a conflict of interest and may influence the deliberations and vote.

15.6.3 Conducting Virtual Meetings

Both the USDA and OLAW allow for the use of telecommunications for IACUC meetings when a convened quorum is required if certain criteria are met. The USDA discusses the use of telecommunications for IACUC meetings in the Animal Welfare Inspection Guide (USDA 2013b). Guidance is provided by OLAW in notice number NOT-OD-06-052, which was released on March 24, 2006 (National Institutes of Health 2006). OLAW's guidance is consistent with the policies of the Office of

Human Research Protections (OHRP), the Food and Drug Administration (FDA), and the Department of Health and Human Services, regarding the use of telephone conference calls for institutional review board (IRB) meetings under their respective regulations for the protection of human research subjects. As stated in the guidance document, OLAW recognizes that the use of telecommunications may facilitate the conduct of business, reduce regulatory burden, are standard practice in many forums, and enhance flexibility without compromising the quality of deliberation and interaction. The IACUC chair is responsible for encouraging member participation and interaction during the meeting. The chair can facilitate member participation and interaction by periodically checking in with those who are not present in the room during the meeting.

The guidance provided by OLAW and the USDA is identical and specifies eight criteria that must be met if telecommunications are used to conduct an IACUC meeting. Examples of acceptable telecommunications include teleconferencing and audio-video conferencing. The use of these communication methods is acceptable for conducting official IACUC business requiring a quorum, provided that the following criteria are met:

1. All members are given notice of the meeting.
2. Documents normally provided to members during a physically convened meeting are provided to all members in advance of the meeting.
3. All members have access to the documents and the technology that is necessary to fully participate.
4. A quorum of voting members is convened when required.
5. The forum allows for real-time verbal interaction equivalent to that occurring in a physically convened meeting (i.e., members can actively and equally participate, and there is simultaneous communication).
6. If a vote is called for, the vote occurs during the meeting and it is taken in a manner that ensures an accurate count of the vote. A mail ballot or individual telephone polling cannot substitute for a convened meeting.
7. The opinions of absent members that are transmitted by mail, telephone, fax, or e-mail may be considered by the convened IACUC members, but may not be counted as votes or considered as part of the quorum.
8. Written minutes of the meeting are maintained as required.

At the start of the meeting, it is important to state who is present in the room and who is on the telephone so that everyone knows who is in attendance. Make sure that those who are not present in the room can hear the discussion, and ask them to speak up and let the group know if they are having difficulty hearing any comments or following the discussion. It is useful for members to state their name prior to commenting so that those who are not present in the room do not have to guess who is speaking based on his or her voice. If the committee is reviewing documents, or if there is a PowerPoint presentation, it is useful to state the page or slide that is being discussed to ensure that all those participating are literally "on the same page." One may also consider the use of an Internet webinar format for presenting documents/slides. Videoconferencing/Skype may also facilitate member interaction, if this type of technology is available to committee members.

15.7 SEMIANNUAL PROGRAM AND FACILITY INSPECTION REVIEW

As part of its oversight responsibilities for the ACUP, the IACUC is responsible for conducting regular assessments of the program and inspections of the facility. The Guide recommends that these activities are conducted at least annually and more frequently if required (NRC 2011). Both the PHS Policy and the AWA require these assessments to be conducted at least once every six months (NIH 2002, USDA 2013a). After conducting the assessment, the IACUC is responsible for compiling the results into a report that is submitted to the IO. This report is one of the primary mechanisms that the IACUC has for communicating the compliance status of the ACUP to the IO, and the chair often has the responsibility of helping to prepare the draft report for committee review. The chair will generally delegate the data compilation and report preparation to the IACUC administrative staff, but he or she may be responsible for reviewing and editing the executive summary, typically two to three pages long.

The executive summary should include a concise description of how and when the facility inspection and program review were conducted, and the date of the convened IACUC meeting when the assessment results were discussed, reviewed, and approved. Other suggested sections in the executive summary include a history/status section where updates are provided on the status of any findings that were identified during the previous semiannual review; a commendations section to inform the IO of positive attributes that were noted during the assessment; a summary of findings (departures from the AWA), with an overview of the number, category, and general type of findings; a section that discusses any IACUC-approved exemptions and exceptions, including any variance/departure from the Guide; a section on any animal welfare concerns; and a summary section that describes how and to what extent the facility meets the AWA standards and regulations, as well as the PHS Policy. The summary section may also include any recommendations that the committee has to the IO regarding any aspect of the ACUP or personnel. The report is signed by a majority of the IACUC members (those present at a convened IACUC meeting where the review and approval occurred). It should also include any minority statements or a comment that there were no minority statements.

15.8 CONDUCTING ANIMAL WELFARE CONCERNS AND COMPLIANCE INVESTIGATIONS

The IACUC is charged by the AWA, the PHS Policy, and the Guide with investigating concerns regarding the care and use of animals within the institution (USDA 2013a, NIH 2002, NRC 2011). Concerns may be raised by staff or employees of the institution, as well as individuals in the community. The institution should develop mechanisms for employees to report animal welfare concerns and educate its employees on their use, as well as the fact that there will be no discrimination against or reprisal for reporting noncompliances or concerns. The ability to maintain confidentiality is critical to the success of an animal welfare concerns investigation process. In addition to the standard means of communication, such as discussing concerns with one's supervisor, human resources, department management, the AV, the IACUC chair, or an IACUC member, consideration should be given to allow for anonymous reporting, either through the use of a third-party-monitored telephone line or through a suggestion-type box where written concerns can be anonymously placed.

The IACUC should develop guidelines or procedures for processing and investigating concerns and allegations of noncompliance. In many cases, a review of the concern or complaint is initially conducted by the IACUC chair or a small subcommittee, which may consist of the IACUC chair, the AV, and potentially a member of human resources or legal counsel or both. As mentioned earlier, the ability to maintain confidentiality throughout the investigation process is important. An allegation of abuse or noncompliance is serious and, if validated, may have an impact on a person's employment or career. The IACUC should consider partnering with appropriate human resource staff and legal counsel when reviewing certain concerns that have the potential to result in disciplinary actions, as it is also important to protect employees rights during these investigations. The IACUC chair plays a pivotal role in these investigations, and he or she must use the utmost discretion in dealing with delicate and confidential matters of this nature.

Once a concern is reviewed and the investigation is complete, it is important to close the loop. This should include communicating the findings to the concerned employee(s); developing and implementing corrective actions as needed; reporting to the IO about the issue, findings, and actions taken; and reporting the noncompliance discovered to OLAW if it involves a PHS-funded study. It is important to remember that if disciplinary action was taken as a result of the reported concern, the specific details of that action remain confidential between the human resource department and the employee's manager. The only comment that can be shared with the reporting employee is that management and human resources were involved with the investigation and appropriate actions were taken. Findings that resulted from an anonymous concern cannot be reported back for obvious reasons. However, some institutions that use a third-party telephone reporting system have a follow-up mechanism built into their anonymous reporting option. At the time that the anonymous report is made, the caller is instructed that he or she may call back after a certain time period and request an update on the status of the investigation into his or her concern.

15.9 SUCCESSION PLANNING: TERM LIMITS OR LIFE SENTENCE?

The role that the IACUC chair plays in the overall success of the IACUC is important but time-consuming, even with a dedicated and experienced IACUC administrative staff to support the chair and the committee. If the IACUC chair is an individual who has some responsibility for institutional animal welfare and regulatory compliance as part of his or her "regular" job responsibilities, then serving as IACUC chair may provide an efficient means for him or her to ensure compliance. However, for the majority of institutions, recruiting a new IACUC chair may be challenging. Most institutions do not have a willing group of eager volunteers ready to take on the chair assignment, and other times, the pool of potential candidates is small due to the size of the institution. In addition, one of the perceived barriers to volunteering to become IACUC chair may be the concern that it will be an assignment with no determined end date. This may happen for a variety of reasons, including the difficulty in recruiting new chairs, the long learning curve that is required of a new chair, and that change is difficult, particularly if the incumbent chair is successful in the role. With all of the challenges, it is easy to see how some institutions end up adopting the philosophy that the IACUC chair role is almost a "life sentence." One can also imagine how that approach would scare away anyone even considering the possibility of volunteering to take on the role of chair.

To address the "life sentence" concern, the institution should consider adopting guidance for term limits of the chair, similar to the processes that are used for executive officer terms in many organizations. Many professional organizations have delineated the roles of president, vice-president, and past-president in overseeing the organization. A similar process could be established within the IACUC, which would include the chair, vice-chair, and past-chair. In such a scenario, a committee member is selected to be vice-chair. The role of the vice-chair is to act as backup to the chair, but he or she is also someone who has been identified (and who has agreed to take on the role) as a future chair. During his or her term as vice-chair, the individual is aware that he or she will be assuming the chair in a defined time period, and that his or her term as vice-chair serves as "on-the job" training. The past-chair is someone who previously served as the IACUC chair, has stepped down from that role, but is still an active voting member of the committee. The role of the past-chair is to provide guidance and counsel to the current chair as that individual steps into the new role. The past-chair also provides continuity of leadership as a mentor for the chair, and can provide a historical perspective to the IACUC and the oversight role of the ACUP. The amount of time that an individual serves in each of the three roles can have some flexibility depending on the experience and background of the individual as well as the needs of the institution. However, it is recommended that maximum term limits of two to three years per role are adopted. Knowing that the commitment for each of the three roles will be limited to a defined time period and that there is a built-in training period will hopefully encourage some individuals to consider volunteering for the role of chair.

15.10 SUMMARY AND CONCLUSION

Hopefully, one has a better understanding of the role that the chair plays in setting the stage for the IACUC to be successful in fulfilling its critical mission of oversight of the ACUP. The chair helps to contribute to the overall institutional culture of humane care and compliance, and reinforces the importance of continual improvement and support of the three Rs. Good animal welfare equals good science and is critical to the success of a self-regulating entity in ensuring and protecting the public's trust in the institutional oversight system. As stated in the beginning of this chapter, I would like to close with the same sentiment. While the chair performs a valuable role in facilitating and enabling the IACUC to fulfill many of the committee's responsibilities, it is also important to remember that the chair has just one vote—the same as any other member. The chair needs to be aware of the influence that his or her actions and comments may have on other members, and to always remember that it is the committee that has the ultimate authority.

REFERENCES

NIH (National Institutes of Health). 2002. Public Health Service policy on humane care and use of laboratory animals. Bethesda, MD: Office of Laboratory Animal Welfare, U.S. Department of Health and Human Services, NIH.

NIH (National Institutes of Health). 2006. NOT-OD-06-052: Guidance on use of telecommunications for IACUC meetings under the PHS policy on humane care and use of laboratory animals. no. 2014. Office of Laboratory Animal Welfare, NIH, Bethesda, MD.

NRC (National Research Council). 2011. *Guide for the Care and Use of Laboratory Animals*. 8th edn. Washington, DC: National Academies Press.

USDA (U.S. Department of Agriculture). 2013a. *Animal Welfare Act and Animal Welfare Regulations* (Animal Care Blue Book). Code of Federal Regulations (CFR), Title 9, Chapter 1, Subchapter A, Parts 1–4.

USDA (U.S. Department of Agriculture). 2013b. *Animal Welfare Inspection Guide*, 1st edn. Washington, DC: USDA. http://www.aphis.usda.gov/animal_welfare/downloads/Inspection%20Guide%20-%20November%202013.pdf.

CHAPTER 16

Perspectives of a Nonaffiliated/ Outside Member

Mark S. Christensen

CONTENTS

16.1 FROM THE OUTSIDE LOOKING IN

A quick glance at the membership roster of any Institutional Animal Care and Use Committee (IACUC) will reveal the inclusion of a nonaffiliated member. The IACUC shares this feature with its counterpart in human subjects research, the Institutional Review Board (IRB), and with hospital ethics committees. It is a simple task to shrug off this observation with the customary comment about government regulations, while shifting one's attention to more important things. Yet, a closer look provides insight into the wisdom behind the requirement of having a nonaffiliated member.

A properly trained and respected nonaffiliated member is a vital and dynamic part of the animal research endeavor. Such a member is uninfluenced by institutional politics and internal pressures and can advocate for the animal without fear of political sanctions. The value of an effective nonaffiliated member extends to the institution, the IACUC, principal investigators (PIs), and individual members of the committee. In this chapter, we will reflect on some ways to groom such a nonaffiliated member.

There is another category of member found on the membership roster of the IACUC. This is the nonscientist member. In some cases, the nonaffiliated member is also the nonscientist member. In other cases, the nonaffiliated member is a scientist and another member from inside the institution is a nonscientist. Some of the discussion in this chapter will involve matters related to both the nonaffiliated and nonscientist categories. I leave it to the reader to make individual distinctions about characteristics and responsibilities appropriate to individual cases.

Ultimately, the effective nonaffiliated member is essential to the welfare of the animal. A key to the effectiveness of the nonaffiliated member is that the member is committed to the well-being of the animal and to the advancement of science. An attitude of getting the greatest amount of benefit from the research while causing the least amount of pain and distress to the animal is a productive mindset for the effective nonaffiliated member.

The singular form, *animal*, rather than the plural form, *animals*, will be used throughout. The purpose of this is as a subtle reminder that our decisions may cause individual sentient beings to experience discomfort.

16.2 ROLES AND RESPONSIBILITIES

The nonaffiliated member makes significant contributions to an effective IACUC. There is good reason for the government to require that every IACUC has at least one such member. When the nonaffiliated member is ineffective, it can negatively impact the effectiveness of the IACUC as a whole. To gain insight into how a nonaffiliated member can perform effectively, let us look at the regulatory documents and begin to construct a mental picture of a nonaffiliated member.

16.2.1 Documents

The requirement for a nonaffiliated member originates in two places. One source is the Public Health Service (PHS) Policy on Humane Care and Use of Laboratory Animals (National Institutes of Health 2002), and the other is the U.S. Department of Agriculture (USDA) Animal Welfare Act and Regulations (AWRs) (USDA 2013). The *Guide for the Care and Use of Laboratory Animals*, 8th edition (NRC 2011), offers additional insight. Collectively, these regulatory documents require that a member who is not affiliated with the institution, and is not a member of the immediate family of a person who is affiliated with the institution, serves on the IACUC to represent general community interests in the proper care, treatment, and use of animals.

Additionally, the Guide specifies that

> Public members should not be laboratory animal users, affiliated in any way with the institution, or members of the immediate family of a person who is affiliated with the institution. The public member may receive compensation for participation and ancillary expenses (e.g., meals, parking, travel), but the amount should be sufficiently modest that it does not become a substantial source of income and thus risk compromising the member's association with the community and public at large. (NRC 2011)

16.2.2 Vocabulary Used and Inferences Drawn

A close examination of the vocabulary in each of the regulatory documents referenced above yields insights into the roles and responsibilities of the nonaffiliated member. Later in the chapter, we will discuss training for the nonaffiliated member. To that end, this reflection on vocabulary might prove valuable to a new nonaffiliated member.

16.2.2.1 Nonaffiliated and Synonyms

The term *affiliated* is used in both the PHS Policy and in the USDA regulations. In both cases, the term is qualified with a negation. In the PHS quote, it reads "not affiliated," while in the USDA quote it is worded, "not be affiliated." Clearly, we find strong precedence for using the title, "nonaffiliated member."

The USDA quote continues by commenting on the secretary's intent for such a member. The wording of interest here is, "provide representation for general community interests." Sometimes, the nonaffiliated member is referred to as the community member, and this is not an error. The Guide uses almost identical language and adds *public member* to the list.

Another commonly used title for the nonaffiliated member is outside member. This humble title does not have the regulatory pedigree of nonaffiliated member, community member, or public member. Simply stated, all four of these labels are quite synonymous. This member must not be connected to the institution in any other way than as a member of the IACUC. Any doubt about this is further emphasized by the clear statements forbidding that such a member even have a familial connection to the institution.

16.2.2.2 Inferences Drawn

There are two inferences that we can draw from the regulatory vocabulary. One relates to representation and the other to detachment or insulation.

This required member is intended to represent the general public concern for how animals are treated. The member is seen as representing something like a broad brushstroke of public opinion. This is different from representing a minority opinion of one type or another. In general, the public is disapproving of unnecessary harm being done to animals and, yet, is in favor of finding cures for medical problems. The nonaffiliated member is present to voice concerns that represent those of the general population.

This member must also be insulated from the effects of institutional politics. To not be affiliated with the institution is to not have what one says in the committee meeting affect one's chances of a promotion next month. The nonaffiliated member can ask difficult and even embarrassing questions without fear of reprisal. The added issue of family connections adds strength to this inference. The committee is most effective in protecting the well-being of the animal only when there is at least one member present who will not hesitate to speak on behalf of the animal. If every member of the committee risks personal reprisal or reprisal against a loved one, then it is not clear that concerns will be voiced.

The idea of this member being sufficiently independent of the institution is further illustrated by the comments in the Guide that discuss compensation. The amount should not distance the nonaffiliated member from the general public or make the nonaffiliated member dependent on the institution as a source of income.

The reader will be left to draw further inferences depending on whether a given nonaffiliated member is also the nonscientist member. The latter is in a sense an outside member in a different way. The nonscientist member is viewing the subject matter from outside the scientific community. Even in cases where the nonscientist member is an employee of the institution, this member represents the broader perspective of a general population made up of people who are often not specifically educated in the sciences.

16.2.3 Purposes of the IACUC

The roles and responsibilities of the nonaffiliated member relate to the overall reason why the IACUC is required. The purpose of the IACUC is to ensure the best possible care and treatment of the animal. Animal welfare oversight is the primary responsibility of the committee. The contributions of the effective nonaffiliated member are fundamentally essential to that end. The other primary purpose of the IACUC is to see that research using live animals does take place, while complying with the appropriate regulatory requirements. It is essential that the nonaffiliated member understands the assumption that research is a beneficial thing, and the IACUC is there to guide and oversee the humane use of the animal in that research.

16.2.3.1 IACUC Responsibilities That the Nonaffiliated
Member Contributes To

The IACUC reviews and takes action on protocols, inspects facilities, develops and approves policies, provides or requires training, and performs various other functions. The active nonaffiliated member brings a general public viewpoint to bear on each of these activities. Such a member also is an ever-present voice; a voice not to be silenced by fear or intimidation. This member participates in the various functions of the IACUC as one who is always mindful of animal welfare, and is always willing to ask the difficult question. Some members of the IACUC are present, in part, to provide information or otherwise contribute given their professional qualifications. The nonaffiliated member may have something of this nature to offer, but this is incidental to the role of the nonaffiliated member. The nonaffiliated member is primarily on the committee to ask questions. When cultivating a new nonaffiliated member, it is good for the chair or another member of the committee to be mindful of influences that may intimidate or otherwise silence the nonaffiliated member.

16.2.3.2 How the Nonaffiliated Member Keeps the IACUC from Failing

As mere regulatory window dressing, the nonaffiliated member is one of three or one of five required members of the IACUC (PHS vs. USDA regulations) (NIH 2002, USDA 2013). In a sense, the IACUC fails to fully exist without the nonaffiliated member. But the functional value of the nonaffiliated member is as the conscience of the committee. This is not meant to imply that the nonaffiliated member is the only member of the committee with a conscience. In so far as the nonaffiliated member represents the general public, this member observes the IACUC and, in essence, holds the IACUC accountable in each of its activities. In short, the effective nonaffiliated member keeps the IACUC honest.

16.3 TRAINING AND RESOURCES FOR THE NONAFFILIATED MEMBER

Training programs have been well covered in Chapter 7, as well as other useful resources that are available in the appendices. Still, training of the nonaffiliated member should not be overlooked, particularly when a member is new to the IACUC process altogether. They cannot be productive as long as they are unclear as to what is going on. The absolute minimum would be a general orientation to what an IACUC is and does, but suggested training at a minimum includes training on regulatory requirements, institutional policies, and protocol review.

16.3.1 Do Not Overlook the Nonaffiliated Member

IACUC-related training is a time-consuming operation. On one hand, it is not productive to require that the nonaffiliated member be required to complete the same training required of research staff doing hands-on work with animals. Consider the case of an IACUC that decided every member of the committee had to take the full battery of online training modules required of various PIs and other institutional personnel with the reasoning that if the IACUC required others to complete the training, that the committee members should do so as well. In this particular case, many of the members of the committee are likely to be animal users and are already required to complete much, if not all, of the training. The only members on the committee that would remain untrained would be the nonaffiliated and the nonscientist members. Taking into account the considerable number of hours dedicated to protocol review and meetings, it is an unreasonable expectation to burden the nonaffiliated member with additional hours of training intended for animal users. Clearly, the nonaffiliated member does not need every type of training that others in the animal research arena are required to have. Given that good nonaffiliated members can be hard to find, this becomes a salient consideration.

On the other hand, it is sometimes the case that the nonaffiliated member receives little or no training or financial means for such training. Considering the significant contributions an effective nonaffiliated member makes to an IACUC, it is short sighted to allow or even cause the nonaffiliated member to be undertrained. Provision should be made by the institution for training opportunities. A balanced approach is a place to start.

16.3.2 Formal and Informal Training

Informal training can be as simple as printed materials for the nonaffiliated member to read or as casual as an occasional lunch with the chair or the AV. Or it can take the form of a pairing of an outgoing nonaffiliated member working with a new nonaffiliated member for several overlapping months. This would imply planning ahead when it becomes known that a nonaffiliated member will be leaving in the foreseeable future. Speed mentoring at conferences can produce a reasonable benefit for a small investment of time. Conference attendance and online training are excellent forms of formal training. Conferences also provide wonderful opportunities for informal training during meals, between sessions and en route to and from the location. The annual IACUC conference put on by Public Responsibility in Medicine & Research (PRIM&R) is likely the most comprehensive conference to provide such training, but the IACUC 101 Series program, the Scientists Center for Animal Welfare (SCAW), and other organizations sponsor regional workshops that provide IACUC member training. The Collaborative Institutional Training Initiative (CITI) organization and the American Association for Laboratory Science (AALAS) Learning Library are world leaders in online animal subject protection training, and subscribing institutions can easily add nonaffiliated members to their list of subscribers, giving them access to a whole host of online coursework. Many states and regions also have associations for biomedical research, and those associations often offer conferences closer to home. An attendee is exposed to so much at such a conference that it is worth the investment on the part of the institution.

New nonaffiliated members do not often come with prior knowledge of the various organizations that support or oversee animal research. There are a number of national and regional conferences and workshops organized by a variety of organizations mentioned elsewhere in this volume. There is also a wealth of literature available that would benefit the nonaffiliated member. Chairs and other experienced members serve their IACUCs well by making such resources available to new nonaffiliated members.

The content of the training most suitable for the nonaffiliated member is not specifically scientific in nature. The nonaffiliated member needs to understand the basics of animal welfare, like the three Rs, the basic needs of the species commonly used at the institution, and a general understanding of the ways in which an animal might experience pain or distress. The nonaffiliated member also needs to become familiar with the IACUC, its various responsibilities, and how it functions. In cases where the nonaffiliated member is not the nonscientist member, the former could already have scientific training, but does not require additional scientific training for the purpose of satisfying the expectations of fulfilling the nonaffiliated role on the committee. It is often discussed as to whether too much scientific training jeopardizes the nonscientist status of a member serving in that capacity.

A well-grounded nonaffiliated member will know to ask other qualified IACUC members questions about technical matters when they arise. The new nonaffiliated member should be introduced to those other members as resources in that capacity.

16.3.3 Value of Mentoring

In the strict sense, mentoring is similar to discipleship or apprenticing. Someone with knowledge, skills, and experience molds someone with less knowledge, skills, and experience in such a way as to bring about a functional change in the latter person. This change grooms and enables the second person to function effectively in an intended capacity. Mentoring is deeper and richer than basic instruction and can include modeling (teaching by example or demonstration) and coaching (instructive and corrective in nature), and can convey attitudes, rationales, and values.

16.3.3.1 Veterinarians as Mentors

Early in my experience, the director of the animal facility arranged a trip to Columbus, Ohio, for myself and a fellow IACUC member. We visited the Columbus Zoo in the morning, where staff charged with the care of large primates provided us with a most informative behind-the-scenes tour. After lunch, we met with one of the veterinarians at the Ohio State University. His instruction to a new nonaffiliated member has had a lasting impression. He instructed that my attitude toward laboratory animals should reflect "dignity, respect, compassion," and that my efforts as a committee member should strive toward keeping animals "free of pain and distress" and giving them the "best quality of life (we are) able to provide." I returned to the IACUC with a richer understanding of why I was on the committee.

16.3.3.2 Other IACUC Members and Nonaffiliated Members as Mentors

In addition to veterinarians, a new nonaffiliated member can learn a lot from an experienced nonaffiliated member. Such learning can be afforded by having more than one nonaffiliated member on the committee concurrently. It could also be useful for several neighboring institutions to arrange for nonaffiliated members from each institution to meet with each other. This could take the form of an informal social reception, or it could be part of an actual training opportunity.

16.3.3.3 Lawyers and Ethicists as Mentors

Early in my experience as a nonaffiliated member, I came across an article from the *ILAR Journal* that introduced me to the idea that Congress "wanted the unaffiliated member to bring a broader values perspective to committee deliberations" and to be a "public witness" (Dresser 1999). The article encourages the nonaffiliated member to represent the outside community, to see the importance of the lay summary, and to not be passive in their role on the IACUC. The article further suggests that, "Two general ethical judgments are implicit ... animal experiences are worthy of some moral consideration ... human interests in promoting new scientific knowledge and the health and welfare benefits ... take priority over laboratory animal welfare" (Dresser 1999).

16.3.3.4 Getting Up to Speed

For many of us it takes some time to get up to speed on something new. It can take even longer to figure out how to perform an unfamiliar task on our own. It has been said that imitation is the highest form of flattery. Many of us catch on to something new much faster if we have the opportunity to observe someone else performing the task prior to attempting it ourselves. The benefit is enhanced when the person serving as the example is attentive to the observer's intent to duplicate the task. The one serving as the example becomes a mentor when he/she assists the observer in imitating him/her.

16.3.3.5 Effective Coaching

When the mentor is both effective at the task being modeled and effective at mentoring, there will be an increased likelihood that the one being mentored will become more effective at the task. Here, the coaching flavor comes to bear. The process is better served when the mentee receives instruction in the form of explanations for the modeled behavior and encouragement and correction (if necessary) as they begin to imitate. Once I am clear on what I was supposed to do and why I was supposed to do it, I felt capable in my IACUC participation. When the new nonaffiliated member becomes confident that they understand their role, they will fulfill that role with confidence.

16.4 IMPORTANCE OF THE LAY SUMMARY

Although there is no regulatory requirement for a *lay summary*, often referred to as the *rationale* or *background*, many IACUC protocol forms ask that the PI provide a description of animal use that is written in nonscientific terms. The lay summary allows all IACUC members to still be able to thoughtfully evaluate the protocol, whether they are a nonscientist, nonaffiliated member, or even a fellow scientist who may have difficulty understanding highly technical information specific to a particular area of scientific investigation (Fish 2004). The importance of the lay summary is intertwined with two facts. The public drives legislation and regulatory policy; and public money funds much of the research involving live animals. The importance of the nonaffiliated member is closely related to the importance of the lay summary— each represents general community interests in the proper care and use of animals. If the public member does not understand, the public will not understand. The lay summary is written for consumption by the general public.

16.4.1 The Lay Summary as a Litmus Test

Nonaffiliated members and nonscientist members are a good test of the effectiveness of the lay summary. The protocol is often a public record document. The current legal and political climate reinforces the need for a clear and understandable lay summary. Sunshine laws and freedom of information legislation afford members of the general public access to documents, including approved protocols. In light of this, the importance of the role of the nonaffiliated member and the nonscientist member as proofreader of the lay summary is clear. The lay summary is the part of the protocol that needs to be clear and understandable to a broad audience. The non-affiliated member is that token representative of the general public who gets to read, comment on, question, and ultimately vote on the lay summary (and protocol) before it becomes available to the general public. Biomedical researchers provide the general public with many life-saving and life-improving discoveries and refinements. If they can communicate what they are doing and establish that they are responsible in the way they use the animal, then the general public will be more accepting and supportive of their work.

16.5 WHAT THE NONAFFILIATED MEMBER DOES OR DOES NOT NEED TO KNOW

16.5.1 They Should Not Vote for It if They Do Not Know What It Is

The nonaffiliated member *is* a voting member of the IACUC.

It is not expected that a nonaffiliated or nonscientist member is going to understand all that is contained in a protocol, however it is expected that such a member will ask questions to compensate for their lack of expertise and be able to vote from an informed position. Many nonaffiliated members would not know if a given drug is best for a particular animal, so they should be encouraged to ask someone who does know. (Christensen 2004)

Other members of the committee have the appropriate scientific and veterinary expertise to evaluate those aspects of the protocol. Protocol by protocol, every nonaffiliated member should be able to answer the question, "Why did I vote the way I did?" The answer should reflect an understanding of what is going to happen to the animal and how the animal will be cared for. It should include a degree of confidence that alternatives have been explored, and that this is the least burdensome (to the animal) way to achieve the desired outcome of the research. The answer should also be supported by a basic understanding of the goal of the research. The nonaffiliated member in essence determines whether the general public would conclude that the animal is treated as well as possible given the nature of the research, and that the goal of the research is important enough to justify the burden to the animal.

16.5.2 They Do Need to Know That a Less Harmful Alternative Is Not Available

The nonaffiliated member should be confident that the pain and distress to be experienced by the animal has been minimized to the highest degree possible. The nonaffiliated member should be confident that alternatives have been considered, and that the burden placed on the animal is the least possible while still accomplishing the purpose of the research. This is typically accomplished through a literature search to identify alternatives to painful and/or distressful procedures and discussion of the three Rs within the protocol form.

16.6 ACTIVE PARTICIPATION IN COMMITTEE DELIBERATIONS

Once the nonaffiliated member is comfortable with the overall protocol, it is time to move on to playing an active role on the committee. Training and mentoring lay a foundation of knowledge, but the nonaffiliated member needs to become a doer.

16.6.1 Two Metaphors

Serving on the IACUC is not just about the nonaffiliated member having the appropriate knowledge. It is about them being empowered and feeling confident in contributing to the process in substantive ways. I interpret the regulations as intending that the nonaffiliated member should feel safe in voicing potentially unpopular concerns. Early in my experience as a nonaffiliated member, I identified two characteristics of a nonaffiliated member that greatly enhanced the effectiveness of such a member. Discussed below are two metaphors that illustrate these characteristics.

16.6.2 Bullet Proof

In relation to internal politics and associated sanctions, the nonaffiliated member is, in essence, bullet proof. Such a member does not experience the pressures felt by an IACUC member who may be reviewing a superior's pet project. They are not subject to the fear, "If I vote against my boss's protocol, I won't get a favorable employee evaluation next month." The wisdom of the requirement that each committee have at least one nonaffiliated member is that there is always someone on the committee that can question things that are politically volatile without fear of reprisal.

The nonaffiliated member is safely outside of the internal institutional political environment and can serve the committee and the animal by using that safe position to ask the questions and make the motions that other members might not feel comfortable with. The nonaffiliated member can also take the pressure off other members of the IACUC.

16.6.3 The Emperor Has No Clothes

There is an old tale of traveling con artists who lead an emperor to believe that they can weave a fabric so exotic that mortal human eyes cannot see it. The emperor commissions them to produce royal robes made of this wonderful cloth. All adults in the realm come to believe the story. A simple child looks at the emperor parading about in his new clothing and says, "Mother, the emperor has no clothes." The nonaffiliated member shares this role with the nonscientist member. The nonaffiliated member is the "child" in a political sense, and the nonscientist member is the "child" in a technical sense. The seventeenth-century Scottish poet Robert Burns said it best, "O wad some Power the giftie gie us. To see oursels as inthers see us! It wad frae monie a blunder free us." An effective nonaffiliated member provides the eyes to "see" and hence prevents the "blunders" (Burns 1936).

16.6.4 About Pain and Distress to the Animal

Even though it is the duty of the IACUC to oversee animal welfare issues, it is often the nonaffiliated member who is willing to intelligently and honestly ask questions about the well-being of the animal. We have already discussed that the nonaffiliated member represents the general public. It is also the case that the nonaffiliated member represents the animal. This role is certainly shared with the attending veterinarian and other members. The key idea here is that the animal cannot represent itself in committee deliberations.

16.6.5 About Alternatives: The Three Rs

We often think of alternatives as alternatives to using live animal models in research. In the place of live animals, we ask if the same findings could come from computer simulations or tissue cultures, for instance. The nonaffiliated member who questions whether such substitutes would suffice is an asset to the committee. The term "alternatives" can also apply to procedures performed on the animal. In a behavioral study, we may inquire as to whether a painful negative reinforcement could be replaced by a positive motivator, for example.

We can apply the concept of refine (one of the three Rs) to diet, housing, and enrichment. One may inquire as to the condition of the animal when it is off study. Nonaffiliated and nonscientist members can learn much and contribute in important ways when included in facility inspections and the program review process. Participation in these IACUC activities will generate many questions.

16.7 POLICY WRITING, PROGRAM REVIEWS, INSPECTIONS

The nonaffiliated member represents the general public when participating in other IACUC functions such as policy writing, program reviews, and inspections. The more of these activities that have the input of the nonaffiliated member, the more the interests of the general public are represented. Here, time becomes a concern. Monthly meetings and a few hours a month given to reading protocols before meetings is probably a reasonable expectation to place on someone. Semiannual program reviews happen twice a year and may involve a couple of hours each time. Facility inspections will vary in the investment of time they require based on the size and type of facility. It is good that the nonaffiliated member participates in each of these activities, but in many cases this places quite a burden on that person. One solution is for the IACUC to have two nonaffiliated members. In such a case, the workload can be divided.

Unless the nonaffiliated member has some needed expertise, it is probably excessive to involve him/her in policy writing. On the other hand, it is good to have the outside eyes look at new policies once they are drafted. This is often done during normal IACUC meetings, and hence does not require additional time.

16.7.1 What Do I Bring to the Table?

During my first year as a nonaffiliated member of an IACUC, a USDA inspector bluntly asked me, "Who are YOU to be a nonaffiliated member?" Although I believe my qualifications as a professor of bioethics and a clinical ethicist at a separate and nonaffiliated institution more than fulfilled the regulatory criteria for a nonaffiliated member, it can be fruitful to do a bit of self-examination and ask, "What about me matches the regulatory requirement that every IACUC have a nonaffiliated member?" "I have made the acquaintance of nonaffiliated members who are attorneys, members of the clergy, foreign language professors, veterinarians, a librarian, and a police officer. Each brings something to the table. Part of becoming a nonaffiliated member is to recognize one's own personal resources and to determine how best to use them in service to the IACUC." (Christensen 2004) Every nonaffiliated member is well served to reflect on what their educational and professional experiences afford them in committee service.

16.7.2 How Can I Advocate for the Animal and Support the IACUC?

Each nonaffiliated member will have a unique set of personal resources. Those resources should be employed to the benefit of the animal. As it is the case that each nonaffiliated member is an individual, it will require some self-examination to determine how one can contribute to the well-being of the animal. The nonaffiliated member is in a sense a teammate of the other IACUC members and plays a supportive role as a member of the IACUC. As the nonaffiliated member does a personal inventory, particular attention should be paid to how one can support one's teammates. The nonaffiliated member is on the IACUC to represent the general public and to advocate for the animal. It is also the case that the nonaffiliated member be there to benefit the committee.

16.7.3 Learn Who Has the Expertise That You Lack

There are a great many things any given nonaffiliated or nonscientist member does not know. It serves such a member well to get to know other committee members. One should become familiar with who to seek out for answers to particular types of questions. Earlier we introduced the idea that you should not vote for it if you do not know what it is. It is beneficial for the nonaffiliated or nonscientist member to seek out the expertise of other committee members. Early in my IACUC experience, I served with an individual who was most knowledgeable about the regulations, as well as veterinary matters. It only took a few meetings for me to realize that I could turn to this individual with a question and be confident of receiving a clear, accurate answer.

16.7.4 Be Willing to Listen to Answers

There are two good reasons for a nonaffiliated or nonscientist member to listen to others. One is to learn that which one does not yet know. The other is to show respect to the speaker. One needs to vote from an informed position. There can be aspects to the protocol that one does not pick up from an initial reading (herein lies the wisdom of not allowing protocols to be voted on via electronic polling!). Each member benefits from hearing the questions and answers that make up active, face-to-face committee deliberations. Often, the answer to an initial question generates subsequent questions. Listening means following the progression of questions and answers as a means of becoming informed.

To be respected is to give respect. It clearly disrespects a person to ask them a question and then not listen to their reply. There is the rare occasion when the non-affiliated or nonscientist member is not thought of with the same esteem as other members. This may stem from an inappropriate attitude on the part of those who may have a condescending view of the nonaffiliated or nonscientist member. It may also be that the given nonaffiliated member has not earned the respect of others. Demonstrating respect for other committee members, including by listening to the contributions each makes during meetings, is a step in the direction of earning that respect.

16.8 CONCLUSION

So, we arrive at the heart of what it is to be a nonaffiliated member. When one combines being a public member with being an advocate for the animal and then blends this with the metaphors of "the emperor has no clothes," and most importantly, with being politically "bullet proof," one becomes empowered to ask the difficult question. The nonaffiliated member is at times the only member who is willing to ask a particularly important question. Whatever this question is, on a particular occasion, it may be the most important moment in the given IACUC meeting. It takes conviction and courtesy to do this well. The nonaffiliated member should respect the animal, respect the law, respect the system, and respect the people involved. The active and effective nonaffiliated member is a great asset to the IACUC, the institution, society at large, and the animal. Others in the animal research community can help prepare and empower the nonaffiliated member, and their efforts will be well rewarded.

REFERENCES

Burns, R. 2000. To a louse, 1786, *The Norton Anthology of English Literature: The Romantic Period*; Vol. 2A, 7th edn, p. 107. New York: W. W. Norton.
Christensen, M. 2004. Becoming a nonaffiliated IACUC member: A work in progress. *Contemporary Topics in Laboratory Animal Science* 43:106.

Dresser, R. 1999. Community representatives and nonscientists on the IACUC: What difference should it make? *ILAR Journal* 40 (1):29–33.

Fish, R. E. 2004. How to work with your institutional animal care and use committee (IACUC). Office of Research Integrity, U.S. Department of Health & Human Services website online tutorial found at the following address: http://ori.hhs.gov/education/products/ncstate/iacuc.htm.

NIH (National Institutes of Health). 2002. Public Health Service policy on humane care and use of laboratory animals. Office of Laboratory Animal Welfare, NIH, Bethesda, MD.

NRC (National Research Council). 2011. *Guide for the Care and Use of Laboratory Animals*. 8th edn. Washington, DC: National Academies Press.

USDA (U.S. Department of Agriculture). 2013. *Animal Welfare Act and Animal Welfare Regulations* (Animal Care Blue Book). Code of Federal Regulations (CFR), Title 9, Chapter 1, Subchapter A, Parts 1–4.

CHAPTER 17

Managing a Proactive Progressive Animal Care and Use Program

Taylor Bennett and Andrew D. Cardon

CONTENTS

The foundation for building an effective process for managing inspections or site visits is to have in place a proactive, progressive Animal Care and Use Program (ACUP). The 8th edition of the *Guide for the Care and Use of Laboratory Animals* (NRC 2011) defines the ACUP as the "activities conducted by and at an institution that have a direct impact on the well-being of animals, including animal and veterinary care, policies and procedures, personnel and program management and oversight, occupational health and safety, [IACUC] functions, and animal facility design and management." To have a proactive, progressive ACUP, the Institutional Animal Care and Use Committee (IACUC) must review all components of the program on a regular basis and implement policies to address changes in the requirements of oversight agencies, in the scientific and management literature, and in the generally accepted standards for the care and use of laboratory animals.

17.1 ONGOING RIGOROUS SELF-ASSESSMENT PROGRAM

A primary component of a proactive, progressive program is to have an ongoing and rigorous process for assessing the program. Collectively, the mandated review requirements of the Animal Welfare Regulations (AWRs) (USDA 2013a), the Public Health Service (PHS) Policy on Humane Care and Use of Laboratory Animals (PHS Policy) (National Institutes of Health [NIH] 2002), and the institutional Program Description required for accreditation by the Association for Assessment and Accreditation of Laboratory Animal Care International (AAALAC International) provide a mechanism for an ongoing self-assessment program. (AAALAC International 2014a)

17.1.1 Utilize the Semiannual Review Process

Both the AWRs and the PHS Policy require the IACUC to conduct inspections of the animal facilities and study areas and to review the ACUP on a semiannual basis. The Office of Laboratory Animal Welfare (OLAW) provides a Semiannual Program Review and Facility Inspection Checklist on their website (NIH 2014b), which includes instructions on how to use the checklist. The checklist covers the major topics found in the Guide and the requirements of the PHS Policy, with endnotes referencing specific requirements of the U.S. Department of Agriculture (USDA) that differ from those in the PHS Policy. There is also a sample document that can be used for creating reports of the findings of the facilities inspection and semiannual program review, which provides a useful format for tracking those items identified and in need of correction.

While checklists are an excellent way of assuring that all the required items are addressed and provide an objective means for identifying and tracking program deficiencies, a narrative description of the inspection and review process provides a mechanism for a more subjective evaluation of the program. It provides the ability to comment on areas where positive changes have been made, to provide positive feedback to those responsible for a facility or an area(s) within the facility, and to identify areas or issues that, while in compliance, could be improved. A narrative description can also be useful in developing the letter that accompanies the report to the Institutional Official (IO) and in preparing annual reports to OLAW and AAALAC International, because it helps put the program in perspective. It is important to highlight the positive aspects of the program and the changes that are being made to improve things, which often get lost in the whole semiannual inspection and review process. It is important to remember that a rigorous self-assessment program should be about not just identifying areas in need of improvement, but also identifying areas where good things are happening and where improvements are being made. This approach helps put the whole process in a more positive light because it puts the program in a more realistic perspective.

17.1.2 Utilize the AAALAC International Program Description

One of the often underrated benefits of the AAALAC International accreditation process is the development of the program description (PD). It requires those involved in the process to conduct a methodical self-assessment process, which, because of the detail required will, by default, be rigorous. The process must be repeated every three years as part of the triennial site-visit process. It is important to have a defined process for doing this, which starts with how to write the institutional description. Some institutions update their description as changes to the program are being made, creating a living document that only requires minor tweaks prior to submission to AAALAC International. Others keep a running file of the program changes, utilizing a semiannual review narrative and inspection reports format, which is ideally suited to this approach. This approach does require more time in updating the description prior to submission to AAALAC International, but this can be time well spent because it highlights the changes and improvements that have been made since the last site visit, a process that might not be as obvious when regular updates are made to the description. It is important to remember that the AAALAC International process is based on peer review and evaluation, and being able to clearly delineate the program changes and improvements within the description and during the site visit should be an important component of managing the AAALAC International site-visit process. A third and less desirable approach is when institutions do neither, which can result in the update of the institutional description becoming a much more stressful process than is necessary.

An important component of updating the institutional description involves determining those responsible for doing it. Involving as many people in the process as possible assures that the description does not omit any essential information and helps develop a sense of ownership of the program by all those involved. This can translate into a very positive experience during the site visit when more people are involved, which will convey to the site visitors that the program described is the program being practiced.

17.1.3 Internal Review and Goal-Setting Process

In addition to the semiannual review and inspection process conducted by the IACUC and the triennial update of the institutional description for AAALAC International, those responsible for managing the animal care support service should have in place an annual review and goal-setting process. This process should involve those with responsibility for managing the various aspects of the program. It should be a bottom-up process with the suggestions for improvements and changes coming from those with daily responsibility for managing the staff. The management should seek input from the staff they manage, as this conveys the message that management respects the employees and makes the whole process participatory in nature. The most proactive, progressive programs are that those that have a sense of ownership by all those involved, and nothing creates that sense of ownership like being part of the annual review and goal-setting process.

Those impacted by any changes to the program should also be part of the process, in that they should be kept informed when changes are proposed that will impact the services they use. This is especially true when such changes might increase the cost of providing a service. The use of user groups to keep all involved informed and to seek early buy-in for changes is an important part of a proactive, progressive program.

In addition to the semiannual review process conducted by the IACUC, some programs have a separate internal review of the IACUC processes and procedures. This is particularly important when it comes to improving the level of service provided to the users. An annual review of forms and documents that are part of the protocol submission and approval process can address issues that will improve the level of service provided. If there are questions on the protocol form that do not consistently elicit the desired response or processes that require repeated explanation, changes should be considered that will make the process as user friendly as possible. As part of the consideration process, the users should be consulted before changes are made and implemented. If the users know what is coming and have been part of the process, the rollout of changes will go more smoothly.

17.1.4 Follow-Through on Areas in Need of Improvement

Another vital step to effectively managing a proactive, progressive ACUP is follow-through. When items and issues are identified during the self-assessment process, a plan for addressing them should be developed. The plan should have a reasonable time frame for completion, and all those involved in carrying out that plan need to be involved in establishing both the plan and the time frame. When the plan involves institution-wide policies and procedures, all those impacted by the changes need to be kept in the loop. Even a simple change in a management process can impact the users. Those responsible for the oversight of the program at the institutional level should also be kept informed, particularly if institution resources are required for the implementation of the proposed changes.

17.1.5 Concentrate on Addressing Issues, Not Finding Fault

A third component to establishing a proactive, progressive ACUP is establishing an environment for open and honest communication, where issues are raised before they become problems. To establish such an environment requires that all those involved feel free to come to those in charge with their issues and concerns. This is most likely to happen in an environment where the emphasis is on addressing issues and not finding fault. Mistakes do happen, and when they do, the key is to identify the cause and then to fix the cause. It is also important to keep things in perspective. In a large, complex ACUP, every animal contact represents a potential for an unforeseen event to occur, and when one does occur, it needs not only to be addressed but also evaluated in terms of the actual incident rate that it represents.

17.2 MAINTAINING AN INSPECTION-READY POSTURE

Pivotal to maintaining an inspection-ready posture is that those responsible for the various components of the program and the areas of the facility know what is going on.

17.2.1 Practice Management by Walking Around

In a large, complex program, the amount of time spent managing the paperwork trail that documents institutional compliance can often leave little time for practicing management by walking around. In a smaller program where those in charge often wear multiple hats, the same thing can happen. It is important that those with direct or delegated responsibility for the welfare of the animals being housed and used within a facility make it a priority to know what is going on within their area of responsibility by seeing it firsthand with some regularity. This will require setting priorities in terms of the level of intensity given to different areas of the facilities and components of the program.

17.2.2 High-Profile Studies

It is important that those studies that have the greatest potential for impacting the welfare of the animals be identified and that their location within the facility is noted so that that they are the most frequently observed. The same can be said when new techniques are implemented or when new studies and staff begin working within the facilities. This allows those with management responsibility to observe firsthand what is happening and to interact with those individuals who are new to the study or studies that have the greatest potential to impact animal welfare. The purpose of this type of activity is to help facilitate the research process and to provide a research support service to the users. When done on a regular basis, it will be seen as such. This type of regular observation and interaction can become an important component of the ongoing review that is required and will not be seen solely as a compliance activity. This is important for establishing the type of environment mentioned previously, which fosters open and honest communication.

17.2.3 Get to Know the Players

One of the recognized benefits of management by walking around is that those who practice it get to know the people working in and using the facilities and services as individuals. It is important to build the type of rapport that is conducive to establishing and maintaining a positive communication environment. Walking around offers those who practice it the opportunity to make suggestions and ask questions that build mutual respect among those involved in the ACUP. It is important that when issues need to be addressed, it is done in a positive manner (finding solutions rather than finding fault) and, when positive things are observed, that they are noted and those responsible are acknowledged for their efforts.

17.2.4 Records Management

Regardless of the size of the research facility, maintaining accurate and sufficiently detailed records is critical to managing an effective ACUP. In addition to being used to monitor the status of research studies and ensure animal welfare, various records are required to be kept by the AWRs, governmental regulatory and funding agencies, and institutional policies. As a program's records are also used during unannounced USDA inspections to determine the facility's compliance with the AWA, establishing an organized and consistent record-keeping system is an integral part of maintaining an inspection-ready posture.

To ensure a properly functioning records management system, it is necessary to establish templates and oversight policies for documents commonly reviewed during inspections. IACUC minutes, research protocols, animal health records, and other commonly reviewed documents should, to the extent practicable, be kept in a standard format in order to prevent necessary information from being omitted and to discourage the inclusion of unnecessary extraneous information. Prior to finalizing IACUC minutes, committee members should carefully review the minutes to ensure they accurately represent the information as well as to determine what information should be maintained in the minutes and what information is best kept in the protocol file. Research facilities should regularly review their existing records to identify records that no longer need to be maintained under their institutional document retention periods or records that do not represent the true state of the ACUP.

17.2.5 Keep FOIA-Ready Records

When creating and reviewing documents, individuals involved in an ACUP should be cognizant of the fact that the record is potentially subject to release under the federal Freedom of Information Act (FOIA) or a state open records law. Any document submitted to, created by, obtained by, or otherwise in the possession of a federal agency at the time a request is made must be disclosed under the federal FOIA, unless part or all of the information falls within one of nine limited statutory exemptions (FOIA n.d.). Individuals employed by or contracting with a public state entity, such as a public university, should also recognize that records kept for internal use as part of the ACUP may also be released.

Records should be kept in such a way that they are FOIA ready, meaning the document is factual, accurately represents the state of the ACUP, and does not include extraneous information. FOIA-ready records generally prevent the inclusion of unnecessary information, such as an individual's opinions, personal information, or other data that was not meant to be released. Standard templates for specific types of documents and review policies that include oversight from individuals familiar with the FOIA and open records laws may not only prevent extraneous information from being included, but also lead to documents that better meet the needs of a proactive, progressive ACUP.

17.2.6 Know What Is Required

It is important that individuals involved in record keeping have a thorough understanding of what documents the ACUP is required by law or institutional policy to maintain and what documents are being maintained either unnecessarily or for the convenience of the ACUP. Such individuals should not only have an understanding of the institutional document retention policies, but should also carefully review the requirements of funding agencies, the AWRs, and other applicable federal and state regulations. For example, under federal law, financial records, supporting documents, statistical records, and all other records pertinent to a grant award are required to be retained by the grant recipient for a period of three years. The three-year period begins from the date of the submission of the final expenditure report or, for awards that are renewed quarterly or annually, from the date of the submission of the quarterly or annual financial report. After this period, documents generally do not need to be retained unless retention is required by state law.

17.2.7 Avoid Extraneous Information

Always be in full compliance with relevant laws, regulations, and institutional policies, but avoid including extraneous information. Extraneous information may be taken out of context, resulting in citations, or it may be released as part of a

FOIA or state open records law request. For example, IACUC minutes do not have to be included as an addendum to the PHS Animal Welfare Assurance, and rats, mice, and birds not covered by the AWA should not be included on USDA Annual Reports. Additionally, institutions may, at their discretion, represent the names of members other than the chair and veterinarian with program authority by using numbers or other symbols in submissions to OLAW (PHS Policy) (NIH 2002). In some cases, templates may help employees with record-keeping responsibilities avoid including extraneous information and ensure that necessary information is included.

17.2.8 Address Issues When They Arise

When issues arise, they need to be addressed in a manner that reinforces that the program's goal is addressing the issues and not finding fault; that is, finding solutions and not placing blame. When issues arise, it is important to get the facts and then address them in a step-by-step manner that minimizes any stress that might develop as a result of both the issue of concern and the steps taken to resolve it. In an environment of open and honest communication, those involved should not hesitate to raise issues or even potential issues because they will be heard and know that appropriate and positive action will be taken.

17.2.9 Do Not Let Issues Become Problems

When issues are addressed in a positive and proactive way as they arise, the number of issues that rise to the level of problems can be minimized. When issues arise that do become problems, the methods used to address them may become more formalized and rise to the level of a reportable event that could lead to repercussions impacting the entire program.

17.2.10 Knowledgeable Inspection Response Team

Regardless of the nature of the inspection—or in the case of AAALAC International, program evaluation—it is imperative that those involved in the process be knowledgeable about the regulations, policies, and relevant references. Not all the members of the response team need to be experts, but a primary member of the team should have a full working knowledge of the regulations and any external policies and guidelines. All members of the response team should have a thorough working knowledge of the internal policies and procedures as they relate to their area of responsibility as well as to the relevant references.

17.2.11 Know the Area and the Projects

Members of the inspection response team need to know what is going on in their area of responsibility and be familiar with the projects that are currently ongoing. For those projects that have the most potential to impact the welfare of the animals, they should be able to convey to those reviewing the program that they are regularly observing the animals and are aware of what has taken place.

17.2.12 Know How to Communicate

Members of the inspection response team must know how to communicate. They need to keep in mind that the purpose of the inspection or site visit is to assess the program and to assure the welfare of the animals cared for and used in the program. All parties have a common goal, and that is the welfare of the animals. Members of the response team need to be able to communicate how the program assures the welfare of the animals and thus complies with the regulations, standards, and guidelines. Matters of disagreement need to be addressed in terms of the requirements of the regulations, standards, and guidelines. It is important that members of the inspection response team convey a sense of ownership and investment in the program and should not take questions about the program personally. It is also important that differences of opinion and differences between personalities do not impact the final outcome of the inspection.

17.2.13 Postinspection Review and Analysis

A postinspection review process should be in place, during which the inspection response team reviews both the inspection report and the overall events. Those events should be summarized, for the purpose, among other things, of reporting to the IO and the IACUC a summary of the steps that have been or will be taken to address any items of noncompliance or any potential for future noncompliance.

17.2.14 Review Issues That Arose

It is important that someone in the response team takes notes of the issues that arise, the questions that are being asked, or both. During most inspections or site visits, those charged with evaluating the program are taking notes, so it is important that the site-visit response team do the same. If, during the process, it is unclear exactly what the issues or questions are, someone needs to ask for clarification. It is important that the team meet to review and clarify these issues as soon as possible after the visitors have left. For multiday visits, this should be at the end of each day while things are fresh in everyone's minds. In the event that not everyone identified the same issues, it is important that clarifications be sought from the inspection or site-visit team the next day.

17.2.15 Review Potential Future Issues

If, during the inspection or site visit, the visitors ask questions or point out things that might become issues in the future, they need to be identified. The same can be said for issues or items that members of the inspection response team notice that might not have been noticed by the inspectors or site visitors.

17.2.16 Develop a Plan to Address Issues

When issues or items have been identified, either in an inspection or site-visit report or through the postinspection and review process, a plan to address each needs to be developed. These plans need to include a realistic schedule for completion and identify those with primary oversight responsibility. Regular follow-ups should be included in the plans to monitor the progress being made and to allow the plan to be adjusted when issues arise that impact the timely completion of the plan. It is important that those responsible for program oversight (the IO and the IACUC) be included in the development of the plan and kept abreast of the progress being made, and this certainly should be the case when the plan needs to be changed or adjusted in any way. It is important to avoid repeat items of noncompliance, since they can trigger further enforcement action. A review of the most commonly reported items of noncompliance each year has shown that many of the repeat items are preventable, and an effective postinspection review and follow-up process should help accomplish this.

17.2.17 Be Prepared to Explain the Program

When issues or items arise during the course of the inspection or site visit, members of the inspection response team need to be prepared to explain the program in terms of how it complies with the regulations or standards or with the recommendations contained within pertinent guidelines. It is important that this be a fact-based approach and that the interjection of feelings and personal opinions not become part of the process. When such issues arise during the inspection or site-visit process, they should whenever possible be addressed at the time they arise, and an attempt to resolve them should be made on the spot. When this is not possible, a carefully thought out response should be prepared prior to the exit interview. When a difference cannot be resolved during an inspection by the USDA, facility representatives have recourse through a formally defined appeal process.

17.3 APPEAL PROCESS

If the members of the site-visit response team are unable to resolve an issue of disagreement during the site visit or the exit interview, the facility can file a written appeal with the Supervising Animal Care Specialist (SACS) for their area. The current appeal process is posted on the Animal and Plant Health Inspection Service (APHIS) website. The appeal should stick to the facts and clearly enunciate how the item(s) cited are in compliance with the published regulations and/or standards. The purpose of the appeal is not to defend the quality of the ACUP but to address a specific item or items that the facility finds are in compliance. While an inspection is under appeal, the report will not be posted on the USDA's website until the appeal is finalized. An appeal can only be filed within 21 calendar days following receipt of the final inspection report (USDA 2014). Facilities should have a process in place in the event that it becomes necessary to file an appeal that has been approved by those with responsibility for institutional oversight of the ACUP.

17.3.1 Legal Counsel

The institution's legal counsel should be integrally involved in appealing disputed citations. The basis for an appeal is that the citation is not justified, as the facility knows it is in compliance with the relevant regulations. The institution's legal counsel can not only assist in determining whether an appeal is warranted but can also assist in drafting the appeal and navigating the process. As potential fines for violation of the AWA have increased, more institutions are involving their legal counsel early in the process rather than waiting to see if the USDA will assess a fine.

17.4 IDENTIFYING AND MANAGING POTENTIAL ISSUES

An important function of the self-assessment program is to identify and manage issues that may potentially lead to the institution being found to be in noncompliance with the regulations and standards or the recommendations of applicable guidelines. Once identified, those responsible for managing the program can make the necessary adjustment to eliminate those issues or prepare a justification for those issues based on the specific needs of the program that have been reviewed and approved by the IACUC.

17.4.1 Protocol Congruence

One circumstance that can often lead to confusion and to a citation is when protocols are designed so that multiple questions address the same or similar issues but do not elicit the same answers. An example of this is where a question requires specific details in the overall description of the project, such as anesthesia, which then must be repeated in a different question in the form. It is important to eliminate this type of confusion. It is also important to review the protocol forms on a regular basis and revise those items that do not consistently elicit the appropriate response.

17.4.2 Records Congruence

One of the circumstances that often leads to a citation is when the medical or research records contain information that is not consistent with the information contained within the approved protocol. It is important that those responsible for maintaining these types of records be familiar with the approved methodology in the protocol and initiate appropriate action when changes to the protocol are needed.

17.4.3 Special Circumstances

Some research projects will require that the IACUC approve exceptions to the regulations and standards, deviations or departures from the Guide, or both, in order to successfully carry out the goal of the study. These special circumstances must be reviewed and approved by the IACUC in accordance with the requirements of the regulations, PHS Policy, or both; and the recommendations of the Guide. It is important that this process be adequately documented and that representatives of the facility can address any questions that may arise about the approval process during an inspection or site visit. It is also important that those who provide day-to-day support for protocols with special circumstances be aware of the reasons for those circumstances; they are best able to address any questions that might consequently be raised in terms of the management of the animals and the potential impact on their welfare.

17.4.4 Unique Situations

Some facilities house species not commonly seen in research facilities or support research projects not commonly found in other facilities. When these unique situations exist, it is important that facility representatives be able to explain how the program has adapted to these unique situations and what steps have been taken to assure the animals' welfare. For example, when species are housed that have unique physiological or behavioral requirements that may not be clearly covered by the requirements of the standards, it is important to have documentation of the sources consulted and used in developing in-house standards that meet or exceed those for more commonly used species. Where unique techniques or project requirements are being used, it is important to have documentation on how the techniques or requirements were evaluated to determine their impact on animal welfare before the actual project was initiated.

17.5 MANAGING USDA INSPECTIONS

Since the USDA inspections are unannounced, it is important to have in place a process for managing the inspection and that all those who will participate in the inspection are aware of this process. This includes those in the front office or at the point of entry to the facility, who will be the first to greet the inspector. It is very important to have the appropriate people available to accompany the inspector. Those people need to be notified when an inspector arrives and announces that they are there to conduct an inspection. The facility should have identified an inspection walk-through team that is familiar with the operation of the areas through which they will accompany the inspector. It is also important to have in place a plan that provides coverage for those individuals on the inspection team so that the operations continue to function normally. The animal care and IACUC support staff should also be notified that an inspection will be taking place. Depending on the defined procedure at your facility, others who also may need to be notified are security staff, legal counsel, public relations personnel, IACUC members, senior management, the IO, the Quality Assurance Unit, and investigators. Finally, a postinspection review process should be in place, through which the inspection team reviews both the inspection report and the overall events that took place. A member of that team should be responsible for summarizing those events for the purpose of reporting to the IACUC and the IO. This will help document things while they are fresh in everyone's minds in the event that the institution elects to appeal the results of an inspection. The veterinarian with programmatic responsibility should report the results of an inspection to the IACUC and the IO, indicating what steps have been or will be taken to address any items of noncompliance contained in the inspection report.

When the inspector first arrives, the person with overall responsibility for managing the inspection process should determine what the inspector plans to review during the process, make arrangements for pertinent records to be available, and arrange that an office or conference room be provided for the inspector to use. This is good time to provide any follow-up on the issues raised during the previous inspection and to highlight program changes that have taken place.

Developing a good rapport with the inspector is important, because when issues arise they need to be discussed in a calm and friendly atmosphere. It is important to discuss issues as they arise during the inspection process so that steps to clarify the situation can be taken immediately. The inspector does have some flexibility in whether to include on the final report an item of noncompliance corrected during the inspection, and having a good working relationship with the inspector can be very important in this regard. It is important to keep in mind that both the inspector and the facility personnel have a common goal, which is to assure the well-being of the animals being cared for and used by the facility.

The inspection process should be viewed as a mutual assessment of the facility's compliance program and should not become adversarial in nature. Those individuals who accompany the inspector must have a detailed working knowledge of the institution's ACUP, and they should know the regulations and standards and the information contained in the Animal Welfare Inspection Guide (USDA 2013b) on conducting inspections and on activities specific to the inspection of research facilities. Should an item of noncompliance be identified, the facility representative should ask for clarification and be prepared to discuss the item in terms of the requirements of the regulations and standards, any relevant policies or guidelines, and the currently accepted practice standards. It should be noted that an Animal Care Policy should never be referred to on an inspection report or used as the sole basis for a citation. If the facility representative feels that an item should not be cited, they need to be prepared to discuss the issue thoroughly and to carefully explain how the facility's program operates and why that operation is consistent with the requirements of the regulations and standards.

If the USDA inspector will be removing copies of research facility records, protocols, or IACUC minutes (photocopies or photographs) from the facility, the facility will be afforded the opportunity to review or redact the records for proprietary business information. The inspector should allow the facility 24–48 hours for this purpose.

Inspectors have specific instructions concerning circumstances that require documentation with photographs. It is important that you be aware of those circumstances, which can be found in the Animal Welfare Inspection Guide. Inspectors are not allowed to share the photographs with the facility, but they should allow the facility to remove any identifiers (cage cards, etc.) that might be seen in the photographs. Upon request, the USDA inspector will show (on the camera viewer) all of the photos that were taken during the inspection. If any identifiers or proprietary information are seen on a photo, the inspector will delete the photo and take a replacement photo that does not contact the identifier or proprietary information. Since the inspector cannot provide copies of photographs, the facility should take their own photographs so that they have a representation of what could be in their file and thus subject to a request under FOIA.

The exit interview is an important part of the inspection process, as it affords the opportunity for the facility representatives to address any areas of disagreement that were not resolved during the actual inspection. In a larger facility where the inspection process may take more than a day, the inspector may be conferring with their supervisor on issues that arose during the inspection, so it is important to make sure that the results of any previous discussions have not changed. If there are still areas of disagreement when the final report is received, accept the report and then proceed with the postinspection review process so that the institution's process for considering and filing an appeal can be implemented. If the facility decides to file an appeal, the appropriate regional office should be notified within 21 days of the inspection in order to prevent the initial inspection report, which contains the disputed citations, from being uploaded to the USDA's website.

17.6 MANAGING AAALAC SITE VISITS

The AAALAC International site-visit process generally occurs every three years, unless a follow-up inspection is required to confirm corrections to deficiencies or to review major program changes. Site visits are conducted by a team of at least two people, consisting of a member of the AAALAC International Council on Accreditation and a consultant to the council. These individuals will have done a thorough assessment of the PD prepared by the facility, and during the site-visit they will confirm that the description accurately reflects the program in place as well as address any issues identified in the initial review or that arise during the site visit.

It is important that the development of the PD consists of a rigorous self-assessment process as previously described, and that all those who are involved in the site-visit process are familiar with the document. The site-visit process starts with a review of the description to address any items that the site visitors would like clarified. At this time, the facility representatives should provide any updates to the program that might have occurred since the PD was submitted.

AAALAC International's assessment process is more performance based than the USDA's process, and this can lead to rather in-depth discussions at times. During these discussions, differences in professional judgment can arise, and when they do, it is important that facility representatives be professional, stick to the facts, and be prepared to discuss in detail the basis for the performance standards that are in place and how those standards are assessed in term of achieving the end goal. Issues should be addressed as they arise. If they cannot be resolved as they occur, they can be addressed in the exit briefing. If they are still unresolved during the exit briefing, they can be addressed in writing following the site visit and prior to a review of the site-visit report by the council.

The AAALAC International program review process may identify two types of actionable items. Mandatory items represent serious issues that do not meet the standards identified by AAALAC International and must be addressed to maintain accreditation. Suggestions for improvement (SFI) are those items that AAALAC International believes will improve a program. It is not necessary to address these issues in either the exit briefing or in any follow-up correspondence. However, it is advisable that careful consideration be given to SFIs and that, either in a response to the letter from the council or in subsequent annual reports, they be addressed so that subsequent site visitors will be aware of any action taken.

Should AAALAC International elect to withhold or revoke accreditation, facility representatives have recourse to a hearing and appeal process, which is described on the AAALAC International website (AAALAC International 2014b).

17.7 MANAGING DEPARTMENT OF DEFENSE (DOD) SITE VISITS

When a facility receives funding from the Department of Defense (DOD), it must demonstrate compliance with the requirements of the branch of the service providing the funding. For the U.S. Army Medical Research and Materiel Command (USAMRMC), it must demonstrate compliance with the USAMRMC Animal Care and Use Policies. It is the responsibility of the Animal Care and Use Review Office (ACURO) to determine this compliance, which includes conducting site visits. Representatives from ACURO will use a site-visit checklist when evaluating the facility's ACUP. The checklist includes topics related to the AWRs and the Guide, as well as a specific review of the protocols and the implementation of those protocols for a DOD-funded project. The site visit will focus on aspects of the program and the facility that are specifically involved in providing support for the DOD-funded research protocol.

17.8 MANAGING OLAW SPECIAL REVIEWS AND SITE VISITS

Section V of the PHS Policy is entitled "Implementation by PHS." Subsection C is entitled "Conduct of Special Review/Site Visits" and indicates that awardee institutions are subject, at any time, to review by PHS personnel and external advisors, which could include a site visit. The purpose of this site visit would be "to assess the adequacy or accuracy of the institution's compliance or expressed compliance with the Policy." The Office of Extramural Research (OER) indicates that one of the major responsibilities of OLAW is that it "evaluates the effectiveness of PHS policies and programs for the humane care and use of laboratory animals through site visits of awardee institutions" (NIH 2014a). OLAW conducts two types of site visits: Assurance site visits conducted by the Division of Assurances and *for cause* site visits conducted by the Division of Compliance Oversight.

As with all site visits, the institution must demonstrate its compliance with the applicable regulations as well as its adherence to the processes described within its Animal Welfare Assurance. OLAW provides a notification of between one and two weeks for assurance site visits, and in preparation for such a site visit, those responsible for representing the institution should review the checklist mentioned previously and be prepared to explain how the program is in compliance with the PHS Policy and the recommendations of the Guide for each of the items on the checklist.

17.9 SUMMARY

Successful management of the inspection or site-visit process includes a proactive, progressive ACUP wherein all aspects of the program are reviewed on a regular basis for the purpose of assessing and improving the overall program. This review and assessment process should involve all those impacted by the program and should concentrate on improving animal welfare and facilitating the institution's research program. With a proactive, progressive program in place, the management of the actual inspection or site-visit process requires that the institutional team be composed of individuals who know the pertinent regulations, policies, and guidelines; the activities taking place at the institution; and the personnel involved in those activities. Management also needs to know how to effectively communicate the various aspects of the programs. With this type of team in place, inspectors or site visitors will recognize the commitment of the institution and all those involved in maintaining a high-quality ACUP.

REFERENCES

AAALAC (Association for Assessment and Accreditation of Laboratory Animal Care International). 2014a. AAALAC home page. AAALAC. http://www.aaalac.org/index. cfm.

AAALAC International (Association for Assessment Accreditation of Laboratory Animal Care International). 2014b. Rules of accreditation. Section 7. Hearings and appeals. Frederick, MD: AAALAC International. http://www.aaalac.org/accreditation/rules. cfm#hearings.

Freedom of Information Act 5 U.S.C. § 552 signed into law 1966, and amended by Public Law No. 104-231, 110 Stat. 3048 in 1996.

NIH (National Institutes of Health). 2002. Public Health Service policy on humane care and use of laboratory animals. Bethesda, MD: Office of Laboratory Animal Welfare, U.S. Department of Health and Human Services, NIH.

NIH (National Institutes of Health). 2014a. OER Office Web Pages (OLAW): OLAW Organizational Chart. http://grants.nih.gov/grants/oer_offices/olaw.htm. Updated July 11, 2014.

NIH (National Institutes of Health). 2014b. Semiannual program review and facility inspection checklist. Bethesda, MD: Office of Extramural Research, NIH. http://grants.nih.gov/grants/olaw/sampledoc/cheklist.htm.

NRC (National Research Council). 2011. *Guide for the Care and Use of Laboratory Animals.* 8th edn. Washington, DC: National Academies Press.

USDA (U.S. Department of Agriculture). 2013a. *Animal Welfare Act and Animal Welfare Regulations* (Animal Care Blue Book). Code of Federal Regulations (CFR), Title 9, Chapter 1, Subchapter A, Parts 1–4.

USDA (U.S. Department of Agriculture). 2013b. *Animal Welfare Inspection Guide*, 1st edn. http://www.aphis.usda.gov/animal_welfare/downloads/Inspection%20Guide%20-%20 November%202013.pdf.

USDA (U.S. Department of Agriculture). 2014. Appeals process. http://www.aphis.usda.gov/ publications/animal_welfare/2014/appeals_process.pdf.

CHAPTER 18

Acronyms and Abbreviations

AAALAC International	Association for Assessment and Accreditation of Laboratory Animal Care International
AALAS	American Association for Laboratory Animal Science
ACLAM	American College of Laboratory Animal Medicine
AHT	animal health technician
ALAT	assistant laboratory animal technician
ALF	Animal Liberation Front
AOR	authorized organizational representative
APHIS	Animal and Plant Health Inspection Service (USDA)
ASLAP	American Society of Laboratory Animal Practitioners
ASR	Academy of Surgical Research
ATA	Animal Transportation Association
AV	attending veterinarian
AVMA	American Veterinary Medical Association
AWA	Animal Welfare Act
AWIC	Animal Welfare Information Center
AWRs	Animal Welfare Regulations (USDA)
BSO	biosafety officer
CAAT	Center for Alternatives to Animal Testing
CCAC	Canadian Council on Animal Care
CDC	Centers for Disease Control and Prevention
CEO	chief executive officer
CFA	complete Freund's adjuvant
CFR	Code of Federal Regulations
CIO	chief institutional official
CPSC	Consumer Product Safety Commission

DEA	Drug Enforcement Administration
DHHS	Department of Health and Human Services
DOD	Department of Defense
DVM/VMD	doctor of veterinary medicine
EAE	experimental autoimmune (or allergenic) encephalitis
eFOIA	Electronic Freedom of Information Act
EHS	environmental health and safety
EPA	Environmental Protection Agency
ESA	Endangered Species Act
ESCRO	Embryonic Stem Cell Research Oversight
FASEB	Federation of American Societies for Experimental Biology
FDA	Food and Drug Administration
FOIA	Freedom of Information Act
GLP	good laboratory practice
Guide	*Guide for the Care and Use of Laboratory Animals*
IACUC	Institutional Animal Care and Use Committee
IATA	International Air Transport Association
IBC	Institutional Biosafety Committee
IFA	Freund's incomplete adjuvant
ILAR	Institute for Laboratory Animal Research
IO	institutional official
IRB	institutional review board (human subjects)
LAT	laboratory animal technician
LATG	laboratory animal technologist
LD50	lethal dose it takes to kill 50% of test animals
mAb	monoclonal antibody production
MOU	memorandum of understanding
MTA	material transfer agreement
MTD	maximum tolerated dose study
MSDS	material safety data sheet
NABR	National Association for Biomedical Research
NAL	National Agriculture Library
NHP	nonhuman primate
NIH	National Institutes of Health
NLM	National Library of Medicine
NRC	National Research Council

NSET	nonsurgical embryo transfer
NSF	National Science Foundation
OBA	Office of Biotechnology Activities
OHRP	Office for Human Research Protection
OHSP	Occupational Health and Safety Program
OLAW	Office of Laboratory Animal Welfare
OSHA	Occupational Safety and Health Administration
PD	protocol director or program description
PETA	People for the Ethical Treatment of Animals
PHS	Public Health Service
PHS Policy	Public Health Service Policy on Humane Care and Use of Laboratory Animals
PI	principal investigator
PRIM&R	Public Responsibility in Medicine and Research
QA	quality assurance
RSO	radiation safety officer
RVT	registered veterinary technician
SCAW	Scientists Center for Animal Welfare
SOP	standard operating procedure
SPF	specific pathogen free
TLI	total lymphoid irradiation
USDA	U.S. Department of Agriculture
VAS	Vertebrate Animal Section
VS	veterinary services

APPENDIX A

Forms, Templates, and Notices

A.1 SAMPLE IACUC PROTOCOL FORM

CONFIDENTIAL
Institutional Animal Care and Use Committee
Protocol for the Humane Care and Use of Live Vertebrate Animals

Information about Using this Form

	Please Leave Blank

- Respond to all questions in this form. If a particular question does not apply to your proposed use of animals, indicate "N/A" in the space provided.

Please Leave Blank
Protocol #:
Approval Date:
Expiration Date:

- Only complete those attachments that apply to your proposed use of animals (you will be reminded to do so throughout the form where applicable).
- Your protocol application will not be considered complete until the signed "Certification of Compliance Assurance" is received.

Preparing Your Protocol for Approval -

- You should consult with a veterinarian for potentially painful procedures, and/or procedures using analgesics, anesthetics, or paralytics.
- Review all current IACUC policies and procedures; these may be referenced in your protocol rather than describing the details associated with these procedures.

For questions, contact the IACUC Coordinator.

Date:

Section 1: General Information

1. Protocol Title (include species and be descriptive of the procedures/surgery involving animals):
2. Does this protocol replace a previously approved protocol? ☐ No ☐ Yes (provide previous protocol number:)
3. Protocol Personnel—List the names of all individuals authorized to conduct procedures involving animals under this proposal and identify key personnel (e.g., Co-Investigator); if the person will not be working with animals (e.g., Administrative Contact), you do not need to answer questions A-D.

Principal Investigator
Name:
Department: Mailstop: Email:
Office Phone: Cell Phone:

Protocol Number
Institutional Animal Care and Use Committee

A.   Have they completed required animal welfare training? ☐ Yes ☐ No

B.   Have they completed required primate biosafety training? ☐ Yes ☐ No ☐ N/A

C.   Have they received Occupational Health clearance to work with species listed? ☐ Yes ☐ No ☐ N/A

D.   Describe experience/training have had or will have with specific animal model(s):

Co-Investigator

Name:

Department: Mailstop: Email:

Office Phone: Cell Phone:

Will this person be working with animals? ☐ Yes ☐ No (if "No," skip A. - D.)

A.   Have they completed required animal welfare training? ☐ Yes ☐ No

B.   Have they completed required primate biosafety training? ☐ Yes ☐ No ☐ N/A

C.   Have they received Occupational Health clearance to work with species listed? ☐ Yes ☐ No ☐ N/A

D.   Describe experience/training have had or will have with specific animal model(s):

Administrative Contact

Name:

Department: Mailstop: Email:

Office Phone: Cell Phone:

Will this person be working with animals? ☐ Yes ☐ No (if "No," skip A. - D.)

A.   Have they completed required animal welfare training? ☐ Yes ☐ No

B.   Have they completed required primate biosafety training? ☐ Yes ☐ No ☐ N/A

C.   Have they received Occupational Health clearance to work with species listed? ☐ Yes ☐ No ☐ N/A

D.   Describe experience/training have had or will have with specific animal model(s):

Other Protocol Personnel (Copy this section and insert required information for Other Protocol Personnel as needed.)

Name:

Department: Mailstop: Email:

Office Phone: Cell Phone:

Will this person be working with animals? ☐ Yes ☐ No (if "No," skip A. - D.)

A.   Have they completed required animal welfare training? ☐ Yes ☐ No

B.   Have they completed required primate biosafety training? ☐ Yes ☐ No ☐ N/A

C.   Have they received Occupational Health clearance to work with species listed? ☐ Yes ☐ No ☐ N/A

D.   Describe experience/training have had or will have with specific animal model(s):

CONFIDENTIAL

Protocol Number

Institutional Animal Care and Use Committee

Section 2: Funding Source, Collaborations, and Conflict of Interest

1. Funding Source (check all that apply):

☐ Grants/Contracts (copy and insert required information for multiple grants/ contracts)

   A. Grant/Contract Title:

      Grant #:   Funded by:

      Funding Administered by:

      Name of Principal Investigator:

      For PHS Funded Projects, are contents of the protocol the same as described in the PHS proposal application? ☐ Yes ☐ No (attach a copy of the PHS-funded grant for congruency check)

      This protocol supports:

         ☐ A single grant and describes all grant supported animal procedures

         ☐ Multiple grants and describes all grant supported animal procedures

☐ Fellowships (copy and insert required information for multiple fellowships)

   A. Fellowship Title:

      Fellowship Reference #:   Funded by:

      Name of Fellow:

      For PHS Funded Projects, are contents of the protocol the same as described in the PHS proposal application? ☐ Yes ☐ No (attach a copy of the PHS-funded grant for congruency check)

☐ Gift Funding (copy and insert required information for multiple gift funds)

   A. Gift Name:

      Gift Account #:

☐ Department Funding (copy and insert required information for multiple department funds)

   A. Department Name:

      Department Account #:

☐ Other Funding (describe):

2. Collaborations (defined as institutional funds used to support off-site animal studies, custom antibody production, etc.)

   A. Have you submitted a copy of the host institution's IACUC protocol/approval letter?

      ☐ Yes   ☐ No

   B. Have you submitted proof of host institution's PHS Assurance?

      ☐ Yes   ☐ No   ☐ N/A

   C. Have you submitted proof of host institution's USDA License?

      ☐ Yes   ☐ No   ☐ N/A

   D. Have you submitted proof of host institution's AAALAC Accreditation?

      ☐ Yes   ☐ No   ☐ N/A

CONFIDENTIAL
_____
Protocol Number
Institutional Animal Care and Use Committee
_____

3. Conflict of Interest
   A. Does anyone who:
      • Is involved with the design, conduct, or reporting of this research;
      • Plans to analyze data;
      • Plans to serve as an author on any papers originating from this research;
      • Is an immediate family member (spouse, dependent child as defined by IRS, domestic partner of any of the above):
         1. Have consulting arrangements, responsibilities or equity holdings in the sponsoring company, vendor(s), provider(s) of goods, or subcontractor(s)? ☐ Yes ☐ No
         2. Have a financial relationship with the sponsoring company, vendor(s), provider(s) of goods, or subcontractor(s) including the receipt of honoraria, income, or stock/stock options as payment? ☐ Yes ☐ No
         3. Serve as a member of an advisory board with the sponsoring company, vendor(s), provider(s) of goods or subcontractor(s)? ☐ Yes ☐ No
         4. Receive any gift funds from the sponsoring company, vendor(s), provider(s) of goods, or subcontractor(s)? ☐ Yes ☐ No
         5. Have an ownership or royalty interest in any intellectual property utilized in this protocol? ☐ Yes ☐ No
   B. To your knowledge, does anyone in a supervisory role to the Principal Investigator have a conflict of interest related to this study? ☐ Yes ☐ No

   If you answer "Yes" to any of the questions in #3 above, you must file a Conflict of Interest (COI) disclosure with the Conflict of Interest Office.

Section 3: Animal Information
   1. Species—Common Name: Scientific Name:
      Sex: Approximate age, weight or size:
      Bacteriological status (e.g., germfree (axenic), defined flora (gnotobiotic), specific pathogen free (SPF), conventional):
      Viral status (e.g., simian immunodeficiency virus, simian retrovirus):
      Surgery performed by vendor: ☐ No ☐ Yes (describe):
      Surgery performed by investigator: ☐ Yes (complete Attachment 2)   ☐ No
      Will live animals be used for teaching? ☐ No ☐ Yes (describe goals of course and intended audience):
      Approximate Daily Census: Housing Location:
      Animal identification methods (check all that apply):
      ☐   Cage card   ☐   Ear tag   ☐   Ear punch/notch
      ☐   Tattoo   ☐   Collar   ☐   Microchip
      ☐   Other (describe:)

   2. Animal Numbers Justification—A key principle in the ethical use of animals in research, testing and teaching is that the number of animals used in each project is the minimum necessary to obtain valid and meaningful results, while avoiding unnecessary duplication. A Biostatistician can assist in the statistical design of your study by performing a power analysis to determine sample size "n," number

CONFIDENTIAL

Protocol Number
Institutional Animal Care and Use Committee

of groups, and/or numbers of experiments necessary to statistically validate your hypothesis (specific aims). In determining the numbers of animals required, which of the following are applicable (check all that apply):

☐ Power analyses indicated that the proposed sample size, number of groups, and/or number of experiments is the lowest required for statistically valid tests of the hypothesis (i.e., 80% power with 0.05 type I error).

☐ Differences from controls are expected to be small, and large sample sizes are necessary to distinguish differences reliably.

☐ Based on previous and/or published data, the numbers of animals requested are the minimum needed to achieve sufficient statistical power.

☐ These animals will be used to produce antibodies or tissues, and numbers are based on yield.

☐ The numbers of animals or group sizes have been established by federal guidelines/requirements.

☐ This is a pilot/feasibility study that uses the minimum number of animals required to provide meaningful, but not statistically significant data (i.e., model development).

☐ This protocol involves breeding of genetically modified rodents. Based on Mendelian genetics, we expect ¼ of all pups to be homozygous and ¼ to be wild type, with the remaining ½ heterozygous. The homozygous and wild type mice will be used to generate data for the experiment, and the heterozygotes will be used to replace the breeding stock or euthanized.

☐ This is a teaching protocol. Animal numbers were determined by a specified student-to-animal ratio and have been minimized to the fullest extent possible without sacrificing the quality of the hands-on teaching experience for students.

☐ Other (describe):

3. Estimate of Animal Numbers Required—(Note: The approved number of animals is an annual allocation which coincides with the approval date of a protocol. On the anniversary approval date, all existing animals will be deducted from the approved number of animals available for the upcoming year.):

A. What is the number of animals per experimental group (group size or "n"):

B. How many groups per study or experiment (including controls):

C. How many studies (experiments/compounds) do you anticipate conducting/ screening each year:

D. Estimated number of animals to be used annually (A x B x C) =

4. Source of Animals (check all that apply):

☐ Procured from outside sources

☐ Use or breeding of genetically modified animals (describe breeding procedures):

Section 4: Purpose and Value of the Research

1. Using non-technical (lay) language that a non-scientist would understand, briefly explain the aim of the study and why the study is important to human or animal health, the advancement of knowledge, or the good of society. Do not use

CONFIDENTIAL

Protocol Number
Institutional Animal Care and Use Committee

scientific jargon or cut and paste paragraphs from grant applications that were written for scientific reviewers. Initially spell out any acronyms or abbreviations used.

Section 5: Rationale for Using Animals and Species Involved

1. Provide a rationale for the use of animals (or their tissues) and describe the characteristics of the chosen species which make it the appropriate model by checking all that apply:

   ☐ The complexity of the processes being studied cannot be duplicated or modeled in simpler systems.

   ☐ There is not enough information known about the processes being studied to design nonliving models.

   ☐ Preclinical studies in living animals are required by federal regulations prior to human testing. Cite the agency, the code of Federal Regulations (CFR) title number, and the specific section number (e.g., APHIS, 9 CFR 113.102):

   ☐ This is a behavioral, learning or developmental study.

   ☐ A large database exists for this species, allowing comparisons with previous data.

   ☐ The anatomy, genetics, physiology or behavior of this species is uniquely suited to the animal use proposed (describe):

   ☐ This is the phylogenetically lowest species that provides adequate size, tissue or anatomy for the proposed animal use.

   ☐ The species provides a particularly good model for duplicating the human situation (describe):

   ☐ This species has unique features that make it the best choice available for the proposed animal use (describe):

   ☐ Previous experiments using this species formed the background of this project.

2. Explain why a "lower order" species or non-animal alternative cannot be used to achieve the desired results:

Section 6: Alternatives Search

The federal Animal Welfare Act and PHS Policy require that researchers evaluate the existence of alternatives when procedures cause more than slight or momentary pain or distress for the animal. Examples of alternatives include less sentient species, computer models, audio-visual training programs, and refinements to proposed procedures, such as the use of pain relieving drugs/treatments for otherwise painful procedures. A search must also be performed for alternatives to prolonged restraint when animals will be restrained continuously for >12 h.

An alternatives search must be conducted for studies in pain categories C, D, and E for regulated species, and D and E for non-regulated rodent (mouse and rat) species.

1. Which database sources or methods were used to evaluate the existence of viable alternatives? (check all that apply) You must include two or more databases in your search. Inadequate searches will result in a delay of IACUC approval. An Alternative Search by an Information Scientist is strongly encouraged.

CONFIDENTIAL

_____
Protocol Number

Institutional Animal Care and Use Committee
_____

☐   AGRICOLA   ☐   Animal Welfare Information Center (AWIC)
☐   Biological Abstracts   ☐   Biosis
☐   CAB   ☐   Current Contents Connect
☐   Embase   ☐   PubMed (Medline)
☐   Tox Line   ☐   Tox Net
☐   Other—list:

2. Which keywords were used in conducting the database search (alternative should be one of the key words)?

3. Date(s) the search was conducted:

4. Years included in the search criteria:

5. Other resources (e.g., attendance at meetings (include seminar titles, dates of attendance, location, and other relevant supportive information), consultation with colleagues):

6. Based on your search, are alternatives to the use of animals available:
   ☐   Yes (describe in question #8. below)   ☐   No

7. Based on your search, are alternatives to painful/distressful procedures available:
   ☐   Yes (describe in question #8. below)   ☐   No

8. If you answered "Yes" in questions # 6. and/or # 7. above, explain why any identified alternatives were rejected and describe how the 3 Rs (Replacing or Reducing the animal numbers used and/or Refining the procedures to eliminate, minimize, or alleviate the level of pain or distress experienced by the animals as a result of painful/distressful procedures in this protocol) have been addressed. If you have previously performed the animal-related procedures contained in this protocol, describe any refinements you have made:

Section 7: Experimental Procedures

1. Briefly explain the experimental design and describe all animal procedures to be employed in this study. This description should allow the IACUC to understand the experimental course of an animal from its entry into the experiment to the endpoint of the study. A flowchart may be an effective presentation of the planned procedure.

2. Experimental procedures that apply to this protocol (check all that apply):
   ☐   Although death is not an endpoint, some mortality is expected as a result of the procedures in this proposal (describe expected cause of death):
   ☐   Animals used in this protocol will develop acute or chronic illness, disease, or physiological deficit spontaneously or through experimental manipulation (describe):
   ☐   Surgery will be performed (complete Attachment 2)
   ☐   Chronic catheterization and/or instrumentation
        Catheter type (vascular or other):
        Maintenance for chronically maintained catheters (list anticoagulants or other catheter maintenance solutions in Attachment 1):
   ☐   Experimental administrations (complete Attachment 1)

CONFIDENTIAL   _____

                                                          Protocol Number
                              Institutional Animal Care and Use Committee
_____

☐   Non-surgical use of anesthetics (complete Attachment 1).
    Purpose:
Criteria for assessing level of anesthesia (check all that apply):
    ☐   Respiratory rate/character   ☐   Toe or tail pinch
    ☐   Color of mucous membranes   ☐   Heart rate
    ☐   Muscular relaxation   ☐   % Expired (end-tidal) CO_2
    ☐   ECG   ☐   Corneal reflex
    ☐   Blood pressure   ☐   Other - specify:
    a. List equipment to be used for anesthesia monitoring, if applicable:
    b. List which assessment criteria you will document, including frequency:
☐   Blood collection (refer to "A Good Practice Guide to the Administration of
    Substances and Removal of Blood, Including Routes and Volumes" (*J. Appl.
    Toxicol.* 21, 15–23 (2001)). Exceptions to this guideline must be scientifically
    justified and you must describe any safeguards for the animals in Section 11
    below).
    Method:
    Frequency:
    Volume of a single blood withdrawal:
    Volume of total blood withdrawn per day and week:
☐   Food or water restriction that departs from the recommendations in the *Guide*.
    Purpose:
    Duration:
    Scientific justification:
    Method for assessing health and wellbeing:
☐   Special or manipulated diets or water (describe:)
☐   Medicated feed or water (complete Attachments 1 and 3)
☐   Tissue harvest
☐   Antibody production—If using ascites production to produce antibodies, pro-
    vide a justification for not using an *in vitro* system:

Section 8: Animal Restraint
Prolonged restraint must be justified and appropriate oversight to ensure it is minimally distressing. Studies requiring continuous restraint beyond 12 h without the
opportunity for a continuous hour of unrestrained activity require a rigorous scientific justification and a search for alternatives to the prolonged restraint. (Examples
of restraint include primate chairs, dog/pig slings, rodent restraint devices/cages
(e.g., Bollman cages).)
    1. Unanesthetized animals will be restrained (exclude momentary procedures such as
        blood draws, injections, dosing, etc.)
        ☐   No
        ☐   Yes (describe below):
            Purpose (restraint methods must be included in the search terms for your
            Alternatives Search):
            Method of restraint:

CONFIDENTIAL
_____

                                                    Protocol Number
                            Institutional Animal Care and Use Committee
_____

     Duration of restraint:
     Frequency of restraint:
     Frequency of observations during restraint:
     Justification for type and duration of restraint:
     Training/habituation/acclimatization procedures:
     ☐ Will follow IACUC procedure for dog, swine, or nonhuman primate restraint
     ☐ Other (describe):

Section 9: Experimental Endpoint Criteria and Veterinary Care

1. Describe the anticipated clinical signs which may develop in this model (e.g., tumors, percentage body weight gain or loss, inability to eat or drink, behavioral abnormalities, or signs of toxicity):
2. What are the proposed study endpoints in regard to the clinical signs and what treatment or action will be initiated for each? (Provide scientific justification for any unrelieved pain/distress or if using death as an endpoint)
3. Early euthanasia criteria (list the criteria that will be used to determine when euthanasia is to be performed. Death as an endpoint must be scientifically justified):
4. Veterinary care (indicate the plan of action in case of animal illness (e.g., initiate treatment, call investigator prior to initiating treatment, euthanize)):

Section 10: Animal Housing and Husbandry

1. Describe the housing and husbandry that will be provided to animals on this protocol (check all that apply):
    ☐ Standard husbandry
    ☐ Non-standardized husbandry, that is, wire-bottom cages (rodents), altered light cycles, etc. (describe):
    ☐ Provided by research group (describe):
    ☐ Animals will be kept in areas outside of animal facilities for more than 12 h or overnight (requires prior approval by the IACUC)
       Describe justification, proposed location (building/room), and attach a copy of the husbandry SOP:
2. Will animals receive enrichment in accordance with species-specific IACUC enrichment policies?
    ☐ Yes
    ☐ No (provide justification for exemption from IACUC enrichment policies):

Section 11: Pain Category

1. Are any of the procedures or experiments in this protocol, or the genetic manipulation or mutations (spontaneous or induced) of the animals used in this protocol, expected to cause more than slight pain/distress of very short duration? (If anesthetics/analgesics will be used to prevent/relieve pain, you must answer "Yes")

CONFIDENTIAL
_____
                                                     Protocol Number
                        Institutional Animal Care and Use Committee
_____

☐   No
☐   Yes—Answer A through B and review the Alternative Search in order to assess
    and evaluate the alternative possibilities.
    A. List the procedures/experiments/genetic manipulation/genetic mutations
        or genotype that are known to cause pain/distress, including death as an
        endpoint or prolonged (>12 h) restraint:
    B. What will be done to alleviate or minimize the pain/distress/discomfort
        (check all that apply):
        ☐   Drugs will be used (complete Attachment 1 for non-surgical proce-
             dures and/or Attachment 2 for surgical procedures)
             What criteria will be used to initiate this care?
        ☐   Habituation or acclimatizing the animal
        ☐   Enrichment opportunities above and beyond standard enrichment
             program (see species-specific IACUC Enrichment Policies for
             approved activities)
        ☐   Other methods will be used (i.e., special bedding, supplemental food,
             heat packs, etc.)
             Describe method and explain how this will provide relief:
             What criteria will be used to initiate this care:
        ☐   No method of relief will be used
             Provide scientific justification for performing painful or distressful
             procedures without appropriate pain relieving or sedating medica-
             tions. State methods or means used to determine that pain and/or
             distress relief would interfere with test results (include article reprint
             or reference, if any, to support the justification):

Section 12: Administration of Paralytics

Federal regulations require that neuromuscular blocking agents (drugs or compounds that cause skeletal muscle paralysis) can be used only in appropriately anesthetized animals. Any drug/compound with paralyzing properties should be listed in
Attachment 1, regardless of whether it is to be used as an experimental agent, control, or adjunct to facilitate testing. The Attending Veterinarian and IACUC office
must be notified by email at least 24 h before the expected date and time of use of
neuromuscular blocking agents.

1. Animals will be subjected to the use of neuromuscular blocking agents (drugs or
    compounds that cause skeletal muscle paralysis):
    ☐ Yes   ☐ No (proceed to Section 13)
2. If yes, what anesthetic agent will be used (complete "non-surgical anesthetics" por-
    tion of Attachment 1 or Attachment 2 if part of a surgical procedure as applicable):
3. How will proper anesthetic depth be evaluated and documented while the animal is
    under the effects of the paralytic agent?
4. How will ventilation be maintained?
5. List all physiologic parameters and clinical signs to be monitored, and frequency
    of monitoring, below. Documentation regarding monitoring for proper anesthetic

CONFIDENTIAL

<u>   </u>
Protocol Number
<u>   Institutional Animal Care and Use Committee</u>

depth must be maintained and available to inspectors (USDA, AAALAC, FDA, and IACUC).

Physiologic parameters/ clinical signs	Frequency of monitoring	Variables to be considered as indicators of inadequate anesthesia

6. If animals are found to be inadequately anesthetized, explain what will be done for the animals:

Section 13: Use of Hazardous Agents

The minimum required personal protective equipment (PPE) for handling novel drug compounds (as well as biohazardous, hazardous, or radioactive materials) includes safety glasses, gloves, and protective clothing (e.g., a lab coat or disposable coveralls). Respiratory protection (e.g., a disposable dust/mist respirator) is also required for working with or around laboratory animals (in most situations), or if novel drug compounds will become airborne. Refer to the PPE Policy and Animal Facility/Animal Lab PPE Policy on the EH&S website.

1. Will hazardous agents besides novel drug compounds or reference compounds be used in this protocol (refer to list of hazardous agents in Attachment 3):
   ☐   Yes (complete Attachment 3)
   ☐   No

Section 14: Final Disposition of Animals

1. Final disposition of all animals in this protocol (check all that apply):
   ☐   Euthanasia for tissue collection with no experimental manipulation of the animal
   ☐   Animals will be euthanized and submitted for necropsy
   ☐   Animals will be euthanized and carcasses properly disposed
   ☐   Animals will be returned to the colony for continuing use on this protocol or transferred to other approved protocols in accordance with the IACUC's Animal Transfer Policy. (Note: <u>Prior</u> approval by the IACUC is required before reassigning animals that have experienced pain or distress or were administered an anesthetic or analgesic to alleviate pain or distress)
   ☐   Other (describe):

Section 15: Euthanasia

<u>All</u> methods of euthanasia must be consistent with the recommendations of the *AVMA Guidelines for the Euthanasia of Animals: 2013 Edition* unless scientific justification for alternative methods is provided and approved by the IACUC. It is not necessary to list methods of euthanasia used by support personnel (i.e., laboratory

_____

animal facility, veterinary services personnel, necropsy) as long as they are consistent with the aforementioned recommendations/policy.

1. Does the method of euthanasia meet the recommendations of the AVMA Guidelines?
   □ Yes
   □ No (provide justification):
2. Animals will be euthanized by (check all that apply):
   □ Support personnel - List groups performing euthanasia:
   □ Principal Investigator/listed personnel
3. Method(s) used to euthanize animals (check all that apply):
   □ Animal may be sedated prior to euthanasia to facilitate handling (list sedative(s) in Attachment 1)
   □ CO_2 via compressed gas cylinder with pressure regulator and flowmeter
   □ Combination pentobarbital sodium solution for euthanasia
     Dose (mg/kg) and route:
   □ Decapitation or cervical dislocation (Note: IACUC approval is required for the application of either technique on unanesthetized mice and rats; cervical dislocation should only be applied to mice, or rats weighing < 200 g; documentation is required to verify that the equipment used to perform decapitation is maintained in good working order and serviced on a regular basis to ensure sharpness of blades.)
   □ Exsanguination under anesthesia (list anesthesia in Attachment 1)
   □ Other: Agent: Dose: mg/kg   Route:
                 Agent: Dose: mg/kg   Route:
4. Describe how death is assured prior to disposal (check all that apply):
   □ Auscultate for heart beat
   □ Bilateral thoracotomy
   □ Decapitation/cervical dislocation
   □ Left in room air for 5–10 min following CO_2 exposure
   □ Other—Describe:

CONFIDENTIAL

Protocol Number
_____

Institutional Animal Care and Use Committee
_____

To be completed by IACUC

☐ This protocol was approved by designated member review   Date:_____

Designated Reviewer Name(s):_____   _____

Signature(s):   _____   _____

☐ This protocol was approved by full committee review   Date:_____

This protocol is in USDA Pain Category:

☐ Category C   No Pain/Distress expected and no pain relieving drugs given
☐ Category D   Potential Pain/Distress alleviated by the use of appropriate drugs
                or other means
☐ Category E   Unalleviated expected Pain/Distress

Rationale for Selecting Reporting Category:

Protocol Approved:_____   _____
                   Signature of IACUC Chair   Date

Receipt of this signed, numbered document serves as IACUC notification of your approved protocol.

CONFIDENTIAL

Protocol Number
Institutional Animal Care and Use Committee

ATTACHMENT 1
EXPERIMENTAL ADMINISTRATIONS

1. List all experimental administrations—attach additional sheets if necessary (refer to IACUC webpage "A Good Practice Guide to the Administration of Substances and Removal of Blood, Including Routes and Volumes").

Agent	Vehicle	Route	Volume (ml/ kg) and Dose Range if Known (mg/kg)	Frequency Expected (times per day/week/ month) (D/W/M)	Duration of Dosing (no. of days/weeks/ months) (D/W/M)
Chemical restraint/sedation/tranquilization for non-surgical procedure:					
Anesthetics/analgesics (non-surgical procedures):					
Neuromuscular blocking agents:					
Other (anti-coagulants, saline, etc.):					
Experimental agents (describe class, novel drug compound, etc.):					

2. Will any of the agents administered, including vehicles, cause pain or distress or dependency?
   ☐   Yes (describe below)   ☐ No
3. If using a biological material/animal product for use in animals (e.g., cell lines, antiserum, etc.), has the material been tested for pathogens?
   ☐   Yes (attach copy of results)   ☐ No

CONFIDENTIAL

Protocol Number

Institutional Animal Care and Use Committee

ATTACHMENT 2
SURGICAL PROCEDURES

The Principal Investigator is responsible for ensuring all individuals listed below are appropriately trained to administer/monitor anesthesia and/or carry out all surgeries listed in the species this protocol covers:

Name & Phone Number	Name & Phone Number

Section 16: Surgical Administrations

1. List all medications to be given immediately pre-, peri- and post-operatively in the table below:

Agent	Dose (mg/kg)	Route	Frequency
PRE-OPERATIVE MEDICATIONS –			
Pre-anesthetics (i.e., for chemical restraint/sedation/tranquilization):			
Pre-emptive analgesics:			
Adjunctive medications (i.e., anticholinergics):			
INTRA-OPERATIVE MEDICATIONS –			
Anesthetic agents:			
Adjunctive medications:			
Fluid support:			
POST-OPERATIVE MEDICATIONS –			
Analgesics:			
Antibiotics:			
Adjunctive medications:			

CONFIDENTIAL

_____

Protocol Number

Institutional Animal Care and Use Committee

Section 17: Surgical Procedures

1. The following describes the proposed surgeries covered by this protocol (check all that apply):
   ☐ Non-survival: Animals euthanized without regaining consciousness
   ☐ Minor survival surgery: No penetration of a major body cavity
   ☐ Multiple minor survival surgical procedures—Provide a rationale for why multiple minor survival procedures must be done:
      What is the maximum number of procedures that the animal would undergo?
   ☐ Major survival surgery (e.g., penetration of a body cavity, production of substantial impairment of physical or physiologic functions, or involves extensive tissue dissection or transection, such as laparotomy, thoracotomy, craniotomy, joint replacement, or limb amputation).
   ☐ Multiple major survival surgical procedures—Provide a rationale for why multiple major survival procedures must be done: (see IACUC Policy on Multiple Major Surgical Procedures)

2. Description of surgical procedures. Refer to the IACUC Policy on Standards for Aseptic Rodent Survival Surgery. This section should include details about patient preparation, approach to the anatomic structure(s), instrumentation, and method of closure.

3. Location where surgery will be performed (check all that apply):
   ☐ Large Animal Surgery Suite
   ☐ Small Animal Surgery Suite
   ☐ Human Patient Areas (List building, room, infection control plan, mode/route of transportation, and scheduling considerations to minimize public patient exposure):
   ☐ Other—Specify location and explain why surgery must be done at this location (requires IACUC approval):

For parts 4-8, documentation must be maintained for all species, particularly for USDA regulated species (e.g., dogs, nonhuman primates, rabbits, guinea pigs, swine, ferrets, and cats), and must be available to inspectors (USDA, AAALAC, FDA, IACUC).

4. Description of animal's pre-surgical work up and pre-operative care
   a. Criteria used to select animals suitable for use in surgical procedures (e.g., health assessment, blood work, etc.):
   b. List any medications to be given immediately prior to anesthetic induction, including sedation, pre-emptive analgesia, and any adjunctive medications in the Surgical Administrations table in Section 16.

5. Description of intraoperative care and treatment
   a. Describe supportive care given during surgery (i.e., external heat source, fluid therapy, etc.):
   b. List the anesthetic agent(s), fluid therapy, and other adjunctive medications in the Surgical Administrations table in Section 16.

CONFIDENTIAL

Protocol Number
Institutional Animal Care and Use Committee

   c. Criteria for assessing level of anesthesia (check all that apply):
      ☐ Respiratory rate/character   ☐ Toe or tail pinch
      ☐ Color of mucous membranes   ☐ Heart rate
      ☐ Muscular relaxation   ☐ % Expired (end-tidal) CO_2
      ☐ ECG   ☐ Corneal reflex
      ☐ Blood pressure   ☐ Other - specify:
   d. List equipment to be used for anesthesia monitoring:
   e. List which assessment criteria you will document, including frequency:
 6. Description of <u>immediate</u> (day of surgery) postoperative recovery monitoring procedures, including duration and frequency (survival procedures only):
 7. Description of postoperative monitoring procedures, including duration, frequency, and date sutures/staples will be removed (survival procedures only):
   a. Surgical recovery to time of study use:
   b. List any therapeutic medications to be given post-operatively, including analgesics, antibiotics, etc. in the Surgical Administrations table in Section 16.
 8. For multiple major survival procedures, describe the length of time between subsequent surgical manipulations:

CONFIDENTIAL

Protocol Number
Institutional Animal Care and Use Committee

ATTACHMENT 3
HAZARDOUS AGENTS

1. Identify the hazardous agent(s) and describe how human exposure to the hazardous agent(s) will be minimized:

Hazardous Agent	Other Panel Approvals (list Protocol #)	Dose and Route of Administration	Risks, Containment Procedures, Animal Biosafety Level, Engineering Control(s)*
Biohazardous/ Infectious agent:			
Naturally-occurring biological toxin:			
Recombinant DNA:			
hESCs or Human Fetal Tissue:			
Volatile anesthetic agent (e.g. Halothane, Isoflurane):			
Chemical agent (highly toxic chemical, carcinogen, nanomaterial, or reproductive toxin):			
Radioactive material:			
Other (specify):			

* If containment procedures/engineering controls are described in another document, you may summarize them here and reference the other document for details.

2. Describe special precautions for animal handlers:

3. Describe special waste or animal disposal procedures:

4. Obtain signature from the Associate Director of the Animal Facilities (or designee) if there is potential risk to the facility personnel (e.g., infectious agents shed by animals).

_____   _____

Associate Director, Laboratory Animal Facilities Signature   Date

CONFIDENTIAL

_____

Protocol Number

Institutional Animal Care and Use Committee

_____

ATTACHMENT 4
CERTIFICATION OF COMPLIANCE ASSURANCE

Protocol Title:

I agree with the following (check the appropriate answer):

Yes   No

☐   ☐   No animals will be used in more than one major operative procedure from which it is allowed to recover unless scientifically justified or required as a veterinary procedure.

☐   ☐   No paralytics will be used without prior approval, appropriate anesthesia and monitoring for proper anesthetic depth.

☐   ☐   Medical care for animals will not be withheld and will be provided or supervised by a veterinarian.

☐   ☐   The animals' living conditions, including housing, feeding, psychological enrichment programs, exercise, and non-medical care, will be appropriate for the species, will maintain their health and comfort, and will not deviate from USDA and the 8th edition _Guide for the Care and Use of Laboratory Animals_ standards.

☐   ☐   Analgesic, anesthetic, and tranquilizing drugs will be used where indicated and where appropriate to minimize discomfort and pain.

☐   ☐   Animals that would otherwise experience severe or chronic pain/distress that cannot be adequately relieved will be euthanized at the end of the procedure, or if appropriate during the procedure.

☐   ☐   Personnel conducting animal procedures will read and agree to comply with this protocol. They will be appropriately qualified and/or trained in those procedures and the training and qualifications of such personnel will be appropriately documented and readily accessible to all regulatory representatives.

☐   ☐   All individuals working on this protocol who are at risk are participating in the institution's Occupational Health and Safety Program.

☐   ☐   This protocol does not unnecessarily duplicate previously reported research.

☐   ☐   Significant additional procedures or changes in procedures not approved by the IACUC will not be performed until an amendment is submitted and approved by the IACUC.

☐   ☐   Any drug or compound to be administered to the animals in this protocol will be pharmaceutical grade when available and appropriate. (See IACUC policy on the use of non-pharmaceutical grade compounds)

For any statement above that is answered "No" justify below:

_____   _____

Signature of Principal Investigator   Date

_____   _____

Signature of Veterinarian consulted in the planning of this proposal   Date

CONFIDENTIAL
_____
                                                    Protocol Number
                                Institutional Animal Care and Use Committee

A.2 SAMPLE IACUC PROTOCOL AMENDMENT FORM

CONFIDENTIAL
Institutional Animal Care and Use Committee
PROTOCOL AMENDMENT

Protocol Title:
Protocol Number:
Principal Investigator:
USDA Pain Category:

Section 1: Procedural Changes
Include a brief explanation, original wording of the section to be changed, and the specific changes (insertions should be in **BOLD** and deletions in ~~strikethrough~~):

Reason(s) for the changes:

Section 2: Personnel Changes (Copy and complete section below for all personnel being added)
1. Name:
   Department: Mailstop: Email:
   Office Phone: Cell Phone:
   A.   Have they completed required animal welfare training? ☐ Yes ☐ No
   B.   Have they completed required primate biosafety training? ☐ Yes ☐ No ☐ N/A
   C.   Have they received Occupational Health clearance to work with species listed?
        ☐ Yes ☐ No ☐ N/A
   D.   Describe experience/training have had or will have with specific animal model(s):
☐ Personnel to be deleted:

Section 3: Changes in Funding
1. Grant/Contract Title: Grant #:   Funded by:
   Principal Investigator:
   For PHS Funded Projects, are contents of the protocol the same as described in the PHS proposal application? ☐ Yes ☐ No (attach a copy of the PHS-funded grant for congruency check)
☐ Grants to be deleted:

_____   _____
Signature of Principal Investigator   Date
_____   _____
Signature of Veterinarian (Applies to Category D & E Protocols) Date
_____   _____
Signature of Principal Investigator (for transferred protocol)   Date

CONFIDENTIAL
_____
Protocol Number
Institutional Animal Care and Use Committee
_____

A.3 SAMPLE PROTOCOL EXPIRATION NOTIFICATION FORM

CONFIDENTIAL
Institutional Animal Care and Use Committee
PROTOCOL EXPIRATION NOTICE

Protocol Title:
Protocol Number:
Principal Investigator:
USDA Pain Category:

The IACUC protocol specified above was approved on (Date) and will be expiring on (Date). Check the appropriate box below, and sign and return to the IACUC office as acknowledgement of receipt of this notice.

☐ Close the protocol. It is no longer being used. (Note: Any remaining animals must be transferred to another approved protocol, or to the lab animal facility's holding protocol.)

☐ I will be submitting a new protocol to the IACUC office for review and approval prior to the above expiration date.

In order to continue activities covered by this protocol, a new protocol must be submitted to the IACUC office for a *de novo* review **at least 2 months** prior the expiration date. A new protocol number will be issued at the time of approval.

_____   _____
Signature of Principal Investigator   Date

CONFIDENTIAL
_____
                                                              Protocol Number
_____ Institutional Animal Care and Use Committee

A.4 SAMPLE ANIMAL LIMITS NOTIFICATION FORM

CONFIDENTIAL
Institutional Animal Care and Use Committee
ANIMAL LIMITS NOTICE

Protocol Title:
Protocol Number:
Principal Investigator:
USDA Pain Category:

This notice is to inform you that you have reached 80% of your annual estimated animal limit for the protocol listed above.

Species:
Limit:
Number of animals used to date:

If you need to increase this number, please submit a Protocol Amendment to the IACUC office with a new estimate of animal numbers required and a revised animal numbers justification.

CONFIDENTIAL

Protocol Number
Institutional Animal Care and Use Committee

A.5 SAMPLE CEASE AND DESIST FORM

CONFIDENTIAL
Institutional Animal Care and Use Committee
PROTOCOL CEASE AND DESIST NOTICE

Protocol Title:
Protocol Number:
Principal Investigator:
USDA Pain Category:

IACUC approval for the above listed protocol expired on (Date). Renewal correspondence was sent to you on (List Dates).

Active funding: (Note: If there is active funding on this protocol, the Grants Office will be notified as well.)

Institutional policy and federal regulations prohibit the use of animal subjects without a current IACUC approval. Check the appropriate box below, and sign and return to the IACUC office as acknowledgement of receipt of this notice.

☐ Close the protocol. It is no longer being used. (Note: Any remaining animals must be transferred to another approved protocol, or to the lab animal facility's holding protocol.)
☐ I will be submitting a renewal to the IACUC office for review and approval. I understand that no animal procedures, including breeding, can be conducted until the renewal has been reviewed and approved by the IACUC, and that any remaining animals will be automatically transferred to the lab animal facility's holding protocol.

_____   _____

Signature of Principal Investigator   Date

CONFIDENTIAL

A.6 SAMPLE ANIMAL EXPOSURE HEALTH
SURVEILLANCE QUESTIONNAIRE

Animal Exposure Health Surveillance Questionnaire

Name (Last, First, MI)	Employee #	Date of Birth	Sex (M/F)
Job Title	Department	Work Phone	E-mail
PI/Supervisor's Name	PI/Supervisor's Phone	PI/Supervisor's E-mail	

This questionnaire is part of an integrated program to protect your health related to any work involving exposures to animals and/or animal materials*. Your responses to the following questions will help guide your training, medical screening, and annual surveillance needs. Your responses will be reviewed by a healthcare professional and kept in your confidential medical record in compliance with the Health Insurance Portability and Accountability Act of 1996 ("HIPAA") regulations, as well as institutional privacy and security policies.

*Animal materials are defined as unfixed tissues, cells, or body fluids (blood, urine, saliva, etc.).

If you have health-related questions while completing this questionnaire, please contact the Occupational Health Department. If you have questions about your clearance and authorization to work with animals or animal materials, please contact the IACUC office.

Part I: Occupational & Environmental Risk Factors - Animal Exposure
1. Choose the statement that best identifies the type of contact you have with animals or animal materials:
   ☐ I am an animal care worker (i.e., veterinarian, RVT, animal caretaker, cage wash operator, vivarium supervisor, necropsy technician).
   ☐ I am a researcher that works with animals and/or animal materials.
   ☐ I do not work with animals or animal materials, but will be in areas where animals are present.
   ☐ I AM NOT exposed to any animals or animal materials.
2. Which of the following animals do you have exposure to, or contact with, while at work?
   Research with Purpose Bred Laboratory Animals:
   ☐ Aquatic Amphibians (axolotls, Xenopus frogs, newts, salamanders, etc.)
   ☐ Aquatic Reptiles (turtles, etc.)
   ☐ Birds (chickens, owls, parrots, hummingbirds, etc.)
   ☐ Cats

CONFIDENTIAL

   ☐ Dogs
   ☐ Ferrets
   ☐ Fish
   ☐ Hooved Mammals (indicate species below)
      ☐ Cattle
      ☐ Goats
      ☐ Horses
      ☐ Sheep (indicate sex/age below)
         ☐ Female/Neonatal
         ☐ Male
   ☐ Nonhuman Primates (indicate species below)
      ☐ Cynomolgus
      ☐ Rhesus
      ☐ Squirrel Monkey
      ☐ Other (specify species): _____
      ☐ Unfixed NHP Tissues Only (specify species): _____
   ☐ Pigs
   ☐ Rabbits
   ☐ Rodents (mice, rats, gerbils, Guinea pigs, hamsters)
   ☐ Other: _____

Field Study with Wild Caught Animals (specify region of world in space provided):
   ☐ Bats: _____
   ☐ Birds: _____
   ☐ Elephants: _____
   ☐ Fish: _____
   ☐ Marine Mammals: _____
   ☐ Reptiles: _____
      ☐ Non-poisonous: _____
      ☐ Poisonous: _____
   ☐ Wild Rodents: _____
   ☐ Other (specify species and region): _____

Part II: Occupational & Environmental Risk Factors - Hazards

Please indicate which additional exposures or hazards may apply to your work. If you answer "Yes," please list the specific chemicals or agents in the space provided.
   1. **Biohazardous Agents** (infectious, viral vectors, rDNA, synthetic nucleic acids): _____
      ☐ Yes
      ☐ No

CONFIDENTIAL

2. **Human Tissues** (unfixed tissues, cells, blood, or other body fluids): _____
   □ Yes
   □ No
3. **Volatile Anesthetics** (i.e., isoflurane):
   _____
   □ Yes
   □ No
4. **Hazardous Chemicals** (toxic agents, chemotherapeutic agents, biological toxins, nanomaterials): _____
   □ Yes
   □ No
5. **Radiological Hazards** (radiation, radioisotopes):
   _____
   □ Yes
   □ No
6. **Other potential hazard to health** (please specify):
   _____
   □ Yes
   □ No

Part III: Environmental Allergies/Asthma

Please answer the following regarding your personal health history.
1. Do you have or experience any of the following?
   a. Seasonal allergies to pollen/grass?
      □ Yes
      □ No
   b. Allergic eye irritation?
      □ Yes
      □ No
   c. Frequent skin rashes?
      □ Yes
      □ No
   d. Frequent sinus infections?
      □ Yes
      □ No
2. Do you have any significant non-animal allergies (i.e., food, medication, latex)?
   □ No
   □ Yes (list in table below)

Item	Typical Reaction (i.e., rash, hives, shortness of breath, etc.)

CONFIDENTIAL

3. Do you have an allergy or sensitivity to any animals (i.e., cats, dogs, rabbits, etc.)?
   □ No
   □ Yes (list in table below)

Species	Typical Reaction (i.e., rash, hives, runny nose, watery or itchy eyes, wheezing, coughing, shortness of breath, etc.)

If you answered "Yes" above, please answer questions 4–6 below:
4. Do you experience any of these symptoms after working with laboratory animal or their cages/bedding, or after others work with animals near your work area?
   □ Yes
   □ No
5. Do you handle animals or clean cages at work on at least a weekly basis?
   □ Yes
   □ No
6. If you develop these symptoms around animals, does the use of personal protective equipment (i.e., fitted respirator, surgical mask, gloves, etc.) eliminate the symptoms?
   □ Yes
   □ No

Part IV: Vaccinations
Please list any vaccinations you have had, and when you were last immunized.

Vaccination	Immunized?			Date
Hepatitis A	□ Yes	□ No	□ Don't know	
Hepatitis B	□ Yes	□ No	□ Don't know	
Influenza (flu)	□ Yes	□ No	□ Don't know	
MMR (measles, mumps, rubella)	□ Yes	□ No	□ Don't know	
Polio	□ Yes	□ No	□ Don't know	
Q Fever (Coxiella)	□ Yes	□ No	□ Don't know	
Rabies	□ Yes	□ No	□ Don't know	
Smallpox (Vaccinia)	□ Yes	□ No	□ Don't know	
Td/Tdap (Tetanus, Diphtheria, Acellular Pertussis)	□ Yes	□ No	□ Don't know	
Tuberculosis BCG Vaccine	□ Yes	□ No	□ Don't know	
Typhoid	□ Yes	□ No	□ Don't know	
Varicella (Chicken Pox)	□ Yes	□ No	□ Don't know	
Yellow Fever	□ Yes	□ No	□ Don't know	

CONFIDENTIAL

Part V: Health Concerns
   1. Is your immune system compromised because of a disease or treatment for a disease?
      ☐ Yes
      ☐ No
   2. Are you currently taking any medication that suppresses your immune system?
      ☐ Yes
      ☐ No
   3. Is anyone living in your home immune-compromised?
      ☐ Yes
      ☐ No
   4. Have you been diagnosed with an autoimmune disorder, such as Lupus or rheumatoid arthritis?
      ☐ Yes
      ☐ No
   5. Have you been diagnosed with diabetes or told you have an elevated blood sugar (glucose) level?
      ☐ Yes
      ☐ No
   6. Have you been diagnosed with chronic liver or kidney disease?
      ☐ Yes
      ☐ No
   7. Have you undergone a splenectomy (surgery to remove the spleen)?
      ☐ Yes
      ☐ No
   8. Do you currently smoke?
      ☐ Yes
      ☐ No
   9. Have you been diagnosed with asthma or COPD?
      ☐ No
      ☐ Yes (list any medications: _____
   10. (Female only) Are you currently pregnant or breastfeeding?
      ☐ Yes
      ☐ No
      ☐ I would prefer to discuss this with the Occupational Health physician

Do you have any health or workplace concerns not covered by the questionnaire that you feel may affect your occupational health?
Answering "Yes" to this question will prompt the Occupational Health clinician to contact you for an in person consultation.
☐ Yes
☐ No

CONFIDENTIAL

Part VI: Additional Questions ONLY for Personnel Working with NHPs/Elephants

Type of TB Tests	Last Date	Result
Skin Test		☐ Positive ☐ Negative ☐ n/a
Blood Test		☐ Positive ☐ Negative ☐ n/a
Chest X-ray		☐ Positive ☐ Negative ☐ n/a

1. Have you ever had a positive skin or blood test for TB?   ☐ Yes ☐ No
2. Have you ever experienced persistent coughing (3 weeks or more)?   ☐ Yes ☐ No
3. Have you ever coughed up blood or bloody sputum?   ☐ Yes ☐ No
4. Have you ever had night sweats (soak the sheets)?   ☐ Yes ☐ No
5. Have you ever had unexplained weight loss?   ☐ Yes ☐ No
6. Have you ever had unexplained, excessive fatigue?   ☐ Yes ☐ No
7. Have you ever had a fever or unknown origin?   ☐ Yes ☐ No

If you answered "Yes" to any of questions 1–7 above, please describe:

_____

8. Have you ever been told by a doctor or healthcare provider that you had active TB?
   ☐ Yes
   ☐ No
9. Have you ever taken medication for TB?
   ☐ No
   ☐ Yes
      Which medication(s)? _____
      What year? _____
10. Have you ever had a BCG vaccine for TB? (This is used where TB is prevalent—BCG is not routinely used in the U.S.)
    ☐ Yes
    ☐ No
11. Have you cared for, or lived with, anyone diagnosed with active TB disease in the past year?
    ☐ No
    ☐ Yes (please describe: _____)
12. Have you worked or volunteered in a setting where TB may be more common, such as a homeless shelter, nursing home, group home, or prison, in the past year?
    ☐ Yes
    ☐ No
13. Have you traveled outside the U.S. in the past year?
    ☐ No
    ☐ Yes (list where: _____)

CONFIDENTIAL

14. In what country were you born? _____

    If not the U.S., when did you first move to the U.S.? _____

15. Have you received a live vaccine in the past 6 weeks (e.g., measles, mumps, rubella, polio, chickenpox, or shingles)?
    ☐ Yes
    ☐ No

Part VII: Additional Questions ONLY for Personnel Working with Sheep/ Hooved Mammals

1. Do you have a history of heart surgery, valvular disease (heart murmurs), congenital heart disease, or a blood vessel graft (aneurysm repair)?
    ☐ Yes
    ☐ No

2. Do you now have or have you ever had Q-Fever?
    ☐ Yes
    ☐ No
    ☐ Don't know

3. Have you ever received Q fever vaccination?
    ☐ Yes
    ☐ No
    ☐ Don't know

Review & Submit Questionnaire

Before submitting your completed questionnaire, please verify that you have answered all required questions. Once this form has been submitted, it will be reviewed by a health care professional, and you will be contacted if a follow-up visit to Occupational Health is needed. You will be prompted to update this questionnaire on an annual basis, however, should your occupational exposures change, or should you have a change in health status, please update the form and/or contact the Occupational Health Department.

By submitting this form I certify that the information I have provided is accurate to best of my knowledge.

_____   _____

Signature   Date

APPENDIX B

Resources for IACUC Information

B.1 POLICIES, LAWS, AND GUIDELINES

AVMA Guidelines for the Euthanasia of Animals, 2013 Edition
American Veterinary Medical Association (Version 2013.0.1)

Animal Law Section
National Association for Biomedical Research (NABR)

Animal Welfare Act Quick Reference Guides
Compiled by Richard L. Crawford, DVM, Animal Welfare Information Center
(In cooperation with the Virginia-Maryland Regional College of Veterinary Medicine)

Biosafety in Microbiological and Biomedical Laboratories (BMBL), 5th Edition
U.S. Department of Health and Human Services, Public Health Service, Centers for
Disease Control and Prevention, National Institutes of Health
HHS Publication No. (CDC) 21-1112 (Revised December 2009)

*Final Report of Environment Enhancement to Promote the Psychological Well-
Being of Nonhuman Primates*
U.S. Department of Agriculture (USDA) Animal and Plant Health Inspection Service
(APHIS) Animal Care (July 15, 1999)

*A Good Practice Guide to the Administration of Substances and Removal of Blood,
Including Routes and Volumes*
European Federation of Pharmaceutical Industries Associations (EFPIA) and
European Centre for the Validation of Alternative Methods (ECVAM)
Journal of Applied Toxicology 21:15–23 (2001)

Guide to the Care and Use of Experimental Animals
Canadian Council on Animal Care (1993)

Guide for the Care and Use of Laboratory Animals, 8th Edition
Institute for Laboratory Animal Research, National Research Council
The National Academies Press, Washington, DC (2011)

Guidelines for Ethical Conduct in the Care and Use of Nonhuman Animals in Research
American Psychological Association (APA) Committee on Animal Research and
Ethics

Guidelines for the Care and Use of Mammals in Neuroscience and Behavioral Research
Committee on Guidelines for the Use of Animals in Neuroscience and Behavioral Research
Institute for Laboratory Animal Research, National Research Council
The National Academies Press, Washington, DC (2003)

Guidelines for the Treatment of Animals in Behavioural Research and Teaching
Association for the Study of Animal Behavior/Animal Behavior Society (ASAB/ABS)
Animal Behaviour 83:301–309 (2012)

Guidelines of the American Society of Mammalogists for the Use of Wild Mammals in Research
The Animal Care and Use Committee of the American Society of Mammalogists
Journal of Mammalogy 88(3):809–823 (2007)

Guidelines to Promote the Wellbeing of Animals Used for Scientific Purposes: The Assessment and Alleviation of Pain and Distress in Research Animals
Australian Government National Health and Medical Research Council, Canberra, ACT (2008)

Guidelines to the Use of Wild Birds in Research, 3rd Edition
The Ornithological Council

Institutional Animal Care and Use Committee Guidebook, 2nd Edition
Applied Research Ethics National Association and Office of Laboratory Animal Welfare
National Institutes of Health, Bethesda, MD (2002)

International Guiding Principles for Biomedical Research Involving Animals
Council for International Organization of Medical Sciences (CIOMS) and the International Council for Laboratory Animal Science (ICLAS) (December 2012)

Monoclonal Antibody Production: A Report of the Committee on Methods of Producing Monoclonal Antibodies
Institute for Laboratory Animal Research (ILAR) and National Research Council (NRC)
National Academy Press, Washington, DC (1999)

Occupational Health and Safety in the Care and Use of Research Animals
Institute of Laboratory Animal Research (ILAR) and National Research Council (NRC)
National Academy Press, Washington, DC (1997)

Public Health Service Policy on Humane Care and Use of Laboratory Animals
Office of Laboratory Animal Welfare, National Institutes of Health (Revised August 2002)

B.2 ADVOCACY GROUPS FOR RESEARCH

Americans for Medical Progress (AMP)
California Biomedical Research Association (CBRA)
California Society for Biomedical Research (CSBR)
Foundation for Biomedical Research (FBR)
Incurably Ill for Animal Research (iiFAR)
Massachusetts Society for Medical Research (MSMR)
Michigan Society for Medical Research (MISMR)
National Association for Biomedical Research (NABR)
National Center for Research Resources (NCRR)
Ohio Scientific Education and Research Association (OSERA)
Pennsylvania Society for Biomedical Research (PSBR)
Texas Society for Biomedical Research (TSBR)

B.3 ALTERNATIVE DATABASES AND WEBSITES

AGRICOLA: National Agricultural Library
AGRIS: International Information System for the Agricultural Science and Technology
Alternatives to Skin Irritation Tests
AnimAlt-ZEBET database (German and English versions)
Animal Welfare Institute (AWI) Refinement and Environmental Enrichment for All
    Laboratory Animals
Aquatic Sciences & Fisheries Abstracts (ASFA)
Bibliography on Alternatives to the Use of Live Vertebrates in Biomedical Research
    and Testing (ALTBIB)
BioMed Central
BIOSIS Previews
CAB Abstracts
Center for Alternative to Animal Testing (CAAT)
Commonwealth Agriculture Bureau (CAB) Abstracts
Defense Technology Information Center (DTIC)
ECOTOX: U.S. Environmental Protection Agency ECOTOXicology Database
ECVAM: European Union Reference Laboratory for Alternatives to Animal Testing
EMBASE Elsevier Life Science Biomedical Database
Education Resources Information Center (ERIC)
Fund for the Replacement of Animals in Medical Experiments (FRAME)
Google Scholar
Interagency Coordinating Committee on the Validation of Alternative Methods
(ICCVAM)
Institute for In Vitro Sciences (IIVS)
INSPEC: Institution of Engineering and Technology Bibliographic Database
MEDLINE National Library of Medicine (NLM)

National Centre for the Replacement, Refinement and Reduction of Animals in
    Research (NC3Rs)
National Institutes of Health Model Organisms for Biomedical Research
Norecopa Norwegian Reference Centre for Laboratory Animal Science and
Alternatives Information on Alternatives Databases
NORINA: Norwegian Reference Centre for Laboratory Animal Science and Alternatives
PsycInfo
PubMed Central (PMC)
PubMed
Registry of Toxic Effects of Chemical Substances (RTECS)
Scopus
Sociological Abstracts
Toxipedia
Toxline
TOXNET: Toxicology Data Network of the U.S. National Library of Medicine
TSAR: Tracking System for Alternative Test Methods Review, Validation and
    Approval in the Context of EU Regulations on Chemicals
University of California, Davis (UCD) Center for Animal Alternatives
Web of Science
Zoological Record

B.4 ANIMAL TRANSPORT ASSOCIATIONS

Animal Transportation Association (ATA)
International Air Transport Association (IATA)

B.5 INTERNET WEBSITES OF INTEREST TO IACUCS

World Wide Web Virtual Library

WWW Virtual Library Biosciences
WWW Virtual Library: U.S. Government Information Services
WWW Virtual Library Veterinary Medicine
WWW Virtual Library Veterinary Medicine Mirror Site in Japan

Veterinary Resources
Consult a Veterinarian Diagnostic Support Program
La Bibliotheque de Medecine Veterinaire (Universite de Montreal; can be translated
to English by Google)
Mosby's Veterinary Guide to the Internet (NetVet)
NetVet Veterinary Resources
The Electronic Zoo
Veterinary Medical Libraries home page

Alternatives Searches
Altweb Alternatives to Animal Testing
National Library of Medicine (NLM)
Searching the Journal Literature for Animal Welfare Information (Welch Medical Journal, Johns Hopkins University)

IACUCs: Academic Websites
CPMCNET Institute of Comparative Medicine, Columbia University
Cornell University IACUC Policy: Care and Use of Animals in Research and Teaching
IACUC, Harvard University
IACUC, Rice University
IACUC, Rutgers New Jersey Medical School
IACUC, University of Arkansas
IACUC, University of California, Santa Barbara
IACUC, University of California, Davis
IACUC, University of Connecticut
IACUC, University of Florida
IACUC, University of Idaho
IACUC, University of Montana
IACUC, Virginia Tech

B.6 LABORATORY ANIMAL JOURNALS

Alternatives to Laboratory Animals (ATLA)
Alternatives to Animal Experimentation (ALTEX)
Animal Welfare
Anthrozoos
Applied Animal Behaviour Science
Comparative Medicine
Institute for Laboratory Animal Research (ILAR) Journal
Journal of Applied Animal Welfare Science (JAAWS)
Lab Animal
Laboratory Animals

B.7 LABORATORY ANIMAL ORGANIZATIONS

American Animal Hospital Association (AAHA)
American Association for Laboratory Animal Science (AALAS)
American Association of Human–Animal Bond Veterinarians
American Association of Laboratory Animal Practitioners
American Board of Veterinary Toxicology
American College of Laboratory Animal Medicine (ACLAM)

American College of Veterinary Anesthesiologists
American College of Veterinary Pathologists
American College of Zoological Medicine
American Committee on Laboratory Animal Disease (ACLAD)
American Fisheries Society
American Society of Animal Science
American Veterinary Distributors Association
American Veterinary Medical Association (AVMA)
Armed Forces Institute of Pathology, American College of Veterinary Pathologists
Association for Assessment and Accreditation of Laboratory Animal Care International (AAALAC International)
Association for Gnotobiotics
Association of Primate Veterinarians
Association of Reptilian and Amphibian Veterinarians
Association of Veterinary Technician Educators
Canadian Association for Laboratory Animal Science (CALAS)
Defense Technical Information Center database
International Council for Laboratory Animal Science (ICLAS)
Laboratory Animal Management Association (LAMA)
Laboratory Animal Science Association (LASA)
Scandinavian Society for Laboratory Animal Science (SCAND-LAS)

B.8 SCIENTIFIC ORGANIZATIONS

American Psychological Association (APA)
American Society of Mammalogists (ASM)
Animal Behavior Society (ABS)
Association for the Study of Animal Behavior (ASAB)
National Academy of Sciences (NAS)
National Institutes of Health Primate Resources for Researchers
Ornithological Council
Primate Information Network (PIN)
Zebrafish Information Network (ZFIN)

B.9 TRAINING RESOURCE ORGANIZATIONS

Academy of Surgical Research (ASR): promotes the advancement of professional and academic standards, education, and research in the arts and sciences of experimental surgery.

American Association for Laboratory Animal Science (AALAS): provides educational materials to laboratory animal care professionals and researchers, administers certification programs for laboratory animal technicians and managers, publishes scholarly journals, supports laboratory animal science research, and serves as a forum for the exchange of information and expertise in the care and use of laboratory animals.

American College of Laboratory Animal Medicine (ACLAM): advances the humane care and responsible use of laboratory animals through certification of veterinary specialists as diplomates of the American College of Laboratory Animal Medicine, professional development, education, and research.

American College of Veterinary Anesthesia and Analgesia (ACVAA): establishes, evaluates, and maintains the highest standards in the practice of veterinary anesthesiology by promoting the establishment of educational facilities and clinical and research training in veterinary anesthesiology. Additionally, the ACVAA establishes the criteria of fitness for the designation of a specialist in the practice of veterinary anesthesiology.

American Society of Laboratory Animal Practitioners (ASLAP): promotes the acquisition and dissemination of knowledge, ideas, and information among veterinarians and veterinary students who have an interest in laboratory animal practice for the benefit of animals and society.

Canadian Association for Laboratory Animal Science (CALAS/ACSAL): sponsors a registry training program for animal technicians, provides continuing education and professional development for animal care professionals, and hosts national symposia.

Laboratory Animal Welfare Training Exchange (LAWTE): global organization for expanding animal welfare and enhancing public understanding through effective training and education of animal research professionals.

B.10 TRAINING SUPPLIES AND PRODUCTS

Animalearn: Science Bank provides over 500 CD-ROMs, models, videos, and manikins as alternatives to animal dissection and experimentation as part of its free humane science loan program.

Digital Frog International: Software company that creates high-quality, computer-based educational programs with an ecological focus, including virtual frog dissection, field trips to the world's most fascinating ecosystems, and a look inside the inner workings of cells.

Ethical Science Education Campaign (ESEC): Alternatives Loan Library provides free access to advanced software, manuals, charts, humane curriculums, and animal resuscitation and intubation models for students at all grade levels—from elementary to veterinary school—to learn about anatomy, physiology, and other sciences.

Froguts Bio-Learning Co.: Computer simulation software for virtual dissection of frogs, squid, starfish, cow eyes, owl pellets, and fetal pigs, as well as virtual genetics laboratories. Uses immersive and interactive three-dimensional (3-D) simulations of anatomy and physiology (K-12 and higher education).

LBL—The Whole Frog Project: Virtual Frog Dissection Kit: Users can generate views of a virtual frog from many different directions, under various stages of dissection. Dissection is done at the major organ level, and by clicking on the image, the user can display the names of organs and their function.

Rescue Critters: Animal training manikins (mouse, rat, dog, and cat), anatomical models, and veterinary training products for teaching cardiopulmonary resuscitation (CPR), hemostasis, suturing, intubation, fracture repair, blood collection, and injections.

Syndaver™ Labs: Manufactures synthetic human tissues and body parts that are used to replace live animals, cadavers, and human patients in medical device studies, clinical training, and surgical simulation. Their replaceable muscles, bones, organs, and vessels are made from materials that mimic the mechanical, thermal, and physicochemical properties of live tissue.

APPENDIX C

Regulatory Agency Contact Information

C.1 OFFICE OF LABORATORY ANIMAL WELFARE (OLAW)

Office of the Director of OLAW
E-mail: olaw@mail.nih.gov
Phone: (301) 496-7163
Fax: (301) 480-3394
Website: http://grants.nih.gov/grants/olaw/olaw.htm

Director, Division of Compliance Oversight
E-mail: olawdco@mail.nih.gov
Phone: (301) 594-2061
Fax: (301) 480-3387

Director, Division of Assurances
E-mail: olawdoa@mail.nih.gov
Phone: (301) 451-0384
Fax: (301) 451-5672
E-mail addresses for document submissions:

- Annual reports: olawarp@mail.nih.gov
- Assurance documents: olawdocs@mail.nih.gov
- Restricted awards: olawra@mail.nih.gov

Director, Division of Policy and Education
E-mail: olawdpe@mail.nih.gov
Phone: (301) 402-4371
Fax: (301) 451-5546

C.2 USDA-APHIS ANIMAL CARE

Headquarters
USDA/APHIS/AC
4700 River Road, Unit 84
Riverdale, MD 20737-1234
E-mail: ace@aphis.usda.gov
Phone: (301) 851-3751
Fax: (301) 734-4978

Eastern Region
USDA/APHIS/AC
920 Main Campus Drive, Suit 200
Suite 200
Raleigh, NC 27606-5210
E-mail: aceast@aphis.usda.gov
Phone: (919) 855-7100
Fax: (919) 855-7123

Western Region
USDA/APHIS/AC
2150 Centre Avenue
Building B, Mailstop 3W11
Fort Collins, CO 80526-8117
E-mail: acwest@aphis.usda.gov
Phone: (970) 494-7478
Fax: (970) 494-7461

Center for Animal Welfare
USDA/APHIS/AC
9240 Troost Avenue
Beacon Facility, Mailstop 1180
Kansas City, MO 64131
E-mail: centerforanimalwelfare@aphis.usda.gov
Phone: (816) 737-4200
Fax: (816) 737-4206

Agricultural Select Agent Program
4700 River Road
Unit 2, Mailstop 22, Cubicle 1A07
Riverdale, MD 20737
E-mail: ASAP@aphis.usda.gov
Phone: (301) 851-3300 (select option 1)
Fax: (301) 734-3652
Website: http://www.aphis.usda.gov/programs/ag_selectagent/

Import/Export Animal and Animal Product Permits
USDA-APHIS-VS-NCIE
4700 River Road, Unit 40
Riverdale, MD 20737
Phone: (301) 851-3300
Website for ePermits: https://epermits.aphis.usda.gov/epermits

C.3 CENTERS FOR DISEASE CONTROL AND PREVENTION

Headquarters
1600 Clifton Rd
Atlanta, GA 30333
Phone: (800) 232-4636

Biosafety
Website: http://www.cdc.gov/biosafety/

Bioterrorism Preparedness and Response
Phone: (404) 639-0385
Website: http://www.bt.cdc.gov/bioterrorism/

Environmental Health
Phone: (770) 488-7100
Website: http://www.cdc.gov/Environmental/

Select Agents and Toxins
1600 Clifton Road NE, Mailstop A-46
Atlanta, GA 30333
E-mail: lrsat@cdc.gov
Phone: (404) 718-2000
Fax: (404) 718-2096
Website: http://www.selectagents.gov/

C.4 U.S. FISH AND WILDLIFE SERVICE

Headquarters
1849 C Street, NW
Washington, DC 20240
Phone: 1 (800) 344-9453
Website: http://www.fws.gov

C.5 U.S. DEPARTMENT OF DEFENSE MEDICAL RESEARCH AND MATERIAL COMMAND

Defense Advanced Research Projects Agency (DARPA)
675 North Randolph Street
Arlington, VA 22203-2114
Phone: (703) 526-6630
Website: http://www.darpa.mil/

USAMRMC Animal Care and Use Review Office (ACURO)
504 Scott Street
Fort Detrick
Frederick, MD 21702-5012
E-mail: USArmy.Detrick.MEDCOM-USAMRMC.Other.ACURO@mail.mil
Phone: (301) 619-6694
Fax: (301) 619-4165

C.6 OCCUPATIONAL HEALTH AND SAFETY ADMINISTRATION (OSHA)

Headquarters
U.S. Department of Labor
Occupational Safety & Health Administration
200 Constitution Avenue
Washington, DC 20210
Phone: (800) 321-6742
Website: https://www.osha.gov/index.html

C.7 FOOD AND DRUG ADMINISTRATION (FDA)

Headquarters
U.S. Food and Drug Administration
10903 New Hampshire Avenue
Silver Spring, MD 20993
Phone: (888) 463-6332

C.8 DRUG ENFORCEMENT ADMINISTRATION (DEA)

Headquarters
Drug Enforcement Administration
Attn: Office of Diversion Control
8701 Morrissette Drive
Springfield, VA 22152
E-mail: DEA.Registration.Help@usdoj.gov
Phone: (202) 307-1000
Website: http://www.justice.gov/dea/contact.shtml

C.9 U.S. GOVERNMENT PRINTING OFFICE (GPO)

Headquarters
GPO Customer Contact Center
723 North Capital Street, NW
Washington, DC 20401-0001
Phone: (866) 512-1800
Fax: (202) 512-2104
E-mail: Contact Center@gpo.gov
Website: http://www.gpo.gov/fdsys/
Electronic Code of Federal Regulations (eCFR) website: http://www.ecfr.gov/cgi-bin/text-idx?c=ecfr&tpl=%2Findex.tpl

APPENDIX D

Guidelines for Blood Sample Withdrawal

Laurie Brignolo and Whitney Petrie

The purpose of these guidelines is

1. To provide researchers with the necessary information to determine the acceptable blood withdrawal volumes for single and multiple collections. These guidelines apply to healthy, adult animals. The use of immature or debilitated animals requires consultation with the veterinary staff.
2. To give IACUC members, during protocol reviews, figures that represent reasonable and acceptable amounts of blood that may be withdrawn.

Excessive blood volume withdrawal can cause increases in cortisol, decreases in prolactin, blood pressure, and tissue/organ perfusion, as well as lactic acidosis, tachycardia, dyspnea, gastrointestinal ulceration, organ failure, and death. Less severe consequences to chronic low-level blood loss such as folic acid/iron deficiency and anemia can also result. Fluids, plasma, resuspended red cells, or iron/vitamin B replacement therapies should be considered when drafting a sampling schedule. For studies requiring multiple blood sampling, the same site should not be used for two consecutive withdrawals.

- The recommended maximum cumulative withdrawal is less than or equal to 15% of blood volume (Table D.1) once every two weeks.
- A single maximum withdrawal should be less than or equal to 15% of blood volume with a 30-day recovery period.

Table D.1 Total Blood Volume

Species	Body Weight (mL/kg)
Mouse	72 (63–80)
Rat	64 (58–70)
Hamster	73 (65–80)
Gerbil	67
Guinea pig	75 (67–92)
Ferret	75
Rabbit	56 (44–70)
Cat	41 (35–52)
Dog (beagle)	85 (79–90)
Macaque, *Rhesus*	65 (44–67)
Macaque, *Cynomolgus*	65 (55–75)
Marmoset	70 (58–72)
Minipig	65 (61–68)
Goat	70 (57–89)
Horse	70

Table D.2   Total Blood and Blood Sample Volumes

Species (weight)	Blood Volume (mL)	7.5% (mL)	10% (mL)	15% (mL)
Mouse (25 g)	1.8	0.1	0.2	0.3
Rat (250 g)	16	1.2	1.6	2.4
Syrian hamster (115 gm)	8.4	0.6	0.8	1.2
Gerbil (75 g)	5.0	0.4	0.5	0.8
Guinea pig (850 g)	64	4.8	6.4	9.6
Ferret (1 kg)	75	5.6	7.5	11
Rabbit (4 kg)	224	17	22	34
Cat (4 g)	160	12	16	24
Dog (10 kg)	850	64	85	127
Macaque, *Rhesus* (5 kg)	280	21	28	42
Macaque, *Cynomolgus* (5 kg)	325	24	32	49
Marmoset (350 g)	25	2.0	2.5	3.5
Minipig (15 kg)	975	73	98	146
Goat (30 kg)	2,400	180	240	360
Horse (500 kg)	35,000	2,600	3,500	5,250
Recovery period single sampling		1 week	2 weeks	4 weeks
Recovery period multiple sampling		1 week	2 weeks	2 weeks

- Animals undergoing the maximum volume blood withdrawal should be evaluated for anemia or iron deficiency before being placed on another study if a sufficient recovery time has not occurred.

Table D.2 is an example of blood volumes and percentages that can be collected at the given weights. It is recommended that individual blood volumes and percentages be calculated for each specific animal. The recommended recovery periods are also listed at the end of Table D.2. It is recommended that animals do not have additional blood collections sooner than the minimum recovery period after the described blood volumes have been collected.

Recommended Blood Collection Sites
Mouse
1. Tail vein
2. Carotid artery
3. Retro-orbital plexus*
4. Jugular vein
5. Cardiac puncture
6. Ear vein
7. Tail tip amputation*

Rat
1. Tail vein
2. Sublingual vein

    3. Retro-orbital plexus*
    4. Cardiac puncture*

Hamster
    1. Retro-orbital plexus*
    2. Jugular vein
    3. Cardiac puncture*
    4. Tail vein
    5. Femoral vein

Gerbil
    1. Tail vein
    2. Lateral saphenous vein
    3. Submandibular vein
    4. Retro-orbital plexus*

Guinea pig
    1. Middle ear vein
    2. Metatarsal vein
    3. Cardiac puncture*
    4. Jugular vein (exsanguination)*

Ferret
    1. Jugular
    2. Cranial vena cava
    3. Cephalic vein
    4. Saphenous vein

Rabbit
    1. Marginal ear vein
    2. Cardiac puncture*
    3. Retro-orbital plexus*

Cat
    1. Jugular vein
    2. Saphenous vein
    3. Cephalic vein

Dog
    1. Jugular vein
    2. Saphenous vein
    3. Cephalic vein

Nonhuman primate
    1. Femoral vein
    2. Tail vein

3. Jugular vein
4. Saphenous vein
5. Cephalic vein

Pig

1. Ear vein
2. External jugular vein
3. Cranial vena cava
4. Brachiocephalic vein

Goat

1. Jugular vein
2. Cephalic vein
3. Saphenous vein

Horse

1. Jugular vein
2. Medial saphenous vein
3. Cephalic vein
4. Transverse facial venous sinus

* Anesthesia required.

BIBLIOGRAPHY

Allen, M.J. and G.L. Borkowski, Experimental methodology. In *The Laboratory Small Ruminant*, pp. 102–105, CRC Press, Boca Raton, FL, 1999.

Baker, H.J., J.R. Lindsey, and S.H. Weisbroth, Appendix 1—Selected normative data. In M.A. Suckow, S.H. Weisbroth, and C.L. Franklin (eds), *The Laboratory Rat*, American College of Laboratory Animal Medicine Series, 2nd edn, p. 883, Elsevier Academic Press, Burlington, MA, 2006.

Diehl, K.-H. et al., A good practice guide to the administration of substances and removal of blood, including routes and volumes, *J. Appl. Toxicol.*, 21, 15–23, 2001.

Hawk, C.T., S.L. Leary, and T.H. Morris, Appendices A.1–A.2. In *Formulary for Laboratory Animals*, 3rd edn. pp. 156–157, Blackwell Publishing, Malden, MA, 2005.

Hoff, J., Methods of blood collection in the mouse, *Lab. Anim.*, 29:10, 47–53, 2000.

Adapted from National Centre for the Replacement, Refinement and Reduction of Animals in Research http://www.nc3rs.org.uk/bloodsamplingmicrosite/page.asp?id=426

Quesenberry, K.E. and C. Orcutt, Basic approach to veterinary care. In K. Quesenberry and J.W. Carpenter (eds), *Ferrets, Rabbits and Rodents, Clinical Medicine and Surgery*, 3rd edn, pp. 17–19, Saunders, St. Louis, MO, 2012.

Walesby, H.A., D.J. Hillman, J.M. Blackmer, and J. Williams, The transverse facial venous sinus: An alternative location for blood collection in the horse, *Equine Vet. Educ.*, 19, 100–102, 2007.

Washington, I.M. and G. Van Hosier, Clinical biochemistry and hematology. In M.A. Suckow, K.A. Stevens, and R.P. Wilson (eds), *The Laboratory Rabbit, Guinea Pig, Hamster, and Other Rodents*, American College of Laboratory Animal Series, p. 92, Elsevier Academic Press, London, 2012.

Volume Guidelines for Compound Administration

Laurie Brignolo and Whitney Petrie

The purpose of these guidelines is

1. To provide researchers with the *maximum* daily volumes of fluids or compounds that may be administered to animals (Table E.1). These guidelines apply for healthy, adult animals. When immature or debilitated animals are used, the veterinary staff must be consulted.
2. To give Institutional Animal Care and Use Committee (IACUC) members, during protocol reviews, figures that represent reasonable and acceptable amounts of fluids or compounds that may be administered.

The administration of excessive dose volumes may produce pain, excitement, and altered physiological parameters (e.g., serum electrolyte imbalance, increased blood pressure, and increased respiratory rate), and cause abnormal compound absorption. A large intramuscular injection into a small muscle mass may force the dose into fascial planes and subcutaneous tissues that may accelerate lymphatic drainage and may also cause pressure necrosis or nerve damage. For parenteral routes of administration (a route other than oral), it may be less irritating to administer the dose halved in two separate locations. For studies requiring repeated parenteral dosing, the same site should not be used for two consecutive administrations.

Table E.1 Compound Administration Volumes Considered Good Practice (maximum)[a]

Species	Oral	Subcutaneous	Intraperitoneal	Intramuscular	Intravenous Bolus (slow injection)
Mouse	10 (50)	10 (40)	20 (80)	0.05[b] (0.1)[b]	5 (25)
Rat	10 (40)	5 (10)	10 (20)	0.1[b] (0.2)[b]	5 (20)
Rabbit	10 (15)	1 (2)	5 (20)	0.25 (0.5)	2 (10)
Dog	5 (15)	1 (2)	1 (20)	0.25 (0.5)	2.5 (5)
Macaque	5 (15)	2 (5)	[c] (10)	0.25 (0.5)	2 ([c])
Marmoset	10 (15)	2 (5)	[c] (20)	0.25 (0.5)	2.5 (10)
Minipig	10 (15)	1 (2)	1 (20)	0.25 (0.5)	2.5 (5)
Fish	2 g/kg[d]	1 ([c])	[c] (10)	[c] (0.05)	5 ([c])

Note: Values are in mL/kg unless otherwise specified.

[a] For nonaqueous injectates, consideration must be given to the time of absorption before redosing. No more than two intramuscular sites should be used per day. Subcutaneous sites should be limited to two or three sites per day. The subcutaneous site does not include Freund's adjuvant administration.
[b] Volumes in milliliters per site.
[c] Data not available.
[d] Administered via gel capsules.

In addition to the volume of administration, one must also consider the character of the solution. Known irritants such as Freund's adjuvant should be delivered according to specific guidelines/protocols. Solutions above pH 8.0 and below pH 4.5 should be diluted or buffered even if this means exceeding guidelines, provided that veterinary and IACUC approvals have been obtained. One must consider any possible effects attributable to the vehicle alone (e.g., dimethyl sulfoxide [DMSO] and polyethylene glycol).

The maximum intradermal dose for all species is 0.05–0.10 mL/site. Volumes listed in Table E.1 are for maximum daily cumulative administrations.

BIBLIOGRAPHY

Diehl, K.-H., Hull, R., Morton, D., Pfister, R., Rabemampianina, Y., Smith, D., Vidal, J.M., van de Vorstenbosch, C., A good practice guide to the administration of substances and removal of blood, including routes and volumes, *J. Appl. Toxicol.*, 21:15–23, 2001.

Morton, D.B., Jennings, M., Buckwell, A., Ewbank, R., Godfrey, C., Holgate, B., Inglis, I., et al., Joint Working Group on Refinement 2001. Refining procedures for the administration of substances. Report of the BVAAWF/FRAME/RSPCA/UFAW Joint Working Group on Refinement. British Veterinary Association Animal Welfare Foundation/ Fund for the Replacement of Animals in Medical Experiments/Royal Society for the Prevention of Cruelty to Animals/Universities Federation for Animal Welfare, *Lab. Anim.*, 35:1–41, 2001.

Turner, P.V., Brabb, T., Pekow, C., Vasbinder, M.A., Administration of substances to laboratory animals: Routes of administration and factors to consider, *J. Am. Assoc. Lab. Anim. Sci.*, 50:5, 600–613, 2001.

Sample IACUC Guideline

Effective Date: January 1, 2014   IACUC Guideline #16, Version 2

ABC UNIVERSITY
INSTITUTIONAL ANIMAL CARE AND USE COMMITTEE

Title: Guideline for Use of Non-Pharmaceutical-Grade Drugs/Chemicals/Compounds in Research Animals

1.0 Purpose

To provide guidance to the research community regarding the use of non-pharmaceutical-grade substances in laboratory animals.

2.0 Background

The ABC University Animal Care and Use Program operates in accordance with federal laws, regulations, and guidelines including the Animal Welfare Act, the Animal Welfare Act Regulations, the Public Health Service Policy on Humane Care and Use of Laboratory Animals, and the *Guide for the Care and Use of Laboratory Animals*. Accordingly, pharmaceutical-grade drugs and other chemicals, when available, must be used, even in nonsurvival procedures, to avoid toxicity or side effects that may threaten the health and welfare of vertebrate animals or interfere with the interpretation of research results or both. However, it is frequently necessary to use investigational compounds to meet scientific and research goals.

3.0 Definitions

Pharmaceutical grade compound

Any active or inactive drug, biologic, or reagent, for which a chemical purity standard has been established by a recognized national or regional pharmacopeia (e.g., the U.S. Pharmacopeia [USP], British Pharmacopeia [BP], National Formulary [NF], European Pharmacopoeia [EP], and Japanese Pharmacopeia [JP]). These standards are used to ensure that products are of the appropriate chemical purity and quality and are in the appropriate solution or compound; they also ensure the products' stability, safety, and efficacy. The Food and Drug Administration (FDA) maintains a database listing of FDA-approved commercial formulations for both FDA-approved human drugs (the Orange Book) and veterinary drugs (the Green Book).

4.0 Procedure

The NIH Office of Laboratory Animal Welfare (OLAW) and the U.S. Department of Agriculture (USDA) have determined that the use of non-pharmaceutical-grade substances should be based on scientific necessity and nonavailability of an acceptable veterinary or human pharmaceutical-grade compound.

4.1 Proposed use of non-pharmaceutical-grade substances in animals must be described in an IACUC protocol.

4.2 Cost savings alone are not considered an adequate justification for the use of non-pharmaceutical-grade substances in laboratory animals.

4.3 If nonpharmaceutical agents are used, the following should be considered: chemical purity, grade, sterility, pH, pyrogenicity, osmolality, stability, storage, site/route of administration, side effects and adverse reactions, physiologic compatibility, pharmacokinetics, and quality control.

4.4 Investigators should consider animal welfare and scientific issues related to the use of the substance including safety, efficacy, potential for contamination, and the introduction of unwanted experimental variables.

4.5 Agents providing sedation, analgesia, anesthesia, or euthanasia must be of an acceptable veterinary or human pharmaceutical-grade product unless the use of an investigational chemical or formulation is scientifically necessary, appropriately justified, and approved by the IACUC.

BIBLIOGRAPHY

NRC (National Research Council). 2011. *Guide for the Care and Use of Laboratory Animals.* 8th edn, p. 31. National Academies Press, Washington, DC.

OLAW (Office of Laboratory Animal Welfare). Frequently asked questions: PHS policy on humane care and use of laboratory animals: May investigators use non-pharmaceutical-grade compounds in animals? NIH, Bethesda, MD. http://grants.nih.gov/grants/olaw/faqs.htm#useandmgmt_4.

USDA. 2014. USDA-APHIS-animal care policy manual; Policy #3: Veterinary care. USDA. Available at: http://www.aphis.usda.gov/animal_welfare/policy.php?policy=3.

APPENDIX G

USDA Pain Categories

USDA Pain and Distress Categories

Pain Category B	Pain Category C	Pain Category D	Pain Category E
Animals being bred, conditioned, or held for use in teaching, testing, experiments, research, or surgery, but not yet used for such purposes. (Example: breeding colonies of any animal species, including parents and offspring.)	*No* pain or distress to animals, and no use of pain-relieving drugs. (Example: routine procedures, e.g., injections and blood sampling.)	Pain or distress to animals for which appropriate anesthetic, analgesic, or tranquilizing drugs are used. (Example: survival surgery under anesthesia with postoperative analgesics given.)	Pain or distress to animals for which the use of appropriate anesthetic, analgesic, or tranquilizing drugs is withheld due to adverse effects on procedures, results, or interpretations. (Example: arthritis study where analgesic or anti-inflammatories would interfere with the testing of novel new therapies.)

Source: Animal and Plant Health Inspection Service (APHIS) Form 7023, August 2009.

Index

Printed in the United States
by Baker & Taylor Publisher Services